Assessing
Attention-Deficit/
Hyperactivity Disorder

Assessing Attention-Deficit/ Hyperactivity Disorder

ARTHUR D. ANASTOPOULOS

and

TERRI L. SHELTON

University of North Carolina at Greensboro
Greensboro, North Carolina

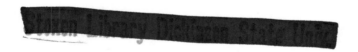
KLUWER ACADEMIC/PLENUM PUBLISHERS
NEW YORK, BOSTON, DORDRECHT, LONDON, MOSCOW

Library of Congress Cataloging-in-Publication Data

Anastopoulos, Arthur D., 1954–
    Assessing attention-deficit/hyperactivity disorder/Arthur D. Anastopoulos and Terri L. Shelton.
      p. cm.
    Includes bibliographical references and index.
    ISBN 0-306-46388-1
      1. Attention-deficit hyperactivity disorder—Diagnosis. 2. Attention-deficit
hyperactivity disorder—Treatment—Evaluation.   I. Shelton, Terri L.   II. Title.

RJ506.H9 A593 2001
618.92′8589—dc21

                                                      00-049780

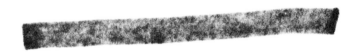

ISBN: 0-306-46388-1

©2001 Kluwer Academic / Plenum Publishers, New York
233 Spring Street, New York, New York 10013

http://www.wkap.nl/

10 9 8 7 6 5 4 3 2 1

A C.I.P. record for this book is available from the Library of Congress

Printed in the United States of America

To Tyler

Foreword

Over the past two decades, the assessment of Attention-Deficit/Hyperactivity Disorder (AD/HD) has evolved into a sophisticated balance of science and clinical judgement essential for arriving at reliable and valid diagnostic decisions. Because of the precarious mix of clinical and empirical skill needed to evaluate children with this disorder, diagnostic practice in this area has been found wanting by many critics. In fact, a 1998 National Institutes of Health consensus panel concluded that "existing diagnostic treatment practices ... point to the need for improved awareness by the health service sector concerning an appropriate assessment, treatment, and follow-up. A more consistent set of diagnostic procedures and practice guidelines is of utmost importance" (p. 21). Drs. Arthur D. Anastopoulos and Terri L. Shelton have designed a book that addresses this need.

A number of themes are highlighted throughout the text. Perhaps the most important is that the assessment guidelines set forth in this book represent a balance between science and practice. The authors account for the realities of clinical practice in an age of managed care while challenging clinicians to heed the lessons of empirical research. Although the use of empirically based assessment procedures may at times fly in the face of cost constraints (e.g., systematic evaluation of medication effects), the authors present a strong argument for them. Further, they call upon their vast clinical experience to provide concrete suggestions for translating research findings into effective evaluations. Anastopoulos and Shelton are not afraid to address the thorny issues that clinicians often face in evaluations, such as inconsistencies in and incompleteness of assessment data. Indeed, incomplete and inconsistent data are the rule rather than the exception, and the authors provide excellent ways to face this challenge.

A second theme pervading the text is an emphasis on not only the content of AD/HD evaluations (*which* assessments should be done), but also on the process used to conduct them (*how* assessments should be done). The authors guide the clinician/researcher through the assessment process step by step, while avoiding a cookbook approach. Stated differently, flexibility in the assessment process is not only allowed for, but it is stipulated by a variety of factors, such as the age of the client and the nature of the practice setting. Anastopoulos and Shelton don't advocate for a single approach to assess individuals with AD/HD, but instead set forth a way to comprehensively plan for and carry out evaluations under a range of circumstances. This emphasis on process is a unique and valuable contribution to the clinical practice literature. In particular, Anastopoulos and Shelton offer clear guidelines for the commonsense application (and re-ordering) of *DSM* criteria when interpreting assessment data, information unavailable in any other text of which I am aware.

A third theme is the multimethod, multi-informant approach. The authors comprehensively review and describe many common assessment procedures, which will be of enormous value to clinicians and researchers operating in a fast-changing environment characterized by the ongoing proliferation of new measures for assessing AD/HD and related disorders. Reasoned, thoughtful recommendations concerning these measures are given to aid clinicians in making informed choices from among the dizzying array of possibilities.

A fourth theme is that the assessment's usefulness does not end with diagnosis. It is also essential for planning and evaluating treatment. Given the heterogeneity of symptomatic presentation and functioning in this population, clinicians must avoid a "one-size-fits-all" approach to treatment design. The authors provide specific guidelines to aid in selecting treatments.

Once interventions are implemented, one must collect data to determine whether they have led to behavioral changes and whether they should be discontinued or modified, and a flexible set of procedures for doing so comprehensively is included. In keeping with their balance of content and process, the authors examine treatment evaluation in detail. For example, they look at treatment integrity, a critical element that must not be ignored, due to the abysmally low rate of treatment adherence typically seen in clinical practice. Case studies are woven into the text to show how assessment data can be used for treatment planning and outcome evaluation.

A fifth theme is the influence of individual and environmental variation and diversity. Age, gender, and ethnicity can have substantial effects on the content, process, and interpretation of assessment data. Also, very few children referred to clinics are purely AD/HD. The authors address this issue of comorbidity in a straightforward and detailed fashion. Symptom assessment in an environmental context is ingrained in the discussion of using assessment data to tailor the treatment to the particular child, family, and system involved. Thus, inherent in the book's philosophy is an understanding of the inextricable link between assessment and treatment.

A final major theme is that responsible assessment practice requires clinicians to collaborate effectively with parents, children, and schools. I know of no other text that offers such clear and extensive information on providing oral and written feedback. How we interact with parents and children is critical to how well they understand the diagnosis and how motivated they are to participate in the treatment.

Clinicians and researchers working with the AD/HD population will find this text invaluable. Drs. Anastopoulos and Shelton are scientist–practitioners of the highest order, and the expertise they share with us here will greatly enhance assessment practice, and ultimately, treatment outcome, for children and adolescents with AD/HD.

George J. DuPaul, Ph.D.
Lehigh University
Bethlehem, Pennsylvania

April 3, 2000

Preface

Professional interest in the topic of Attention-Deficit/Hyperactivity Disorder (AD/HD; American Psychiatric Association, 1994) has increased dramatically over the past decade. Nowhere is this more evident than in scientific journals, where literally hundreds of AD/HD-related articles have appeared. Further evidence of this increased interest is found in many recently published pediatric and child psychology texts, which now routinely include chapters dealing with AD/HD. Along with these trends, there has been a rapid proliferation of professional texts, practitioner guidebooks, and self-help books on the topic, as well as an increase in the number of instructional and informational videotapes available for personal and professional use.

Following closely on the heels of this shift within professional circles is the recent surge of media interest in AD/HD. At the local level, AD/HD has been the focus of countless newspaper stories and radio talk shows. Periodically, it has also been in the national spotlight, including coverage by *Time*, *Newsweek*, the *Wall Street Journal*, *60 Minutes*, *20/20*, *Dateline*, *PBS*, the *Today Show*, *Good Morning America*, and *Sally Jesse Raphael*.

With all that has been written and said about AD/HD, one might legitimately question why anyone would want to write yet another book on the topic. Our reasons for doing so are as follows.

First, as we thought about the written material currently available to assist students and professionals in their clinical work, it occurred to us that something very important was missing. There were indeed many journal articles, book chapters, and professional texts dealing with AD/HD assessment. Many included relatively detailed descriptions of the various procedures for conducting an evaluation. A few recommended which procedures to use, and some even went so far as to explain how one might interpret the results. None, however, provided specific guidelines on how to *integrate* or *interpret* the type of clinical data that usually emanates from an AD/HD evaluation—that is, individual case data—drawn from multiple sources, procedures, or both.

Finding nothing that dealt systematically with the *process* of conducting AD/HD assessments, we developed our own set of interpretive guidelines. Such guidelines have served us well in our clinical practice. Moreover, they have proven to be exceptionally valuable teaching tools. We have routinely shared this assessment knowledge with the many child health-care professionals and educators to whom we have provided consultation over the years. We have also regularly disseminated this information during our clinical supervision of students, including graduate students in clinical psychology, psychology interns, postdoctoral fellows in child psychology, fellows in child psychiatry and pediatrics, and residents in psychiatry, pediatrics, and family practice. Our efforts have been well received, leading us to believe that we have developed an effective way of teaching professionals how to conduct AD/HD evaluations, whether for the purpose of establishing a diagnosis, generating treatment recommendations, or assessing treatment outcome.

Several other considerations also influenced our decision to write this text. For example, we have repeatedly heard parents, teachers, and child health-care professionals voice their concerns about the inconsistent manner in which AD/HD is assessed. Some have expressed discontent with what they perceive as the underidentification of this disorder, which can lead to delays in initiating treatment. Others have been concerned with the overidentification of this disorder, which can result in children and adolescents receiving special-education services or being placed on stimulant medication after being mistakenly identified as having AD/HD. Such a concern has also been evident in the media. Recent allegations have surfaced suggesting that exceedingly high numbers of children and adolescents are being identified as having AD/HD in order to justify controlling their behavior with medication. Although there is little basis for such claims, there is merit in considering some of the clinical and ethical issues inherent in them. Foremost among these issues is the notion that proper treatment flows from accurate diagnoses.

In our opinion, both overidentification and underidentification stem in large part from the highly variable manner in which AD/HD is evaluated. Thus, by making an assessment text available to independent practitioners and students in training, we hope to promote greater uniformity in the delivery of AD/HD assessment services.

This need for greater consistency is especially critical in view of events that have transpired over the past decade. In September of 1991, the United States Department of Education put forth a policy clarification memorandum, indicating that children with AD/HD may qualify for special education and related services under P.L. 94-142/Part B of the Individual with Disabilities Education Act (IDEA) or through Section 504 of the Federal Rehabilitation Act of 1973. Thus, proper identification of students with AD/HD is of tantamount importance to school systems, whose ever-diminishing budgets make it increasingly more difficult to provide special-education services. Another major event was the arrival of the *Fourth Edition of the Diagnostic and Statistical Manual of Mental Disorders* (*DSM-IV*; American Psychiatric Association, 1994), which, among other things, brought with it new criteria for establishing an AD/HD diagnosis. Although far more specific than the criteria set forth previously, the *DSM-IV* guidelines for AD/HD still leave much room for subjectively interpreting how they should be employed.

Our concern for establishing diagnostic uniformity is by no means limited to clinical matters. We also contend that greater adherence to a common set of diagnostic guidelines will go a long way toward reducing the variability in subject selection so often found in AD/HD research. Some studies define AD/HD on the basis of teacher-completed child behavior ratings, whereas others define it exclusively on the basis of parental responses to interview questions. What this has led to, of course, is the proverbial "apples and oranges" problem. The more similar the diagnostic tools and criteria employed in AD/HD studies, the more similar will be the participants across studies. Such uniformity would greatly facilitate cross-study comparisons, thereby allowing for more-rapid accumulation of scientific knowledge.

For these reasons, we decided that there was ample justification for adding another AD/HD professional text to the market. We do not wish to suggest that our assessment approach is *the* correct or only way to assess AD/HD. There are many possible avenues for conducting such evaluations. At the same time, our extensive experience over the past 15 years has afforded us a unique perspective on an extremely complicated process. As part of this experience, we have regularly consulted with experts in the field on extremely difficult and challenging cases. We have also routinely utilized findings from the AD/HD research literature to guide us in our clinical work. The end result is that we have been able to identify useful interpretive guidelines, including those for handling the inconsistencies that commonly arise in our assessment data. This clinical insight combined with what we know from the pertinent research literature has proven indispensable—not only in our diagnostic formulations, but also in our efforts to develop and implement clinically appropriate AD/HD interventions.

Because this approach to assessment has worked so well for us and for those with whom we have worked, we would like to share it with others in the field. The overall goal of this text, therefore, is to provide child health-care professionals and educators with a comprehensive set of practical, case-oriented, yet empirically based, guidelines for evaluating children and adolescents who exhibit symptoms of AD/HD. These guidelines may be used not only for diagnostic purposes, but also for treatment planning and for the ongoing evaluation of treatment outcome. Being process-oriented in nature, this text should be useful not only to seasoned practitioners wishing to sharpen their clinical skills, but also to students just learning such skills, including those in psychology, psychiatry, social work, counseling, education, pediatrics, neurology, and family practice medicine.

Our approach to evaluating children and adolescents with AD/HD is very much grounded in the scientific method of hypothesis testing. In this same spirit, we encourage our readers to put this approach to test in their own clinical practice. Our hope, of course, is that what has worked so well for us will do the same for them. This in turn should serve to enhance the quality of care that we all strive to provide for the many children and adolescents whose lives are affected by AD/HD.

Arthur D. Anastopoulos
Terri L. Shelton

May 17, 2000

Contents

Introduction

"Once he learned how to walk, all hell broke loose."

At some point in their careers, most child health-care professionals and educators hear comments like these, uttered by parents who are frustrated by an inability to control their child's behavior. Although there are many possible explanations for viewing a child in this way, such statements often come from parents whose children display features of Attention-Deficit/Hyperactivity Disorder (AD/HD; American Psychiatric Association, 1994). Some parents do not know a great deal about the disorder and therefore are not inclined to attach such a label. Nevertheless, they know that something is wrong or, at the very least, "different" about their child's behavior. They might then turn to pediatricians, psychologists, psychiatrists, school counselors, or other child health-care professionals for further insight and guidance. Unfortunately, the advice that they receive very often depends upon the source, as illustrated by the following case.

Jason is an 8-year-old boy whose parents and second grade teacher shared mutual concerns about the negative effect that his behavior was having on his performance at home and at school. Although he was of normal intelligence and in good physical health, his academic productivity and achievement were well below grade level expectations. According to his teacher, it was difficult to get him to complete assigned work unless an adult was standing right next to him. Even when he appeared to be attending, he would often rush through an assignment, resulting in careless errors. Another problem was his excessive talking, which was disruptive not only to his teacher but to many of his classmates as well. He had little trouble making friends, but keeping them was problematic due to his silly and immature behavior. At home he rarely followed through on parental requests to complete chores or do homework, which led to family conflict. His parents were also concerned about his low self-esteem and unusually low tolerance for frustration.

With his parents' approval and consent, Jason's teacher contacted the special-education department and requested a school-based evaluation to deter-

1

mine whether he had special education needs requiring services. This assessment, which transpired over a 2-month period, included individually administered intelligence testing, educational achievement testing, projective testing, screening for learning disabilities, a hearing screening, and a speech and language assessment. The end result of the work-up confirmed that Jason was not achieving at grade level, despite the fact that he was of average intelligence and had no specific learning disabilities. No evidence of AD/HD emerged. On the basis of such findings, special-education services were deemed unnecessary.

Somewhat surprised by this appraisal, Jason's parents decided to get a second opinion from their pediatrician. This particular physician had provided excellent medical care to all their children over the years, and therefore was someone whom they trusted and respected. Within a few days of calling, they were able to take Jason to the pediatrician's office for further assessment. This evaluation included a standard pediatric examination, a neurodevelopmental screening, informal observations of Jason in the examining room, and a review of his recent home and school difficulties via parental responses to interview questioning. All of this information was gathered during a 15-minute office visit. Contrary to what the parents described during the interview, neither the medical examination nor the office-based observations of Jason produced any clear-cut evidence of AD/HD. Faced with this inconsistency, the pediatrician did not feel comfortable attributing Jason's reported problems to AD/HD. He suspected that these difficulties were typical for a boy Jason's age. Yet this perception ran counter to the concerns expressed by Jason's parents, whom he had come to trust over the years.

In an effort to resolve the discrepancy, the pediatrician decided that it might be in the family's best interests to have Jason evaluated by an AD/HD specialist. Thus, he referred them to a nearby AD/HD specialty clinic where they met with a clinical child psychologist, who used multiple methods and sources of information as a basis for assessing AD/HD. As part of this multimethod evaluation process, Jason's parents provided extensive information about his psychosocial functioning during a structured diagnostic interview and through their responses to several child behavior questionnaires. The psychologist also obtained a perspective on Jason's school performance and behavior from informal school-based observations, from an interview with his teacher, and from the teacher's responses to various child behavior rating scales. In addition to being interviewed, Jason underwent a brief battery of psychological tests. The psychologist also reviewed prior medical and school records. Although the data obtained from interviewing Jason and from formal testing failed to produce any clear evidence of AD/HD, the information derived from Jason's parents and his teacher suggested that these behavioral difficulties were consistent with an AD/HD diagnosis. Hence, the psychologist recommended a combination of home- and school-based AD/HD treatment services, which, over several months, brought significant improvements in his psychosocial functioning both at home and at school.

What this case illustrates is by no means rare or uncommon. From one professional to the next, strikingly different assessment procedures may be used, resulting in conflicting diagnostic conclusions and treatment recommendations for the same child. Although it was a clinical child psychologist who correctly identified Jason as having AD/HD, it could just as easily have been the pediatrician, the school-based assessment team, or some other child health-care professional.

Why does so much variability exist in AD/HD evaluations? Some of this diversity stems from differences in professional training. But knowing whether a person holds an M.D., a Ph.D., an M.Ed., or an M.S.W. tells little about the type of evaluation a person is likely to employ. One's beliefs about the causes of psychopathology in general, and of AD/HD in particular, exert a strong influence on his or her approach to the assessment process. So too does the level of experience in working with children and adolescents who have AD/HD. Although less obvious, another important element is the degree to which clinicians incorporate methodological rigor into their clinical evaluations. Further complicating matters is that the marketplace is now saturated with child behavior questionnaires, psychological tests, and other products that purportedly measure AD/HD symptomatology. Thus, for many professionals, deciding which tools to employ can be confusing, even intimidating.

As stated in the preface, we have written this text as an AD/HD assessment resource that will enable professionals of various disciplines to deliver more consistent clinical services to children and adolescents with AD/HD. To meet this objective, we have divided the book into eight chapters.

The first two chapters provide the background information necessary for understanding AD/HD as a disorder. These chapters cover the history of AD/HD; the current diagnostic criteria used to identify it; its etiology, epidemiology, and developmental course; its clinical presentation; its impact on psychosocial functioning; and its comorbid features. In the next two chapters we shift our attention to assessment issues. In chapter 3 we present our rationale for using a multimethod, multi-informant assessment procedure. Chapter 4 gives a comprehensive review and critique of many assessment tools commonly used in AD/HD evaluations, such as interviews, rating scales, psychological tests, and observational coding systems.

Chapter 5 begins with some general suggestions for selecting appropriate combinations of such tools, after which we describe the multimethod assessment approach that we have been using over the past 15 years in AD/HD specialty clinics at the University of North Carolina at Greensboro and at the University of Massachusetts Medical Center. With this multimethod battery in mind, we then detail the process of establishing an AD/HD diagnosis. As part of this, we provide suggestions for identifying various comorbid conditions and we examine clinically relevant parent and family issues that have bearing on the child's diagnosis and treatment planning.

In Chapter 6 we illustrate how these assessment findings translate into practical, clinically meaningful, and cost-effective treatment plans, emphasizing a multimodal treatment approach. This includes a discussion of how to select treatment strategies that address not only the concerns about the child, but also any concerns manifested by other family members, which may influence the child's response to treatment. Chapter 7 outlines how to give feedback to parents and children. Suggestions for summarizing such findings in a written report are presented as well, along with a sample report.

The final chapter demonstrates how these same assessment strategies can be used later to evaluate treatment outcome. This is discussed in the context of the three most commonly employed interventions for AD/HD—namely, stimulant medication therapy, school-based interventions, and parent training.

1

Diagnostic Criteria:
A Historical Perspective

"Isn't this just the disorder of the 90s?"

In any professional presentation on the topic of Attention-Deficit/Hyperactivity Disorder (AD/HD; American Psychiatric Association, 1994), there is a good chance that the above question, or one like it, will arise from the audience. Depending on the nature and tone of the presentation, one answer might be, "That's right, it is the disorder of the 90s—the 1990s, the 1890s, the 1790s," and so on. The point is, AD/HD is not a new clinical phenomenon. It is, however, a relatively new diagnostic label to describe individuals who display developmentally inappropriate levels of inattention, impulsivity, and/or hyperactivity.

From the early 1960s until the mid 1980s, children displaying many of these same behavioral features might have been labeled as having Minimal Brain Dysfunction, Hyperkinetic Reaction of Childhood, or Attention Deficit Disorder with Hyperactivity. Even earlier, these same children may have received other diagnostic labels, including Minimal Brain Damage Syndrome and Hyperkinetic Impulse Disorder.

Given the large number and variety of terms that have been applied to what is now known as AD/HD, it is no wonder that confusion about this disorder so often exists—not only in the mind of the general public, but within professional circles as well. Adding to this confusion is the fact that there is no universally agreed upon set of criteria for diagnosing AD/HD. Within North America, child health-care professionals and educators have traditionally followed the guidelines set forth by the American Psychiatric Association (APA), whereas in other parts of the world, the classification system of the World Health Organization (WHO) has been adopted. As a first step toward clarifying some of these diagnostic issues, this chapter reviews the major historical events that have shaped the evolution of AD/HD within the United States and Canada. This is followed by a detailed description of the current APA criteria for establishing an AD/HD diagnosis. Although it is beyond the scope of this text to present the worldwide historical events that have helped to shape thinking on this matter, readers need a better understanding of how the current North American system differs from that used elsewhere. Therefore, also included is a brief description of the WHO diagnostic criteria.

PREVIOUS DESCRIPTIONS AND LABELS

Earliest Account

The first published case reports of children exhibiting AD/HD-like difficulties appeared in the mid-1800s. Not until the turn of the century, however, was any attempt made to view such problems scientifically. In what is often credited as the first such attempt, Still (1902) described a group of children whose behavior was characterized by symptoms of inattention and overactivity, began in early childhood, persisted over time, and deviated significantly from expectations for same-aged peers. As conceptualized by Still, these and similar problems reflected serious deficiencies in the "volitional inhibition" of behavior, as well as "defects in moral control" that presumably stemmed from underlying neurological factors.

Etiologically-Based Descriptions

Around the time of the First World War, there was a large-scale outbreak of encephalitis. Most children who survived this epidemic displayed behavioral, emotional, or cognitive sequelae, including impaired attention span, impulse control, and motor activity regulation (Ebaugh, 1923). The fact that so many of these children displayed this particular pattern of behavioral symptoms led to the widespread use of the term Postencephalitic Behavior Disorder (Hohman, 1922) to describe their condition. This provided further support for the notion that underlying neurological deficiencies might be responsible for the childhood behavior problems that had been described by Still (1902).

Descriptions of children with similar behavioral features continued to appear in the clinical research literature over the next decade. Although the children were not necessarily the victims of encephalitis, or any other clearly defined neurological illness or injury, the prevailing belief was that such behavior problems were caused by underlying organic factors. Reflecting this thinking, Kahn and Cohen (1934) attributed the symptoms to brain stem damage and labeled the condition Organic Driveness.

This presumption of an organic etiology was also apparent in the work of Strauss and associates (Strauss & Kephart, 1955; Strauss & Lehtinen, 1947). Based on research showing that inattention, impulsivity, and hyperactivity appeared more often among developmentally delayed children with brain damage than among developmentally delayed children without such damage, Strauss reasoned that any child exhibiting these behavioral difficulties probably had brain damage. Hence, the term Brain-Injured Child Syndrome came into use, later evolving into Minimal Brain Damage Syndrome.

Although Strauss's assertions dominated the thinking of many in the field, not everyone shared this point of view. Birch (1964) in particular was very vocal in challenging the logic of attributing a causal role to brain damage, given that so many of the behavior-disordered children that he had studied showed no evidence whatsoever of organic involvement. Such challenges very likely influenced the thinking of Clements and Peters (1962), who began using the term Minimal Brain Dysfunction (MBD) to describe children who exhibited symptoms of inattention, impulsivity, and hyperactivity. This terminology was significant, because it reflected increasing disenchantment with the idea that brain *damage* was a major cause of AD/HD-like behavior. At the same time, this new label preserved the notion that the brain was somehow involved in the etiology of this disorder, albeit in a less well-defined role.

Symptom-Based Descriptions

As is evident from the preceding discussion, the early history of AD/HD was replete with descriptive labels highlighting its presumed etiology. Yet despite their firm allegiance to an organic viewpoint, some researchers did not employ etiologically based terminology in their descriptions of children with AD/HD-like symptoms. Childers (1935), for example, emphasized hyperactivity features. So too did Levin (1938), who coined the phrase Restlessness Syndrome. Although Laufer and associates adhered strongly to the belief that AD/HD-like behavior resulted from damage to diencephalic structures, they nevertheless used such terms as Hyperkinetic Impulse Disorder (Laufer, Denhoff, & Solomons, 1957) and Hyperkinetic Behavior Syndrome (Laufer & Denhoff, 1957) to highlight what they saw as the cardinal features of this condition.

This emphasis on motor restlessness was also apparent in Chess's (1960) symptom-based description of the condition, which she referred to as Hyperactive Child Syndrome. Unlike many of her colleagues, Chess did not believe that brain damage was a major cause of these symptoms. She proposed instead that such behavioral difficulties might represent the extreme end of the normal variability that occurs within child populations.

Formal Diagnostic Classification Era

From the time of Still's account until the early 1960s, no less than 10 diagnostic labels had been used to describe the behavior of children who today would probably be identified as having AD/HD. Having so many labels was not conducive to clinical research. A uniform system for categorizing children with AD/HD-type difficulties was clearly needed to ensure that researchers were investigating similar populations.

Although a formal system for classifying mental disorders was already available in the first edition of the *Diagnostic and Statistical Manual of Mental*

Disorders (*DSM-I*; APA, 1952), nowhere in *DSM-I* were there any developmentally appropriate guidelines for diagnosing child or adolescent problems. The absence of such guidelines was no accident; many in the field of psychiatry at that time did not believe that children had the psychological capacity—lacking superegos, as it were—to experience mental health problems.

As the 1960s unfolded, adherence to this viewpoint diminished with the increasing recognition that children and adolescents could indeed have psychiatric difficulties. This shift in thinking greatly influenced the development of the second edition of the *Diagnostic and Statistical Manual of Mental Disorders* (*DSM-II*; APA, 1968), which for the first time included a section called "Behavior Disorders of Childhood and Adolescence." A total of six child diagnostic categories appeared in this new section. Among these was the classification, Hyperkinetic Reaction of Childhood (or adolescence).

The *DSM-II* Criteria

A description of Hyperkinetic Reaction of Childhood (code 308.0) appears in Table 1.1. It shows that its essential features were hyperactivity and inattention. Its inclusion in *DSM-II* was no surprise, given that children with these behavioral features had been described in the research literature for many years. Its name was also very much a product of the times, reflecting both the diminished etiological importance attached to brain damage (Birch, 1964; Clements & Peters, 1962) and the rapid ascendance of symptom-based descriptions, particularly with respect to motor restlessness (Chess, 1960; Laufer & Denhoff, 1957).

By today's standards, the *DSM-II* guidelines for Hyperkinetic Reaction of Childhood would not be considered adequate diagnostic criteria. Especially problematic was their lack of specificity and detail, which increased the likelihood that professionals would disagree on when this diagnosis was warranted. Of additional concern is that the guidelines did not require the presence of impulsivity, which according to many experts in the field today (Barkley, 1998), is AD/HD's hallmark feature.

Although limited, *DSM II*'s introduction of Hyperkinetic Reaction of Childhood was nevertheless the first time that uniform guidelines for identifying children with AD/HD-like features had appeared in a preeminent publication. As such, it afforded the first opportunity for using standardized diagnostic terminology.

TABLE 1.1.   Diagnostic Criteria for
Hyperkinetic Reaction of Childhood (or Adolescence)

This disorder is characterized by overactivity, restlessness, distractibility, and short attention span, especially in young children; the behavior usually diminishes in adolescence.
If this behavior is caused by organic brain damage, it should be diagnosed under the appropriate non-psychotic organic brain syndrome.

Note: Reprinted with permission from the *Diagnostic and Statistical Manual of Mental Disorders, Second Edition* (p. 50). Copyright 1968 American Psychiatric Association.

The *DSM-III* Criteria

Many clinicians and researchers chose not to embrace *DSM-II*'s guidelines. Some thought that the criteria were too vague to be of any practical value. Others were reluctant to let go of what they thought were more accurate, etiologically based accounts of this condition. At the forefront of this resistance was Wender (1973), who continued to use the term MBD.

Douglas (1972) was another prominent expert who had serious misgivings about the manner in which *DSM-II* characterized this disorder. What troubled Douglas was the primary importance that *DSM-II* placed on hyperactivity. Based on her own extensive research and that of others (Werry & Sprague, 1970), Douglas contended that the deficits in sustained attention shown by hyperkinetic children were equal to or greater than their motor restlessness.

So compelling was this contention that professionals increasingly came to regard inattention as the hallmark feature of the disorder. By the time the diagnostic criteria for Hyperkinetic Reaction of Childhood were being revised for the third edition of the *Diagnostic and Statistical Manual of Mental Disorders* (*DSM-III*; APA, 1980), a consensus had emerged that the name of this condition, as well as its defining features, should be modified to reflect this. The symptom-based label ultimately selected for the revised diagnostic category was thus Attention Deficit Disorder with Hyperactivity" (ADDH; APA, 1980).

A summary of the *DSM-III* guidelines for ADDH (314.01) in Table 1.2 illus-

TABLE 1.2.   Diagnostic Criteria for Attention Deficit Disorder with Hyperactivity

A. **Inattention**. At least three of the following:
   (1) often fails to finish things he or she starts
   (2) often doesn't seem to listen
   (3) easily distracted
   (4) has difficulty concentrating on schoolwork or other tasks requiring sustained attention
   (5) has difficulty sticking to a play activity
B. **Impulsivity**. At least three of the following:
   (1) often acts before thinking
   (2) shifts excessively from one activity to another
   (3) has difficulty organizing work (this not being due to cognitive impairment)
   (4) needs a lot of supervision
   (5) frequently calls out in class
   (6) has difficulty awaiting turn in games or group situations
C. **Hyperactivity**. At least two of the following:
   (1) runs about or climbs on things excessively
   (2) has difficulty sitting still or fidgets excessively
   (3) has difficulty staying seated
   (4) moves about excessively during sleep
   (5) is always "on the go" or acts as if "driven by a motor"
D. Onset before the age of seven
E. Duration of at least six months
F. Not due to Schizophrenia, Affective Disorder, or Severe or Profound Mental Retardation

Note: Reprinted with permission from the *Diagnostic and Statistical Manual of Mental Disorders, Third Edition* (pp. 43–44). Copyright 1980 American Psychiatric Association.

trates this dramatic change in diagnostic criteria. Particularly noteworthy was *DSM-III*'s introduction of an impulsivity component. Although impulsivity had been acknowledged in earlier descriptions (Laufer et al., 1957), this represented the first time that it was given a prominent place alongside inattention and hyperactivity. Together with the other two primary features, impulsivity thus formed what is now regarded as AD/HD's "holy trinity."

Another important change was the order in which the criteria were addressed. As might be expected from the new name, the guidelines for meeting the inattention requirements of ADDH were placed ahead of those for hyperactivity. Less readily anticipated was that the impulsivity criteria also went before hyperactivity. That hyperactivity took a back seat to both inattention and impulsivity clearly signaled its declining importance in overall clinical presentation.

In addition to conceptual modifications, *DSM-III* introduced methodological changes to reduce subjectivity and thereby increase the reliability of this diagnostic category. The changes included listings of several behaviors as manifestations of each primary symptom. Also specified were minimum numbers of symptoms that had to be endorsed from each list to determine whether clinically significant levels of inattention, impulsivity, or hyperactivity were present. *DSM-III* further stipulated onset and duration criteria to highlight the chronic nature of this disorder. Following the precedent set by *DSM-II*, there was also a requirement for ruling out alternative explanations before establishing an ADDH diagnosis. Unlike its predecessor, *DSM-III* did not include organic brain syndrome on its list of exclusionary conditions. Instead, the list comprised several mental health conditions and developmental disorders, yet another indication of the diminished role of brain damage in the disorder's etiology.

Further attesting to the elevated importance of the inattention component was the appearance of a completely new diagnostic category, or *subtype*, known as Attention Deficit Disorder (ADD) without hyperactivity (APA, 1980). The *DSM-III* description of ADD (314.00) appears in Table 1.3. The classification was used for children who met all but the hyperactivity criteria for ADDH. Although the intent of the ADD category was to highlight the inattentiveness of such children, this category was not as pure a disorder of inattention as its name implied, because children meeting its criteria also had to display clinically significant impulsivity. We now know that the pairing of inattention with impulsivity does not accurately reflect how these primary symptoms cluster, but when ADD was first conceived, many viewed inattention and impulsivity as intertwined.

Another *DSM-III* contribution was its creation of the subtype category Attention Deficit Disorder, residual type (ADD-RT; APA, 1980; Table 1.4). Although

TABLE 1.3. Diagnostic Criteria for Attention Deficit Disorder without Hyperactivity

---

The criteria for this disorder are the same as those for Attention Deficit Disorder with Hyperactivity except that the individual never had signs of hyperactivity (criterion C).

Note: Reprinted with permission from the *Diagnostic and Statistical Manual of Mental Disorders, Third Edition* (p. 44). Copyright 1980 American Psychiatric Association.

TABLE 1.4. Diagnostic Criteria for Attention Deficit Disorder, Residual Type

A. The individual once met the criteria for Attention Deficit Disorder with Hyperactivity. This information may come from the individual or from others, such as family members.
B. Signs of hyperactivity are no longer present, but other signs of the illness have persisted to the present without periods of remission, as evidenced by signs of both attentional deficits and impulsivity (e.g., difficulty organizing work and completing tasks, difficulty concentrating, being easily distracted, making sudden decisions without thought of the consequences).
C. The symptoms of inattention and impulsivity result in some impairment in social or occupational functioning.
D. Not due to Schizophrenia, Affective Disorder, Severe or Profound Mental Retardation, or Schizotypal or Borderline Personality Disorders.

Note: Reprinted with permission from the *Diagnostic and Statistical Manual of Mental Disorders, Third Edition* (pp. 44–45). Copyright 1980 American Psychiatric Association.

it was not explicitly stated in *DSM-III*, the ADD-RT subtype seemed designed primarily for use with adolescents and adults, making it the first formal attempt to acknowledge that ADD features—in this case, inattention and impulsivity— might persist beyond childhood. Compared with the criteria for ADDH and ADD, the guidelines for ADD-RT were vague and unclear, thereby leaving them open to subjective interpretation. Such subjectivity notwithstanding, an interesting and unique aspect of the ADD-RT criteria was the requirement for social or occupational *impairment* resulting from the inattention and impulsivity symptoms.

From a historical perspective, the modifications that *DSM-III* made with respect to what had been known as Hyperkinetic Reaction of Childhood were dramatic, so dramatic in fact, that ADDH and its various subtypes bore little resemblance to their *DSM-II* predecessor. Especially noteworthy was *DSM-III*'s introduction of clearly delineated decision-making guidelines, which greatly facilitated clinical research and practice with this population. Of additional historical importance was the extent to which the new criteria influenced subsequent revisions of this diagnostic category.

The *DSM-III-R* Criteria

When *DSM-III* was released, it was expected to remain in use until *DSM-IV* was developed. Unfortunately, problems surfaced in many of the clinical and research applications of *DSM-III*, so an interim diagnostic classification system was put together, leading to publication of the revised third edition (*DSM-III-R*; APA, 1987).

The diagnostic criteria for ADDH and its subtypes underwent revision as well. The end result was the creation of two new categories, Attention-Deficit Hyperactivity Disorder (ADHD; APA, 1987) and Undifferentiated Attention-Deficit Disorder (UADD; APA, 1987). Based solely upon a consideration of their names and assigned code numbers, ADHD (314.01) and UADD (314.00) certainly appeared to be the *DSM-III-R* versions of ADDH and ADD in *DSM-III*. In many ways they were, but there were also many important conceptual and methodological differences between these disorders and their *DSM-III* counterparts.

The criteria for ADHD appear in Table 1.5. Unlike ADDH, ADHD did not employ separate symptom listings for inattention, impulsivity, and hyperactivity. Instead, it used a single list of 14 items, thereby addressing all three primary symptoms as a group. This was a direct by-product of an ongoing debate over how these symptoms clustered. Some believed that the three symptoms were distinct clinical entities and should therefore be dealt with accordingly, as had been done in *DSM-III*. Others viewed inattention–impulsivity as intertwined, distinct from hyperactivity. In contrast, factor analytic studies showed a clustering of impulsivity–hyperactivity, distinct from inattention (Achenbach & Edelbrock, 1983; Milich & Kramer, 1984). Because this situation was still unresolved prior to *DSM-III-R*'s release date, its unidimensional symptom listing approach remained in place pending further research.

Another way in which the criteria for ADHD and ADDH differed was in terms of their item content, especially for the hyperactivity component. For example, ADHD did not include *moves about excessively during sleep* or any other symptom pertaining to sleep disturbance, as had been the case for ADDH. It further redefined hyperactivity by including the symptom *often talks excessively*. This represented the first acknowledgement within the field that excessive verbal behavior could be a manifestation of hyperactivity.

TABLE 1.5.   Diagnostic Criteria for Attention-Deficit Hyperactivity Disorder

Note: Consider a criterion met only if the behavior is considerably more frequent than that of most people of the same mental age.

A. A disturbance of at least six months during which at least eight of the following are present:
   (1) often fidgets with hands or feet or squirms in seat (in adolescents, may be limited to subjective feelings of restlessness)
   (2) has difficulty remaining seated when required to do so
   (3) is easily distracted by extraneous stimuli
   (4) has difficulty awaiting turn in games or group situations
   (5) often blurts out answers to questions before they have been completed
   (6) has difficulty following through on instructions from others (not due to oppositional behavior or failure of comprehension), e.g., fails to finish chores
   (7) has difficulty sustaining attention in tasks or play activities
   (8) often shifts from one uncompleted activity to another
   (9) has difficulty playing quietly
   (10) often talks excessively
   (11) often interrupts or intrudes on others, e.g., butts into other children's games
   (12) often does not seem to listen to what is being said to him or her
   (13) often loses things necessary for tasks or activities at school or at home (e.g., toys, pencils, books, assignments)
   (14) often engages in physically dangerous activities without considering possible consequences (not for the purpose of thrill-seeking), e.g., runs into street without looking
B. Onset before the age of seven.
C. Does not meet the criteria for a Pervasive Developmental Disorder.

Note: Reprinted with permission from the *Diagnostic and Statistical Manual of Mental Disorders, Third Edition—Revised* (pp. 52–53). Copyright 1987 American Psychiatric Association.

In addition to these modifications, *DSM-III-R* stipulated that ADHD-like behaviors had to occur to a greater degree than would be expected of "most people of the same mental age," meaning that it was no longer appropriate to arrive at either an ADHD or UADD diagnosis merely on the basis of the presence or absence of symptoms. To warrant diagnostic consideration, such symptoms had to be displayed to a degree that was *developmentally deviant*. Unfortunately, *DSM-III-R* did not give clear guidelines for determining developmental deviance, thus leaving it open to interpretation. Despite this limitation, the new mental-age requirement called attention to the need for assessing ADHD symptoms within a developmental framework—both for normal children and for those with developmental delays, which helped to ensure that only children with clinically significant behavioral difficulties would be diagnosed with ADHD or UADD. Conversely, it lessened the chance that normally functioning children would receive an erroneous diagnosis.

Following the precedent set by *DSM-II* and continued in *DSM-III*, the *DSM-III-R* criteria required ruling out certain alternative explanations before arriving at an ADHD diagnosis. Unlike its predecessors, however, *DSM-III-R* did not list affective disorder or mental retardation as rule-out conditions, instead paring its exclusionary list to a single developmental condition, Pervasive Developmental Disorder (PDD).

The other new *DSM-III-R* classification, UADD (Table 1.6), emphasized inattention. This characteristic alone suggested that UADD might be comparable to its *DSM-III* counterpart, ADD, but closer inspection showed that these disorders had less in common than their names implied. The most important difference between them was the way in which they addressed impulsivity: ADD required the presence of impulsivity, UADD did not. Not having an impulsivity requirement in its criteria made UADD a purer disorder of inattention.

Although this distinction set the stage for UADD to have a meaningful impact on the field, it did not occur for a variety of reasons. Foremost among these was that the diagnostic guidelines for UADD were extremely vague, making it hard to diagnose consistently. Also limiting its use were findings suggesting that UADD might have more in common with various anxiety disorders than with ADHD (Carlson, 1986; Lahey, Schaughency, Strauss, & Frame, 1984). As a result of this conceptual uncertainty, UADD was not presented alongside ADHD, as ADD had been alongside ADDH, but was instead relegated to a much

TABLE 1.6. Diagnostic Criteria for Undifferentiated Attention Deficit Disorder

This is a residual category for disturbances in which the predominant feature is the persistence of developmentally inappropriate and marked inattention that is not a symptom of another disorder, such as Mental Retardation or Attention-Deficit Hyperactivity Disorder, or of a disorganized and chaotic environment. Some of the disturbances that in *DSM-III* would have been categorized as Attention Deficit Disorder without Hyperactivity would be included in this category. Research is necessary to determine if this is a valid diagnostic category and, if so, how it should be defined.

Note: Reprinted with permission from the *Diagnostic and Statistical Manual of Mental Disorders, Third Edition—Revised* (p. 95). Copyright 1987 American Psychiatric Association.

less visible placement within a loosely defined portion of *DSM-III-R* known as "Other Disorders of Infancy, Childhood, or Adolescence."

To the extent that ADHD and UADD replaced ADDH and ADD, one might have expected a counterpart to ADD-RT as well, but nowhere in *DSM-III-R* was there any classification even vaguely resembling ADD-RT. Elimination of this category did not imply that adolescents and adults could no longer receive a diagnosis pertaining to such problems. They still could, as long as they met criteria for either ADHD or UADD. Unfortunately, arriving at these diagnoses was not easily achieved.

In addition to this complication, there were other diagnostic difficulties associated with the new *DSM-III-R* categories. Especially problematic was *DSM-III-R*'s unidimensional symptom listing for ADHD. Although the criteria for this disorder stipulated that 8 of its 14 symptoms had to be present, there were no restrictions as to which combinations of the 3 primary symptoms might meet this requirement. Thus, some children could be labeled ADHD primarily due to inattentiveness, whereas others could be given the very same label due mainly to impulsivity or hyperactivity. Such discrepancies in clinical presentation greatly diminished this diagnostic category's reliability.

CURRENT DIAGNOSTIC CRITERIA

The *DSM-IV*

Although later than planned, the fourth edition of the *Diagnostic and Statistical Manual of Mental Disorders* (*DSM-IV*; APA, 1994) finally arrived in the spring of 1994. With its arrival came Attention-Deficit/Hyperactivity Disorder.

As can be seen in Table 1.7., AD/HD uses many of the same conceptual and methodological features that were a part of ADHD. For example, it encompasses the same 3 primary symptoms: inattention, impulsivity, and hyperactivity. Its symptom description for each bear close resemblance to the 14 items that had been listed for ADHD. Of additional importance is that AD/HD requires evidence of developmental deviance, again highlighting the importance of developmental factors in the assessment process. It also has the same onset criteria, the same duration criteria, and the same exclusionary requirement for ruling out PDD.

But there are also many new features. Among them is AD/HD's introduction of several new symptom descriptions, raising the total to 18 (9 inattention symptoms, 6 hyperactivity symptoms, and 3 impulsivity symptoms). In and of itself, this small increase in the number of symptoms available for consideration is not of any particular diagnostic significance. What is significant, however, is the manner in which this new total is organized and presented. Instead of being grouped together in a unidimensional listing, the items are subdivided into two groups. In one group are the 9 inattention symptoms, in the other are the remaining 9 hyperactivity-impulsivity concerns.

As noted, a similar two-group arrangement had been considered for *DSM-III-R*, but there was insufficient empirical evidence to justify its adoption at that

TABLE 1.7.   Diagnostic Criteria for Attention-Deficit/Hyperactivity Disorder

A. Either (1) or (2)
 (1) **Inattention**: six (or more) of the following symptoms of inattention have persisted for at least
    6 months to a degree that is maladaptive and inconsistent with developmental level:
     (a) often fails to give close attention to details or makes careless mistakes in schoolwork,
        work, or other activities
     (b) often has difficulty sustaining attention in tasks or play activities
     (c) often does not seem to listen when spoken to directly
     (d) often does not follow through on instructions and fails to finish schoolwork, chores, or
        duties in the workplace (not due to oppositional behavior or failure to understand
        instructions)
     (e) often has difficulty organizing tasks and activities
     (f) often avoids, dislikes, or is reluctant to engage in tasks that require sustained mental
        effort (such as schoolwork or homework)
     (g) often loses things necessary for tasks or activities (toys, school assignments, pencils,
        books, or tools)
     (h) is often easily distracted by extraneous stimuli
     (i) is often forgetful in daily activities
 (2) **Hyperactivity-Impulsivity**: six (or more) of the following symptoms of hyperactivity-
    impulsivity have persisted for at least 6 months to a degree that is maladaptive and inconsis-
    tent with developmental level:
    Hyperactivity
     (a) often fidgets with hands or feet or squirms in seat
     (b) often leaves seat in classroom or in other situations in which remaining seated is
        expected
     (c) often runs about or climbs excessively in situations in which it is inappropriate (in
        adolescents or adults, may be limited to subjective feelings of restlessness)
     (d) often has difficulty playing or engaging in leisure activities quietly
     (e) is often "on the go" or often acts as if "driven by a motor"
     (f) often talks excessively
    Impulsivity
     (g) often blurts out answers to questions before they have been completed
     (h) often has difficulty awaiting turn
     (i) often interrupts or intrudes on others (e.g., butts into conversations or games)
B. Some hyperactive-impulsive or inattentive symptoms that caused impairment were present
   before age 7 years.
C. Some impairment from the symptoms is present in two or more settings (e.g., at school [or work]
   and at home).
D. There must be clear evidence of clinically significant impairment in social, academic, or occupational functioning.
E. The symptoms do not occur exclusively during the course of a Pervasive Developmental Disorder, Schizophrenia, or other Psychotic Disorder and are not better accounted for by another
   mental disorder (e.g., Mood Disorder, Anxiety Disorder, Dissociated Disorder, or a Personality
   Disorder).

Note: Reprinted with permission from the *Diagnostic and Statistical Manual of Mental Disorders, Fourth Edition*
(pp. 83–85). Copyright 1994 American Psychiatric Association.

time (Achenbach & Edelbrock, 1983; Milich & Kramer, 1984). As more studies were done, it became increasingly clear that hyperactivity–impulsivity did cluster together, apart from inattention (Bauermeister, Alegria, Bird, Rubio-Stipec, & Canino, 1992; DuPaul, 1991; Edelbrock, 1991; Healey et al., 1993; Lahey et al., 1988). Such findings provided the additional justification necessary for including separate symptom listings in the new criteria for AD/HD.

Presenting the primary symptoms in this way allows for meaningful subtyping to occur. Although this had been possible in *DSM-III*, it was no longer just an option in *DSM-IV*. According to the new guidelines, *all* AD/HD diagnoses must now be accompanied by a subtyping distinction.

Appearing in Table 1.8. are the criteria for the three major subtype classifications in *DSM-IV*. What distinguishes one from another is whether the criteria for one, or from both, primary symptom lists are met. For example, if 6 or more symptoms from both lists are present, and if all other AD/HD criteria are met, AD/HD, Combined Type (314.01) is the diagnosis. Given that this new category encompasses numerous features of inattention, along with some combination of hyperactivity–impulsivity, it seems to be *DSM-IV*'s version of what had been ADHD in *DSM-III-R*.

Subtyping options also exist for situations wherein enough symptoms are present for one listing but not for the other. This might occur, for example, when there are 6 or more inattention symptoms, but fewer than 6 hyperactivity-impulsivity symptoms. When this situation arises, and all other AD/HD criteria are met, a diagnosis of AD/HD, Predominantly Inattentive Type (314.00) is in order. Given its emphasis on inattention, this particular category seems conceptually related to what *DSM-III-R* had termed UADD.

The other possible scenario that might unfold is when there are 6 or more hyperactivity-impulsivity symptoms but less than 6 inattention symptoms. Assuming that all other AD/HD criteria are met, the proper diagnosis for this is AD/HD, Predominantly Hyperactive-Impulsive Type (314.01). This, of course, is a completely new subtype category. Although this new category came mainly from the results of numerous factor analytic studies (DuPaul, 1991; Lahey et al.,

TABLE 1.8. Diagnostic Criteria for Combined, Predominantly Inattentive, and Predominantly Hyperactive-Impulsive Types of Attention-Deficit/Hyperactivity Disorder

Subtype category	Diagnostic criteria
Combined	Six (or more) symptoms of inattention and six (or more) symptoms of hyperactivity-impulsivity have persisted for at least 6 months.
Predominantly Inattentive	Six (or more) symptoms of inattention (but fewer than six symptoms of hyperactivity-impulsivity) have persisted for at least 6 months.
Predominantly Hyperactive-Impulsive	Six (or more) symptoms of hyperactivity-impulsivity (but fewer than six symptoms for inattention) have persisted for at least 6 months.

Note: Reprinted with permission from the *Diagnostic and Statistical Manual of Mental Disorders, Fourth Edition* (pp. 80). Copyright 1994 American Psychiatric Association.

1988), such statistical considerations were not the only grounds for its appearance in *DSM-IV*. Findings from various clinical investigations, which showed that symptoms of hyperactivity and impulsivity were critical in determining current and future psychosocial functioning (Barkley, Fischer, Edelbrock, & Smallish, 1990; Loeber, Keenan, Lahey, Green, & Thomas, 1993), were also influential.

Along with these subtyping changes, many other novel features are found in the criteria for AD/HD. One such modification is that there is now a requirement for establishing evidence of cross-situational pervasiveness, meaning that symptom-related impairment must exist in at least two settings. Another new feature, at least with respect to children, is that there must now be evidence that these symptoms interfere with developmentally appropriate social, academic, or occupational functioning.

Although *DSM-IV*'s requirement for ruling out exclusionary conditions is by no means new, its listing of such conditions is by far the most expansive to date. Going well beyond *DSM-III-R*'s sole requirement, ruling out PDD, this new list requires consideration of schizophrenia, psychotic disorder, mood disorder, anxiety disorder, dissociative disorder, and personality disorder before arriving at an AD/HD diagnosis. This alone is a meaningful addition to the criteria for AD/HD. Making it even more unique is the diagnostic flexibility. Whereas some conditions, such as PDD, automatically preclude having AD/HD, others, such as a mood disorder or an anxiety disorder, do not. Thus, the new guideline recognizes that although there are times when particular disorders better account for the presence of AD/HD-like symptoms, at other times these same disorders can co-exist with AD/HD.

Other important changes are found in how *DSM-IV* addresses the needs of adolescents and adults. Many of *DSM-IV*'s new symptom descriptions include wording that is more developmentally appropriate for an older group. This is evident, for example, in the phrase *may be limited to subjective feelings of restlessness*, which is parenthetically inserted alongside the hyperactivity item, *runs about or climbs excessively*.

Such phrasing adjustments are not the only way in which *DSM-IV* addresses the diagnostic needs of the older end of the age continuum. Table 1.9. shows two new subtype categories for this purpose. The first is AD/HD, In

TABLE 1.9.   Diagnostic Criteria for In Partial Remission
and Not Otherwise Specified Types of Attention-Deficit/Hyperactivity Disorder

Subtype category	Diagnostic criteria
In Partial Remission	Clinically significant symptoms remain but criteria are no longer met for any of the subtypes.
Not Otherwise Specified	Symptoms do not currently meet full criteria for the disorder and it is unclear whether criteria for the disorder have previously been met.

Note: Reprinted with permission from the *Diagnostic and Statistical Manual of Mental Disorders, Fourth Edition* (pp. 80). Copyright 1994 American Psychiatric Association.

Partial Remission, which most often applies to adolescents and adults who, as children, probably met criteria for one of the three major AD/HD subtypes, but who no longer do. Defined in this way, In Partial Remission bears close resemblance to what was known as ADD-RT in *DSM-III*. What makes it different is that a numerical coding option now allows for identifying which of the three major subtypes previously existed. For example, for someone with a history of either the Combined Type or the Predominantly Hyperactive-Impulsive Subtype, the code 314.01 is used. For those who previously met the Predominantly Inattentive Criteria, this In Partial Remission label is used again, but the numerical code is 314.00.

The other new category in *DSM-IV* is AD/HD, Not Otherwise Specified (314.9). This too is primarily intended for adolescents and adults whose symptoms do not currently meet the criteria for any of the three major AD/HD subtypes, but unlike In Partial Remission, Not Otherwise Specified does not assume an earlier AD/HD diagnosis. Instead, it might be used when there is uncertainty about the onset of AD/HD symptoms, a common complication when evaluating adults. Occasionally it arises when evaluating children too, especially children whose early histories are unclear due to chaotic home environments, multiple foster care placements, and so forth.

What should be apparent by now is that *DSM-IV* contains many new conceptual and methodological features. Although it is too early to judge their historical impact, most of these modifications seem to be an improvement over what was used in *DSM-III-R*. Perhaps most important are the three major subtyping options, especially the new Predominantly Hyperactive-Impulsive subtype. That it has been given equal status with the Combined and Predominantly Inattentive subtype reflects the increased conceptual and clinical importance of these behavioral characteristics, particularly impulsivity (Barkley, 1998).

Many other enhancements are also evident in *DSM-IV*'s approach to subtyping. For example, the rules for establishing the three major subtyping diagnoses are clear and specific, which greatly increases their reliability. Another advantage is the manner in which the diagnostic needs of adolescents and adults are addressed: No longer is it necessary for them to meet the same criteria as do children to receive a diagnosis, though this is still a possibility. Other diagnostic options exist, in the form of either the In Partial Remission or the Not Otherwise Specified classifications.

Other *DSM-IV* improvements include the requirement for evidence of psychosocial impairment resulting from AD/HD symptoms and the requirement that the symptoms show cross-situational pervasiveness. Another strength is the manner in which exclusionary issues are addressed. Not only is there an expanded listing of potential rule-out conditions, but *DSM-IV* now allows the use of certain categories on this list in either an exclusionary or a comorbid capacity.

Additional strengths are found in some of the diagnostic criteria that *DSM-IV* carried over from earlier *DSM* editions. Foremost among these is its retention of *DSM-III-R*'s developmental deviance requirement. Such continuity calls further attention to the role of developmental factors in the diagnostic process. *DSM-IV* also uses the same onset and duration criteria that appeared in *DSM-III-R* and in *DSM-III*, again highlighting this disorder's early appearance and chronicity.

Amidst these many advantages, certain aspects of the new diagnostic criteria are problematic, particularly the lack of an operational definition of what constitutes developmental deviance. How this guideline is met is therefore open to interpretation, so clinicians and researchers are more likely to disagree about who does, and who does not, meet this criterion.

Another developmentally related concern is that the same symptom cut-points are used for all ages. Although there are no published reports to challenge its validity, preliminary data suggest that requiring 6 or more symptoms of either inattention or hyperactivity-impulsivity is too restrictive for adolescents and adults (Barkley & Murphy, 1995). For individuals at this end of the age continuum, 4 or 5 symptoms from either list may be all that is needed to establish a level of statistical deviance corresponding to that of children. Under the current guidelines, many adults and adolescents might not receive one of the three major subtyping diagnoses even when it is clinically indicated. To compensate for this, *DSM-IV* offers AD/HD, In Partial Remission, and AD/HD, Not Otherwise Specified for adolescents and adults—clearly a step in the right direction. Unfortunately, both categories contain vague language in their criteria, reducing their clinical utility and reliability.

Similar problems exist for very young children. When *DSM-III-R* was in use, there was evidence that the requirement of 8 symptoms was far too inclusive for preschoolers (DuPaul, 1991). To be sure that only those preschoolers displaying clinically significant levels of AD/HD would receive this diagnosis, some (Barkley, 1990) advocated a cutoff score of 10 symptoms. Whether this same developmental complication applies to the *DSM-IV* criteria for AD/HD remains to be seen. If the current guidelines are too inclusive, many preschoolers may be mistakenly identified as having AD/HD. Further, the wording for many of the inattention symptoms (e.g., *often has difficulty organizing tasks and activities*) is developmentally inappropriate for preschoolers, thereby effectively eliminating these items from clinical consideration. Of additional diagnostic concern is that the duration requirement of 6 months may not be sufficient for differentiating normal preschoolers from those with clinically significant behavioral problems (Campbell, 1987).

Yet another potential problem is that some members of the professional and lay community may inappropriately regard the Predominantly Inattentive and Predominantly Hyperactive-Impulsive subtypes as pure categories. Although they can be, their actual definition suggests that this is not *DSM-IV*'s primary intent. To understand this situation more fully, consider how these subtypes might apply to two children with very similar behavioral features. One child, for example, might display 6 inattention symptoms but only 5 hyperactive-impulsive symptoms and carry a diagnosis of AD/HD, Predominantly Inattentive. Another child, with 5 inattention symptoms and 6 hyperactive-impulsive symptoms, would receive an AD/HD, Predominantly Hyperactive-Impulsive diagnosis. To think of the former child as having pure inattention difficulties and the latter as having pure hyperactive-impulsive concerns is obviously inaccurate. In view of this, clinicians and researchers must bear in mind that both categories include symptoms that go beyond what their labels suggest. Thus, although the Predominantly Inattentive Type refers to a condition in which there are *predominantly* inattention concerns, it can also encompass features of hyperactivity-impulsivity. Likewise, the Predominantly Hyperactive-Impulsive Type pertains to a condition in which there are *predominantly* hyperactive-impulsive symptoms, but it can also include elements of inattention.

The *ICD-10*

Although educators and child health-care professionals in many parts of the world outside of North America would agree that symptoms of inattention, hyperactivity-impulsivity, or both constitute a diagnostic condition, they would not refer to it as AD/HD, nor would they follow the *DSM-IV* diagnostic guidelines. If a diagnosis was made at all, it would be Hyperkinetic Disorder, the criteria for which appear in the *International Classification of Diseases, 10th edition* (*ICD-10*; WHO, 1993). Somewhat akin to *DSM-IV*, the *ICD-10* uses separate symptom listings comprising 18 symptoms. Unlike *DSM-IV*, the *ICD-10* utilizes a 9-item inattention list, a 5-item hyperactivity list, and a 4-item impulsivity list. Each list also differs in the symptom cut-points employed. For example, at least 6 inattention symptoms, 3 hyperactivity symptoms, and 1 impulsivity symptom must be present before considering a Hyperkinetic Disorder diagnosis. The *ICD-10* requires that these symptoms: (1) have an onset no later than 7 years of age; (2) have a duration of at least 6 months; (3) be developmentally deviant; and (4) not be due to PDD or certain other psychiatric conditions.

What should be apparent by now is that the *DSM-IV* and *ICD-10* diagnostic guidelines are similar. This is not a chance occurrence; systematic efforts were made during the development of *DSM-IV* to create a system that allowed direct comparison with equivalent *ICD-10* disorders. Thus, their symptom lists overlap. Their criteria for onset and duration, as well as some of their exclusionary criteria, are essentially identical, and both require cross-situational pervasiveness.

But there are significant differences. For one thing, *ICD-10* does not allow for subtyping. Thus, any comparison between *DSM-IV* and *ICD-10* must necessarily be limited to a consideration of AD/HD, combined type and Hyperkinetic Disorder, respectively. Also, because only one form of Hyperkinetic Disorder is available for consideration, fewer individuals would be expected to receive this diagnosis, which has clinical and research implications, especially for adolescents and adults. Another difference between *ICD-10* and *DSM-IV* is in the exclusionary criteria. In *ICD-10*, the co-occurrence of a depressive episode or an anxiety disorder automatically precludes a diagnosis of Hyperkinetic Disorder. Although *DSM-IV* recognizes that such conditions can preclude an AD/HD diagnosis, it also allows for comorbidity.

CONCLUSION

There is little justification for claiming that AD/HD is merely a "disorder of the 90s." More accurately, it is the most recent diagnostic label for a long-observed phenomenon: children who display developmentally inappropriate levels of inattention, impulsivity, and/or hyperactivity. Although confusing, these earlier labels were reflective of the many ways in which this disorder has been conceptualized over time.

Figure 1.1. shows the two major trends that have characterized the history of AD/HD in North America. The first trend pertains to diagnostic uniformity. From Still's (1902) account until the late 1960s, few agreed on what to call this condition. As it became apparent that the continued use of multiple labels would seriously impede scientific progress, clinicians and researchers acknowl-

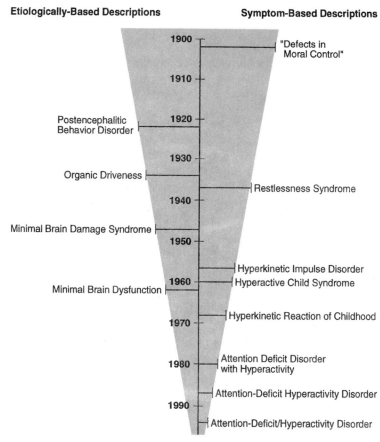

Etiologically-Based Descriptions   **Symptom-Based Descriptions**

1900 — "Defects in Moral Control"

1910

Postencephalitic Behavior Disorder — 1920

1930

Organic Driveness — Restlessness Syndrome

1940

Minimal Brain Damage Syndrome — 1950

Hyperkinetic Impulse Disorder
Minimal Brain Dysfunction — 1960 — Hyperactive Child Syndrome

1970 — Hyperkinetic Reaction of Childhood

1980 — Attention Deficit Disorder with Hyperactivity

Attention-Deficit Hyperactivity Disorder
1990 —
Attention-Deficit/Hyperactivity Disorder

FIGURE 1.1. Historical trends in diagnosing AD/HD.

edged the need for a common diagnostic terminology. The arrival of *DSM-II* (APA, 1968) afforded the first real opportunity for this through its presentation of Hyperkinetic Reaction of Childhood. This commitment to diagnostic uniformity has since gained widespread acceptance; most professionals now use uniform diagnostic language in their descriptions of AD/HD.

The second trend pertains to *how* this disorder has been labeled. With the exception of Still's account, most early names for this condition, such as post-encephalitic behavior disorder (Hohman, 1922), reflected its presumed etiology. During the mid-1930s, a competing trend emerged in the form of various symptom-based descriptions, which included such terms as "restlessness syndrome" (Levin, 1938). Although these competing trends remained in evidence for the next 3 decades (Chess, 1960; Clements & Peters, 1962), etiologically based descriptions eventually declined as symptom-based descriptions gained wider acceptance. When Hyperkinetic Reaction of Childhood appeared in *DSM-II*, it marked the beginning of a new era in which only symptom-based descriptions were used.

As for the *DSM* diagnostic criteria, they too have undergone numerous transformations, a summary of which appears in Table 1.10. What began as a simple text description in *DSM-II* has now evolved into a complex, multifaceted depiction. Along the way there have been major shifts in conceptual emphasis, dramatic changes in how symptoms are listed, and increased awareness of the importance of subtyping. There have also been many modifications in the diagnostic procedures themselves, greatly increasing their accuracy. These include the recently incorporated requirements for establishing developmental

TABLE 1.10.   Summary of Major Changes in *DSM* Criteria

Diagnostic criteria	DSM-II	DSM-III	DSM-III-R	DSM-IV
Symptoms groupings	1-factor	3-factor	1-factor	2-factor
Subtyping options	—	ADDH, ADD, ADD-RT	ADHD, UADD	C, I, HI, IPR, NOS
Symptom onset	—	<7 years	<7 years	<7 years
Symptom duration	—	6 months	6 months	6 months
Developmental deviance	—	—	Yes	Yes
Cross-situational pervasiveness	—	—	—	Yes
Functional impairment	—	—	—	Yes
Exclusionary conditions	OBD	Sx, Aff, MR	PDD	PDD, Sx, Psy, MD, Anx, DD, PD

Note: DSM = Diagnostic and Statistical Manual; ADDH = Attention deficit disorder with hyperactivity; ADD = Attention deficit disorder (without hyperactivity); ADD-RT = Attention deficit disorder, residual type; ADHD = Attention-deficity hyperactivity disorder; UADD = Undifferentiated attention-deficit disorder; C = combined type; I = Predominantly inattentive type; HI = Predominantly hyperactive-impulsive type; IPR = in partial remission; NOS = Not otherwise specified; OBD = Organic brain damage; Sx = Schizophrenia; Aff = Affective disorder; MR = Mental retardation; PDD = Pervasive developmental disorder; Psy = Psychotic disorder; MD = Mood disorder; Anx = Anxiety disorder; DD = Dissociative disorder; PD = Personality disorder.

deviance, for documenting functional impairment, and for considering various exclusionary conditions.

If nothing else, what this history teaches us is that AD/HD's assessment is a dynamic process. Only time will tell how well the current criteria will hold up under empirical scrutiny. In the meantime, as we use the new guidelines in clinical practice and research, it is our responsibility to adhere as closely as possible to them as they are set forth in *DSM-IV*. To the extent that we do this, our field will be in an excellent position to judge which *DSM-IV* features should be retained in any subsequent revisions.

2

Primary Characteristics
and Associated Features

*"I heard about the terrible two's. My son's 10 now.
When is he going to grow out of them?"*

Although the *DSM-IV* criteria have been available since 1994, only in the past few years has research using these criteria made its way into the scientific literature. Thus, gaps remain in our understanding of AD/HD, particularly in terms of the new subtyping classifications. Mindful of these limitations this chapter provides an overview of AD/HD topics that have direct bearing on the assessment process, including primary symptoms, etiology, epidemiology, developmental course, psychosocial impact, and comorbidity. Throughout this review the term "AD/HD" will be employed. Though this label thus far has been used to signify only the *DSM-IV* version of the disorder, it will now be applied to all *DSM* citations.

PRIMARY SYMPTOMS

Clinical Presentation

Most child health-care professionals would agree that developmentally inappropriate levels of inattention, impulsivity, and hyperactivity are the primary symptoms of AD/HD. Despite this consensus, individuals are sometimes unclear about what constitutes an AD/HD diagnosis. For example, when asked to identify the behaviors that lead them to believe that a child might have AD/HD, parents and teachers may cite noncompliance, emotional immaturity, or unsatisfactory academic progress. Such characteristics are often associated with an AD/HD diagnosis, but they are not its essential or defining features. To counter such confusion, clinicians and researchers must be thoroughly familiar with the items that make up the *DSM-IV* symptom lists. Moreover, they must also be familiar with the various ways these symptoms can manifest in everyday life.

Inattention

Descriptions of children with AD/HD frequently include complaints of not listening to instructions, not finishing assigned work, daydreaming, becoming bored easily, and so forth. Common to all of these referral concerns is a diminished capacity for vigilance, that is, difficulties sustaining attention to task (Douglas, 1983). Such problems can occur in free-play settings (Routh & Schroeder, 1976), but most often they surface in situations demanding sustained attention to dull, boring, repetitive tasks (Milich, Loney, & Landau, 1982). Where competing activities provide more immediate and meaningful gratification, children with AD/HD frequently shift "off-task" to engage in them. Although off-task behavior may stem from heightened distractibility, it can also result from diminished persistence in responding to tasks that have little intrinsic appeal or delayed rewards for completion (Barkley, 1990).

How inattentiveness is expressed can vary a great deal, in part as a function of the child's age. Some parents report that their child's earliest displays of inattention occurred during infancy. Descriptions of these infants typically involve such comments as, "He could never entertain himself. Somebody always had to be there keeping him busy." One of the most frequently mentioned ways in which toddlers with AD/HD exhibit inattentiveness is through their inability to watch more than a few minutes of a television program or videotape, even when it is of some interest (e.g., *Sesame Street*). Many preschoolers begin to display inattentiveness in day care or preschool settings, which might manifest as excessive shifting from one activity center to another or as not listening during story time.

Entrance into kindergarten and the early elementary grades typically brings with it a variety of new demands for self-regulation, thereby greatly increasing the number of opportunities for inattentiveness. For a child with AD/HD, this might mean doing tasks incorrectly because of not listening to all of the teacher's instructions, or finishing only 5 of 10 assigned math problems due to daydreaming or being distracted by the movements of other students in the classroom. Further examples of inattentiveness in school include keeping a messy desk, losing pencils and papers, and forgetting to bring home teacher notes. At home, these children might forget to do what they're told, fail to remember where they left their shoes, misplace favorite toys, or lose hats and gloves when playing outside. Often they will start an activity, such as getting dressed, but then, distracted by something of greater interest, stop before the task is completed. For many parents, the only way to be sure that the job gets done is to hover over the child and issue constant reminders to stay on task. Although inattentiveness is more likely to occur during completion of chores, it can also occur during play. Some children with AD/HD shift frequently from one toy to the next, leaving behind a messy trail on the floor. There is also a good chance that young elementary school children will not be able to attend long enough to complete even the simplest of board games, such as *Candyland* or *Sorry*.

As children get older, even greater demands for self-regulation and responsibility arise. During the middle and high school years, many students with AD/HD have trouble remembering to bring books home or to turn in assignments. Just finishing homework assignments is perhaps the biggest challenge, especially when the work is long term in nature and requires careful planning and organization. College entrance exams pose additional problems for many teens with AD/HD, who can't pay attention long enough to do well or who lose track of where they are and fill in the wrong circles on the answer sheet. Other problems exhibited by adolescents include forgetting to show up for work and getting into automobile accidents as a result of not paying sufficient attention to their driving (Barkley, Guevremont, Anastopoulos, DuPaul, & Shelton, 1993).

Impulsivity

Sometimes defined as rapid, inaccurate responding (Brown & Quay, 1977), impulsivity also refers to poor sustained inhibition of response (Gordon, 1979), poor delay of gratification (Rapport, Tucker, DuPaul, Merlo, & Stoner, 1986), and impaired adherence to commands requiring inhibition of behavior in social contexts (Kendall & Wilcox, 1979). Clinic-referred children with AD/HD may show impulsivity in a variety of ways, such as talking out of turn or taking unnecessary risks, or blurting out remarks with no regard for social consequences.

As with inattentiveness, the expression of impulsivity is subject to developmental influences. When something of interest captures a preschooler's attention, he or she may go after it with little regard for what might be in the way, sometimes bumping into tables, chairs, or other objects. Preschoolers with AD/HD are also prone to taking toys away from other children, mainly because they are unable to wait.

Elementary school teachers frequently see children with AD/HD cutting in front of other children in line, beginning tasks before directions are completed, or calling out inappropriate remarks that lead to a reputation as the class clown. Careless mistakes in schoolwork are of additional concern, often resulting from a preference for speed over accuracy, or a failure to stop and check work. At home, elementary school children have a hard time refraining from interrupting a parent who is on the phone, making dinner, reading a newspaper, or visiting with company. Perhaps the best example of this comes from a mother who announced that 10 years had elapsed since she last went to the bathroom without being interrupted by a knock on the door! Many other expressions of impulsivity can occur within the home setting as well. When given a choice by their parents, most children with AD/HD prefer an immediately available small reward to a larger one later. These same children may get into dangerous situations, as did the 5-year-old boy who climbed to the top of a tree before realizing that he had no way of getting back down. Regardless of whether danger is involved, most displays of impulsivity at home are stressful and inconvenient for parents. This was certainly true for the parents of an 8-year-old boy who, in a moment of scientific curiosity, decided to see what would happen if he emptied a container of baby powder in front of a moving fan.

By the time they reach middle school or high school, many teens with AD/

HD are adept at playing the role of class clown. Impulsively talking back to parents, teachers, friends, and employers is yet another problem for the adolescents. Also, such teens may not think through the consequences of their actions. This seemed to be the case with a 15-year-old boy, who pulled a school fire alarm on a dare from a classmate who promised to pay him $50 for his effort. Disregard for consequences also seems to be responsible for many risk-taking behaviors of teens with AD/HD, including sexual indiscretions and reckless experimentation with alcohol or illicit drugs (Mannuzza, Klein, Bessler, Malloy, & LaPadula, 1993).

Hyperactivity

Symptoms of hyperactivity are usually displayed physically, but they can be expressed verbally as well. In extreme cases, hyperactive children appear to be in constant motion, always on the go, driven by a motor, unable to sit still, and so forth. Although most people think of hyperactivity in this way, it can also present itself in less severe forms, such as fidgeting or talking excessively. Whether mild or severe, what makes these behaviors manifestations of hyperactivity is their task-irrelevant, extremely frequent, and developmentally inappropriate nature.

Numerous studies have shown that children with AD/HD are more active, restless, and fidgety than children without this disorder (Porrino et al., 1983). Such differences are commonly attributed to greater-than-normal absolute levels of movement, but many investigators have challenged this assumption, arguing instead that it is the pervasiveness of the hyperactivity across settings that most distinguishes children with AD/HD from other child populations (Taylor, 1986). Implicit in this is the notion that children with AD/HD often fail to regulate their motor activity in response to situational demands (Routh, 1978).

Again, developmental factors influence the manner in which hyperactivity symptoms appear. According to one mother, "all hell broke loose" when her son learned how to walk. Another parent recalled that her daughter had on many occasions jumped out of her crib in a daredevil fashion, long before she even knew how to walk. The toddler of another family used to open drawers to climb on top of dressers and counters. Additional problems with hyperactivity can occur in day care or preschool settings, where the child with AD/HD cannot sit in one place for circle time, lie down on a mat for the duration of rest time, or refrain from running when asked to walk in line.

Walking in line can also pose major challenges for elementary school children with AD/HD, as can remaining seated at a desk. But of all the places where staying seated is required, the school bus is perhaps the most challenging. Even when they manage to stay seated, children with AD/HD continue to exhibit hyperactivity, albeit in a different form, such as noisily tapping fingers on a desk, swinging feet to and fro, or rocking a chair back and forth until it tips over.

Displays of hyperactivity are not limited to school, however. At home, elementary school children are often adept at jumping from one piece of furniture to the next. Sitting at the dinner table for the whole meal can also be difficult. Problems with remaining seated may arise in church, at movie theaters, or in restaurants. Many parents also find it hard to keep their child with them as they walk through grocery stores, department stores, or shopping malls. As one parent said, "These kids are a lot like helium balloons. You let go of them for one second and they're all over the place." In addition to physical restlessness, many children with AD/HD exhibit verbal hyperactivity, which can be just as disruptive and annoying. As a mother once said of her 6-year-old son, "He goes to bed talking and then wakes up talking." In a similar vein, a couple recalled how nerve racking it was to take long car rides with their 9-year-old daughter, a proverbial motormouth who "doesn't stop talking the whole time."

For many reasons, including developmental maturity, most teens with AD/HD display fewer physical features of hyperactivity than do younger children, and such symptoms typically appear in the form of restless leg movements or finger tapping. Even when there are no obvious signs of motor restlessness, some teens experience subjective feelings of restlessness, often described in terms of racing thoughts. Clinical experience would also seem to suggest that many teens are more inclined to exhibit verbal, rather than physical, forms of hyperactivity. Thus, it is common to hear complaints of incessant talking in class and not letting others get in a word edgewise during social conversations.

Situational Variability

Contrary to what many believe, AD/HD is not an all-or-none phenomenon. Its primary symptoms fluctuate significantly in response to situational demands (Zentall, 1985). One of the main determinants of this is how interested the child is in what he or she is doing. Symptoms are much more likely in repetitive, boring, or familiar situations versus novel or stimulating situations (Barkley, 1977). Another determinant of situational variability is the amount of imposed structure. In many free-play or low-demand settings, where children with AD/HD can do as they please, their behavior is indistinguishable from that of other children (Luk, 1985). Significant AD/HD problems may not arise until others place demands on them or set rules for their behavior. Presumably due to increased demands for behavioral self-regulation, group settings are far more problematic for children with AD/HD than are one-on-one situations. Symptoms are also more likely to arise when feedback is dispensed infrequently or on a delayed basis (Douglas, 1983).

In view of this situational variability, it is not surprising that children with AD/HD often display inconsistency in their task performance, in both productivity and accuracy (Douglas, 1972). Variability may show up in daily schoolwork or in their test scores (e.g., getting a grade of 90 one day, 60 the next), or it may involve fluctuations in completing homework or routine home chores. Though all children display some variability in these areas, it is clear from clinical experience and research findings that children with AD/HD exhibit it to a much greater degree. Thus, instead of reflecting "laziness," the inconsistent performance of children with AD/HD represents yet another manifestation of the disorder.

How might such variability come into play during clinical evaluations? Mothers and fathers commonly differ in their observations of AD/HD symptoms. Awareness of the different caretaking responsibilities of each parent is the first step in understanding why this is so. Mothers are often primarily responsible for getting children clean, fed, ready for school, and so on, while fathers often have fewer of these caretaking chores and may engage in more recreational activities that their children enjoy. To the extent that mothers impose repetitive, familiar, and boring caretaking demands, they will observe AD/HD symptoms more often than will fathers. For similar reasons, it is fairly easy to see why the perceptions of parents sometimes differ from those of grandparents, who traditionally shower grandchildren with lots of love, affection, money, trips to the toy store, and the like.

Parental perceptions may differ from those of teachers as well. Some mothers and fathers are surprised when a kindergarten or first grade teacher tells them that their child has been exhibiting AD/HD symptoms. But given the different demands imposed on the child in each setting and the different circumstances under which such demands are addressed, differences between teacher and parent perceptions are understandable. For some children, the subject matter at school is far less interesting than the toys or games available at home, and they rarely have to remain seated and quiet, as they often do in school. Moreover, nearly all school activities take place in a group, which is known to exacerbate AD/HD symptoms.

Differences of opinion are not limited to parents and teachers. Disagreements over the presence or absence of AD/HD symptoms may also surface between teachers and from one grade to the next, or even within the same academic year. When this last situation arises, it is often at least partly related to differences in class size, amount of adult supervision, or both. This helps to explain why regular-education teachers are more likely to observe AD/HD symptoms in a class of 25 students than are special-education teachers, who often receive assistance from an aide in a classroom with substantially fewer (usually 8–10) students.

ETIOLOGY

Dating back to Still's 1902 account, there has been a tremendous amount of public and scientific interest in the causes of AD/HD. For the most part, biological explanations have dominated the discussions, though psychological and psychosocial explanations have been put forth as well. Despite the fact that such efforts have increased our awareness of what might cause AD/HD, just how it arises is still unclear. Thus, what we currently believe about AD/HD etiology is more theoretical speculation than established fact.

Biological Explanations

Neurochemistry

It is commonly assumed that AD/HD is caused by chemical imbalances in the brain. Although intuitively appealing, this assumption has not been well established empirically; relatively few investigations have actually addressed it.

Among those that have, the findings were inconsistent. Some studies have reported abnormalities in one of the monoaminergic systems, involving either dopamine (Raskin, Shaywitz, Shaywitz, Anderson, & Cohen, 1984) or norepinephrine (Arnsten, Steere, & Hunt, 1996). Others have implicated serotonin deficiencies (Nemzer, Arnold, Votolato, & McConnell, 1986).

Due to the variable manner in which AD/HD has been defined, it is likely that the samples in these studies differed in their clinical presentation, which may be the explanation for their discrepancies (Halperin et al., 1997a). According to one recently proposed model (Pliszka, McCracken, & Maas, 1996), norepinephrine dysregulation would be seen in those whose primary difficulties are attentional in nature, whereas dopamine deficiencies would be predicted for those whose hyperactivity and impulsivity are prominent. In addition to these subtyping considerations, certain comorbidity differences may come into play. This point was recently emphasized by Halperin and associates, who detected serotonin abnormalities in an AD/HD sample, but only when co-occurring aggressive features were present (Halperin et al., 1997b).

Technological limitations may have also contributed to the inconsistencies. Because there is no direct way of measuring chemicals in the brain, researchers must rely on indirect estimates, inferred from levels of these neurotransmitters and their metabolites in blood, urine, and cerebral spinal fluid. Such measurements are imprecise and unreliable, and their use may have introduced variability that accounts for the different results across studies.

Neuroanatomy

Abnormalities in the structure of the brain have also been suspected of causing AD/HD (Zametkin & Rapoport, 1987). Early support for this was inferred from clinical observations suggesting that the behavior of individuals with AD/HD was similar to that of people with brain lesions. The recent arrival of new neuroimaging devices has made it possible to address this matter more directly, but little such research has been conducted with children. Moreover, mixed results have emerged from the few studies that have been conducted, presumably due to sampling differences, small sample sizes, and other methodological factors.

In research using coaxial tomographic (CT) scans, structural differences in the brains of AD/HD versus control children have not usually been detected (Shaywitz, Shaywitz, Byrne, Cohen, & Rothman, 1983). Studies using higher-resolution magnetic resonance imaging (MRI) devices have found differences in brain structure, but not consistently. There have been reports that children with AD/HD have a smaller corpus callosum than do children without AD/HD (Baumgardner et al., 1996; Hynd et al., 1991), but some investigators found no anatomical distinction (Castellanos et al., 1996). MRI studies have raised the possibility that the caudate nucleus and other prefrontostriatal areas may be smaller in children with AD/HD (Castellanos et al., 1996; Filipek et al., 1997; Hynd et al., 1993). Whether these anatomical differences are functionally important has not been adequately addressed. Preliminary findings suggest that they probably are, given that the size of the prefrontostriatal area was, on one psychological test of behavioral inhibition, significantly correlated with performance (Casey et al., 1997).

Neurophysiology

Brain function in children with AD/HD has been addressed primarily using cerebral blood flow (CBF) and positron-emission tomography (PET) studies. Although few, CBF investigations have consistently found decreased blood flow in the prefrontal regions of the brain and in the various pathways connecting these regions to the limbic system, including the caudate nucleus (Lou, Henriksen, & Bruhn, 1984; Sieg, Gaffney, Preston, & Hellings, 1995). These blood flow deficits were reversed when stimulant medication was administered. In PET scans on adults, there has been evidence of diminished cerebral glucose metabolism in the prefrontal and cingulate regions, as well as in the caudate and in other subcortical structures (Zametkin et al., 1990). Similar PET results were initially reported for adolescent girls with AD/HD (Ernst et al., 1994; Zametkin et al., 1993), but recent efforts to replicate this finding were unsuccessful (Ernst, Cohen, Liebenauer, Jons, & Zametkin, 1997). Likewise, PET scan abnormalities have yet to be found among adolescent boys (Zametkin et al., 1993).

Genetics

Assuming for a moment that neurochemical, neuroanatomical, and/or neurophysiological abnormalities exist, it becomes necessary to ask how they arose. The best answer seems to involve multiple pathways, among which genetic mechanisms likely play a prominent role.

Findings consistent with a genetic hypothesis have emerged from comparisons between biological and adoptive relatives of children with AD/HD (Deutsch, 1987; Morrison & Stewart, 1973). High rates of AD/HD have also been detected among immediate and extended biological relatives of children with AD/HD (Biederman et al., 1987). Among biological siblings, anywhere from 11–32% may have this disorder (Biederman et al., 1992; Levy, Hay, McStephen, Wood, & Waldman, 1997). An even higher degree of concordance exists for twins, with rates of 29–38% for dizygotic pairs and 51–82% for monozygotic pairs (Gilger, Pennington, & DeFries, 1992; Goodman & Stevenson, 1989; Levy et al., 1997). Further analyses of twin data yielded consistently high heritability estimates, ranging from .64–.91 (Edelbrock, Rende, Plomin, & Thompson, 1995; Gillis, Gilger, Pennington, & DeFries, 1992; Goodman & Stevenson, 1989; Levy et al., 1997; Zahn-Waxler et al., 1996). Additional genetic support comes from research that took a somewhat different perspective—namely, from the point of view of the parent. This type of research has shown that when a parent has AD/HD, there is a 50% chance that at least one of the offspring will also have it (Biederman et al., 1995).

Taken together, these findings suggest, but do not prove, that a genetic connection exists for AD/HD. A more direct link needs to be established, however. Chromosomal evidence could certainly be this link, but therein lies a major problem. Should researchers be looking for just one gene, or multiple genes?

This question makes the genetic search more difficult than looking for the proverbial needle in a haystack.

Based upon the results of a large-scale quantitative genetic analysis, some investigators speculate that a single gene may account for the expression of AD/HD (Faraone et al., 1992). Although single-gene defects have been identified, three different locations are implicated: a dopamine transporter gene on chromosome 5 (Cook et al., 1995), a dopamine D4 receptor gene on chromosome 11 (LaHoste et al., 1996), and the HLA site on chromosome 6 (Cardon et al., 1994). Again, procedural variation may account for some of the differences. Alternatively, there may be multiple genes involved, with specific genes or gene combinations leading to the expression of specific AD/HD subtypes.

Prenatal Complications

Another way in which the chemistry, structure, and functioning of the brain might be altered is through prenatal complications. Research shows an increased incidence of AD/HD among the offspring of pregnancies complicated by excessive maternal consumption of alcohol or nicotine (Bennett, Wolin, & Reiss, 1988; Streissguth, Bookstein, Sampson, & Barr, 1995). As with the genetic findings, these results are highly correlational, which limits the etiological inferences that can be drawn. A more convincing argument would require controlling for maternal AD/HD to rule out genetic influences, and documenting a physiological connection between maternal alcohol or nicotine consumption and abnormal brain development in the fetus. Only one study has addressed either of these stipulations. In that investigation, the risk for AD/HD was high for children prenatally exposed to maternal nicotine, independent of whether or not maternal AD/HD was present (Milberger, Biederman, Faraone, Chen, & Jones, 1996).

Other Biological Factors

There have been reports that damage to certain parts of the brain, such as the prefrontal limbic areas, can lead to AD/HD (Heilman & Valenstein, 1979). Because less than 5% of the AD/HD population has a history of this (Rutter, 1983), brain damage is generally not considered a major cause of the disorder. Investigators have also found a relatively higher incidence of AD/HD among children with elevated lead levels (Gittelman & Eskinazi, 1983), but the physiological mechanisms responsible for this association have yet to be identified. Moreover, most children with AD/HD do not have histories of lead poisoning, so elevated lead levels are at best a minor cause. Despite their widespread public appeal, there is also little empirical support for the assertions of Feingold (1975) and others that the ingestion of sugar or other food substances directly causes AD/HD (Wolraich, Wilson, & White, 1995).

Biological Variation

Periodically, the notion of biological variation is put forth as an explanation for AD/HD (Chess, 1960; Kinsbourne, 1977). Resting on the assumption of individual differences, rather than deficits, this account suggests that AD/HD characteristics, like those of intelligence, are distributed in a normal, or bell-shaped, manner within the general population. In this context, children with AD/HD are labeled as such simply because their levels of inattention, impulsivity, and hyperactivity lie at the extreme end of normal. Many experts today would agree with this assertion of developmental deviance (Levy et al., 1997), but many would not attribute this to normal biological processes (Barkley, 1997).

Psychological Theories

Over the years numerous psychological theories have also been put forth to explain how AD/HD affects psychosocial functioning. Early accounts, which often lacked the benefit of neurobiological findings, focused almost exclusively on the attentional processes thought to be at the core of AD/HD. Although attentional hypotheses were intuitively appealing and were compatible with the diagnostic criteria of the day (i.e., *DSM-III*; APA, 1980), investigators soon began to question whether attentional deficits were truly a core problem, partly because they failed to account for why children with AD/HD displayed appropriate levels of attention in some situations and not in others. To address this, investigators put forth alternative explanations, implicating core deficiencies in the regulation of behavior to situational demands (Routh, 1978), in self-directed instruction (Kendall & Braswell, 1985), in the self-regulation of arousal to environmental demands (Douglas, 1983), and in rule-governed behavior (Barkley, 1981). Though differing somewhat, each explanation saw poor executive functioning as a core problem.

Building on what is now known about the biology of AD/HD, recent theories have taken on a distinctive neuropsychological flavor, emphasizing impulsivity. For example, Quay (1997) proposes that AD/HD stems from an impairment in a neurologically based behavioral inhibition system. In an extensive elaboration of this same theme, Barkley (1998) contends that a deficit in behavioral inhibition leads to impairment in four major areas of executive functioning, which in turn sets the stage for the cognitive, behavioral, and social deficits that occur within AD/HD populations. Many others in the field share the view that behavioral inhibition deficits lie at the core of many AD/HD problems (Schachar, Tannock, & Logan, 1993; Sergeant, 1995).

Psychosocial Theories

Although environmental theories have also been proposed to explain AD/HD (Block, 1977; Jacobvitz & Sroufe, 1987; Willis & Lovaas, 1977), there is little empirical evidence that poor parenting, chaotic home environments, or poverty *cause* AD/HD. The results of twin studies in particular have highlighted this limited role by showing that less than 5% of the variance in AD/HD symptomatology can be accounted for by environmental factors (Levy et al., 1997; Sherman, McGue, & Iacono, 1997; Silberg et al., 1996). When AD/HD is found among children from chaotic family circumstances, one could reasonably speculate that the parents may themselves have AD/HD, which might explain why their homes are chaotic, and at the same time support a genetic explanation for the child's AD/HD condition. Under this same scenario, the resulting chaos in the home could be viewed as exacerbating, but not causing, the child's inborn AD/HD (van den Oord & Rowe, 1997).

Summary

Considering the widespread interest, relatively few studies have actually addressed the causes of AD/HD. Among those that have, findings have been inconsistent, presumably due to cross-study differences in defining AD/HD samples, small sample sizes, and other methodological limitations. As a result, what we know about the etiology of AD/HD is largely theoretical.

Several lines of evidence point toward biological factors. In particular, research has pointed to abnormalities in brain chemistry, structure, and/or function. Multiple pathways presumably lead to such abnormalities, as depicted in Figure 2.1. Among them, genetic mechanisms and certain pregnancy complications likely account for the largest percentage of children who have AD/HD. Some children may acquire AD/HD after birth due to head injury, elevated lead levels, or other biological complications.

Although exactly how these biological pieces fit together is far from clear, recent findings offer some interesting leads, especially the recently identified dopamine gene defects (Cook et al., 1995; LaHoste et al., 1996) that may be precursors to the dopamine deficiencies reported in the neurochemical literature (Pliszka et al., 1996; Raskin et al., 1984). These deficiencies may in turn be linked to some of the structural and functional abnormalities that have been observed, particularly in the frontostriatal region (Castellanos et al., 1996), where dopamine systems are at work.

With further advances in medical technology, our understanding of these biological mechanisms should increase dramatically. In the meantime, it is important to continue integrating biological theories with psychological con-

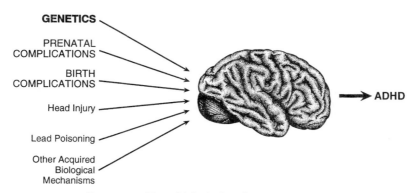

FIGURE 2.1. Neurobiological pathways to AD/HD.

ceptualizations in order to arrive at a more complete understanding. Recently, there have been signs of increased interest in developing and testing such theoretical models (Barkley, 1998; Quay, 1997). At the very least, these contemporary viewpoints may spark further theoretical discussion, which in turn will guide research and inform clinical practice in the future.

EPIDEMIOLOGY

Prevalence

At face value, estimating the prevalence of AD/HD appears relatively straightforward. You simply gather a certain number of children and then calculate the percentage who meet the criteria for AD/HD. Unfortunately, it's not so simple; many things can affect AD/HD prevalence estimates.

One factor is the *composition of the sample*. For a prevalence estimate to be reasonably accurate, the sample must be representative of its population. In most cases this means a sample whose demographic characteristics closely approximate those found in the geographic area under consideration in terms of age, gender, socioeconomic status, ethnicity, and cultural diversity. Small samples seldom achieve this. Samples drawn from clinic referral pools typically fall short as well. In contrast, large samples drawn randomly from the community usually provide fairly good demographic representation, and it is from these, therefore, that the most accurate prevalence estimates are obtained.

Another factor in determining the accuracy of AD/HD prevalence rates is the *manner in which the disorder is diagnosed*. Although most epidemiological research is done in accordance with *DSM's* conceptualization of AD/HD, it is not uncommon to find studies using some, rather than all, of its diagnostic criteria in their prevalence calculations. In many such studies, prevalence rates are determined solely on the basis of how many children meet symptom frequency requirements. Thus, if a child often displays 6 or more inattentive and/or hyperactive-impulsive symptoms, he or she is considered to have AD/HD. This approach is overly inclusive, however, thereby increasing the risk for false positives—that is, for incorrectly identifying children as having AD/HD when in fact their symptoms might be better explained by other diagnostic conditions, such as learning disabilities or child maltreatment. In light of this, such estimates are best viewed as upper limits on the true prevalence of AD/HD within the general population.

Additional variability in AD/HD prevalence rates can arise from *differences in the assessment procedures* used to determine whether *DSM* criteria are met. This might be seen in studies utilizing assessment procedures that are categorically different from one another (e.g., clinical interviews versus child behavior rating scales). It might also arise among investigations using different forms of the same procedure (e.g., structured versus semistructured interviews). Even studies employing identical assessment procedures might use different cut-points (e.g., scores above the 93rd percentile versus those above the 98th percentile).

Having *different informants* can also affect prevalence calculations. As a function of the different demands that they place on children, different informants may have very different perceptions of whether AD/HD symptoms are present, which poses an interesting problem for epidemiological researchers: From whom should the information be gathered? Although there is no definitive answer to this, one should simply bear in mind that the prevalence rates of AD/HD can be influenced by the source.

In view of the many circumstances that can affect the outcome of AD/HD epidemiological research, it is no wonder that prevalence rates vary tremendously. Among the many studies using *DSM-III* and *DSM-III-R* conceptualizations of AD/HD, prevalence rates have ranged from 2–3% to 25–30% of the general child population. Whether this same pattern will hold true for the *DSM-IV* version of AD/HD is unknown, because little research has thus far addressed it, but interesting results have begun to emerge from the few *DSM-IV* studies that have been done.

According to the *DSM-IV* manual itself, the overall prevalence of AD/HD among children—that is, the sum total of all subtyping categories—is 3–5% (APA, 1994). As might be expected, higher estimates have been reported for community samples in which only the symptom frequency criterion was used to define AD/HD. In one such study, DuPaul and associates (DuPaul, Anastopoulos, et al., 1998) found an overall prevalence rate of 7.5%, derived from a large, nationwide sampling of parent ratings of children and adolescents 5–18 years of age. In line with these results was the 8.1% prevalence rate reported by Gaub and Carlson (1997a), calculated from teacher ratings drawn from a large, local community sample. Higher prevalence rates, ranging from approximately 11–21%, were evident in three additional investigations employing teachers as informants (Baumgaertel, Wolraich, & Dietrich, 1995; DuPaul, Power, et al., 1997; Wolraich, Hannah, Pinnock, Baumgaertel, & Brown, 1996). The variability across these studies is not well understood. One explanation is that it may be due to differences in how the symptoms were tabulated. In the Gaub and Carlson study, symptoms were counted only if they were rated as occurring *very often*. In the other studies (DuPaul, Power, et al., 1997; Wolraich et al., 1996), both *often* and *very often* were considered sufficient for making this same determination.

As for subtyping, the Combined category emerged most often in the *DSM-IV* clinical field trials, outnumbering Inattentive and Hyperactive-Impulsive by 2:1 and 3:1, respectively (Lahey et al., 1994). Perhaps due to the nonclinical nature of their samples, community-based studies addressing these same subtypes had different results. In particular, community-based studies have consistently identified the Inattentive subtype as the one most likely to be present (DuPaul, Anastopoulos, et al., 1998; DuPaul et al., 1997; Gaub & Carlson, 1997a; Wolraich et al., 1996). Among the studies using teachers as informants, prevalence rates have ranged from 4.5–10% for the Inattentive type, from 1.7–3.2% for the Hyperactive-Impulsive type, and from 1.9–8.4% for the Combined type. This pattern was also evident when parents served as informants, with rates of 3.2%, 2.1%, and 2.2% occurring for the Inattentive, Hyperactive-Impulsive, and Combined subtypes, respectively (DuPaul, Anastopoulos, et al., 1998).

Age and Gender

From a purely epidemiological point of view, the above findings are indeed interesting. From a clinical practice perspective, these same results are of limited value, because they shed no light on individual differences. Of the many differences that might be considered, age and gender can exert an especially powerful influence on prevalence estimates.

In their analysis of teacher-generated data, DuPaul and associates (1997) found overall prevalence rates of approximately 25% for children 5–7 years old, 23% for children 8–10 years old, 21% for 11–13 year olds, and 15% for youths 14–18 years old. When parents served as informants, the overall prevalence rates were roughly 9% for 5–7 year olds, 6% for 8–10 year olds, 8% for 11–13 year olds, and 5% for adolescents 14–18 years of age (DuPaul, Anastopoulos, et al., 1998). These results raise the possibility that the prevalence of AD/HD, as defined by *DSM-IV* symptom frequency criteria, declines with age.

As shown in Table 2.1., developmental trends are also evident among the subtyping categories, but the exact manner in which they unfold varies with the informant. In teacher ratings, children 5–10 years old are much more likely to be identified with the Combined subtype, followed in order by the Inattentive and Hyperactive-Impulsive subtypes (DuPaul et al., 1997). For students 11–18 years of age the picture changes. The Inattentive subtype becomes the most prevalent, followed in order by the Combined and Hyperactive-Impulsive subtypes. In contrast, parent ratings have suggested that the Hyperactive-Impulsive subtype occurs more often than the other two categories among children 5–7 years old (DuPaul, Anastopoulos, et al., 1998). That this category would be so prevalent among younger children is by no means unusual; it has been reported by other

TABLE 2.1. Prevalence of AD/HD across Development in a Community Sample

	Age group				
Informant	5–7 years	8–10 years	11–13 years	14–17 years	Total
Parents					
Overall	9.1%	6.4%	8.3%	5.8%	7.5%
By subtype	HI > C > I	I > C > HI	I > C > HI	I > C > HI	I > C > HI
Teachers					
Overall	25.3%	23.8%	21.5%	15.0%	21.6%
By subtype	C > I > HI	C > I > HI	I > C > HI	I > C > HI	I > C > HI

Note: AD/HD = Attention-deficit/hyperactivity disorder; C = Combined type; I = Predominantly inattentive type; HI = Predominantly hyperactive-impulsive type. From DuPaul, Power, Anastopoulos, & Reid (1998).

investigators, including those using clinical samples (Lahey et al., 1994; McBurnett, Pfiffner, Tamm, & Capasso, 1996). For reasons that are not entirely clear, the prevalence of the Hyperactive-Impulsive subtype decreases sharply among children 8 years and older, making it the least likely subtype to occur after age 7 (DuPaul, Anastopoulos, et al., 1998). For this same age group, the prevalence of the Inattentive category increases, thereby making it the most frequently encountered subtyping classification for children over 7 years old (DuPaul, Anastopoulos, et al., 1998).

Implicit in the preceding discussion is the notion that AD/HD changes in its clinical presentation across development. Although this seems reasonable, these findings are derived solely from cross-sectional investigations. Whether these developmental trends would be evident in longitudinal studies is unknown. Until research of this sort is completed, the possibility remains that developmental trends exist.

Along with age-related effects, gender influences have also been noted. In particular, the overall prevalence of AD/HD is consistently much higher among boys than among girls (APA, 1994; Arnold, 1996; Lahey et al., 1994). According to *DSM-IV*, boys outnumber girls by approximately 4:1 to 9:1 (APA, 1994). But recently, lower ratios have emerged from two community-based investigations, with boys outnumbering girls by only 2.2:1 in parent-generated samples (DuPaul, Anastopoulos, et al., 1998) and 2.3:1 in teacher-based input (DuPaul et al., 1997). Boys outnumber girls across all three major subtyping categories (Lahey et al., 1994), but the exact magnitude of these differences seems to depend on both the informant and the subtype. Parent-based research conducted by DuPaul and associates found the ratio of boys to girls to be 1.4:1 for the Inattentive type, 3.1:1 for the Hyperactive-Impulsive type, and 3.3:1 for the Combined type (DuPaul, Anastopoulos, et al., 1998). A similar pattern emerged from the teacher ratings, with boy:girl ratios of 2:1 for the Inattentive, 3.2:1 for Hyperactive-Impulsive, and 2.6:1 for Combined (DuPaul et al., 1997).

Socioeconomic Status

To date, researchers have not systematically addressed the effect of socioeconomic status on the prevalence of AD/HD as defined in accordance with *DSM-IV*. To the extent that earlier research indicates what might be found, one would expect AD/HD to occur across the entire socioeconomic spectrum (Barkley, 1990). Although there are indications that AD/HD appears more often among those from lower socioeconomic backgrounds (Szatmari, 1992), its exact distribution is not well understood.

Ethnic and Cultural Diversity

In the *DSM-IV* clinical field trials, ethnicity was not a major factor influencing the prevalence of AD/HD (Lahey et al., 1994), nor did it seem to affect prevalence rates in the community-based study by Gaub and Carlson (1997a), in which 92% of their sample came from minority backgrounds. Ethnicity did, however, appear to play a role in the community-based findings reported by DuPaul and associates (1997). In the teacher-based study, approximately 6% of Caucasian children and adolescents were identified as having one of the three major subtypes of AD/HD versus a rate of roughly 12% among those from minority backgrounds. From a different perspective, of the total number of children and adolescents identified with any type of AD/HD—approximately 43% were from minority backgrounds, even though minority children and adolescents made up only 34.8% of the total teacher-generated sample. Similar findings emerged from the parallel investigation using parent-generated data (DuPaul, Anastopoulos, et al., 1998).

Why ethnic differences were found in some studies and not others is puzzling. Further complicating this situation is that little published AD/HD research has addressed ethnic diversity. Additional research of this type would be needed to establish a definitive connection between ethnicity and the prevalence of AD/HD.

Only one study has examined the prevalence of the *DSM-IV* version of AD/HD outside of North America. In that investigation, which used a large number of teacher-completed ratings of public school children in Germany, an overall prevalence rate of 17.8% was obtained (Baumgaertal et al., 1995). Although these results clearly diverge from the findings reported in one North American-based study (Gaub & Carlson, 1997a), they are consistent with those of another (DuPaul et al., 1997). Such variability is not unusual; it was also evident in cross-cultural investigations using earlier *DSM* formulations of AD/HD. In one such community-based study using public school teachers in Puerto Rico as informants, approximately 16% of the Spanish-speaking students were identified as having AD/HD (Bauermeister, Berrios, Jimenez, Acevedo, & Gordon, 1990). A relatively lower prevalence rate of 9.9% was reported in another community study based on teacher ratings of Chinese public school students in Taiwan (Wang, Chong, Chou, & Yang, 1993). Whether these discrepancies reflect cross-cultural differences in AD/HD prevalence, cross-cultural differences in expectations for behavior, or just differences in scientific methodology, is unknown. What is readily apparent from these studies and others like them (Bhatia, Nigam, Bohra, & Malik, 1991; O'Leary, Vivian, & Nisi, 1985) is that AD/HD is found throughout the world and is therefore not just an artifact of the American lifestyle and culture.

Summary

Epidemiological studies of AD/HD as defined by *DSM-IV* have recently begun to surface. Although few, they have already produced some interesting findings. Community-based estimates of overall prevalence have ranged from roughly 7% to 21% in both parent- and teacher-generated samples. That these rates are higher than the 3–5% rates listed in *DSM-IV* is not surprising, given that they were derived primarily from symptom frequency counts alone. Having been determined in this way, such figures likely include many children for whom AD/HD would not be diagnosed in clinical practice because they would not meet all of the other *DSM-IV* criteria. Thus, such estimates are best viewed as upper limits on the true prevalence of AD/HD within the general population.

In clinic-based samples, the Combined type is the most commonly encountered subtype, whereas the Inattentive subtype occurs most often in community samples, suggesting that a more severe AD/HD presentation is what prompts clinical referrals. This raises the possibility that many children with milder forms of AD/HD are not receiving services that might decrease their risk of more serious problems later on. In addition to these referral considerations, many other factors may affect the prevalence of these subtypes. According to teachers, younger children display the Combined subtype most often, whereas older children and adolescents are more likely to display the Inattentive classification. Similar findings come from parent ratings of older children and adolescents, but parents more often rate very young children as having the Hyperactive-Impulsive subtype. Of additional interest is that the overall prevalence of *DSM-IV*-defined AD/HD—that is, the total for all three major subtypes—seems to decline with age. Although these findings point toward the existence of developmental trends, such a conclusion is limited by the fact that it comes from investigations using cross-sectional, rather than longitudinal, designs.

In terms of gender, boys outnumber girls across all subtypes, with ratios ranging from 6:1 to 9:1 in clinic samples and 1.3:1 to 3.3:1 in community samples, depending on the informant and subtype under consideration. Because there are mixed results on the moderating influence of ethnicity, few conclusions can be drawn about it. Likewise, not much can be said about socioeconomic factors due to the dearth of research on them.

As mentioned at the outset of this discussion, these epidemiological findings are preliminary in nature and in need of replication. When such research is conducted, close attention should be paid to the various methodological factors that can influence prevalence estimates. Future researchers will also need to examine the effect of different combinations of variables (e.g., Age × Gender × Ethnicity) on the prevalence of AD/HD.

DEVELOPMENTAL CONSIDERATIONS

One of the most consistent findings in the preceding discussion is that age has a significant effect on the prevalence of AD/HD and its major subtypes. This implies that AD/HD expresses itself across development in a dynamic, rather than static, manner. Thus it is important to learn how and when these developmental changes occur. As the first step in addressing this, we will now consider the manner in which AD/HD symptoms first arise.

Onset

Most of what is known about the onset of AD/HD symptoms comes from research using *DSM-III* and *DSM-III-R* guidelines. In one such study, the mean age of onset for a group of 158 hyperactive children was 3.5 years (Barkley et al.,

1990). In a similar investigation involving 177 clinic-referred boys, the mean age of onset was 6 years, with hyperactive-impulsive symptoms appearing somewhat earlier than inattentive symptoms (Green, Loeber, & Lahey, 1991). Recognizing that there can be a great deal of individual variation within group means, McGee, Williams, and Feehan (1992) conducted an individual analysis of their onset data. About a third of their sample had an onset before 3 years of age, consistent with prior research (Hartsough & Lambert, 1985). Another third first showed symptoms prior to 5 or 6 years. The remaining third first displayed their symptoms sometime between 6 and 7 years.

Of what clinical significance are these onset differences? Some researchers believe that the earlier the onset, the more likely the child will have secondary or comorbid conditions and greater psychosocial impairment (McGee et al., 1992). In line with this assertion, the research findings of August and Stewart (1983) showed that hyperactive children with conduct problems had an earlier onset of AD/HD symptoms (2.8 years) than did "pure" hyperactive children (3.8 years). Further support for this was evident in preliminary analyses of our own clinic data, which showed a mean age of onset of 3.4 years for children with a dual diagnosis of AD/HD and Oppositional-Defiant Disorder versus 4.0 years for children with AD/HD alone.

At face value, these findings suggest that AD/HD symptoms do indeed arise in early childhood, thereby justifying *DSM*'s requirement of an onset prior to 7 years of age. Although longstanding and widely held, this assumption has recently been challenged. As pointed out by Barkley and Biederman (1997), there is circularity of reasoning that leads to this conclusion. Specifically, if you use a 7-year cut-off requirement in defining your AD/HD sample, then it should come as no great surprise that all children with AD/HD would have an onset before age 7. These researchers also questioned the accuracy of parent reports of symptom onset. Based on research showing that such reports are only moderately reliable from one year to the next (Green et al., 1991), Barkley and Biederman (1997) argue that using a precisely defined cut-off age is ill-advised. Moreover, they do not believe that existing data (e.g., McGee et al., 1992) support the claim that those with an onset of AD/HD symptoms before age 7 have different patterns of comorbidity and functional impairment than do those with a later onset. Thus, they recommend either abandoning the age of onset requirement or redefining it to allow onset at any point during childhood. They contend that this would lessen the chance that needed treatment services would be withheld from someone who met all the *DSM-IV* criteria for AD/HD except the onset requirement.

Barkley and Biederman (1997) raise interesting clinical and theoretical points. We fully agree with their contention that *DSM-IV*'s recommended use of a 7-year age of onset criteria is not as empirically well established as it should be. At the same time, we would argue that there is also insufficient empirical justification for making drastic changes in the current criteria. Until the situation alters, we believe it best to continue using the 7-year cut-point for establishing an AD/HD diagnosis.

This brings us to yet another problem. How does one determine when AD/

HD symptoms first began? Should all early displays of inattention, impulsivity, and hyperactivity be considered symptoms of AD/HD? Or should they be considered symptoms only when they become problematic, or when they are accompanied by functional impairment as required by *DSM-IV*? Clinical experience suggests that parents are often aware of their child's AD/HD-like behaviors long before they decide that such behaviors are deviant or problematic. Some parents retrospectively report that "all hell broke loose" when their children learned how to walk, because their nonstop explorations required constant parental monitoring. Others recall that their children seemed to take longer to go through the "terrible two's" than they expected. Although tuned in to such behaviors, they did not label them deviant or problematic at the time, largely because they did not have a clear sense of what was, and what was not, normal development. Such a distinction became more apparent when their children began attending school, which afforded increased opportunities for comparisons with other, normal-functioning children.

Recent research findings are consistent with this clinical observation. Based on further analyses of the *DSM-IV* field trial data, Applegate et al. (1997) noted that nearly all children with an AD/HD diagnosis had a parent-reported onset of symptoms prior to 7 years. This was true for 96% of the children with a Combined diagnosis, 100% of the children with a Predominantly Hyperactive-Impulsive diagnosis, and 85% of those with a Predominantly Inattentive diagnosis. Many of these same children showed no evidence of functional impairment until after 7 years, especially the Predominantly Inattentive group, 43% of whom did not show any impairment until after 7 years of age. Up to 18% of those in the Combined group and 2% of the Hyperactive-Impulsive group showed a similar delay. On average, there was a 2-year difference between when parents first noticed AD/HD symptoms and when they labeled them problematic. On the basis of these and related findings, Applegate and associates acknowledged that *DSM-IV*'s decision to include *impairment* as part of its age of onset requirement may have been a mistake. To address this in subsequent versions of *DSM*, two possible solutions have been put forth. One is to retain 7 years as the cut-off for detecting the presence of any AD/HD symptoms. The other is to increase the cut-off to 9 years and require evidence of functional impairment as well.

Developmental Course

According to most experts in the field, AD/HD is a chronic condition that persists across the life span (Barkley, 1998; Weiss & Hechtman, 1986). This suggests a constancy in its clinical presentation, but long-term follow-up studies have consistently shown that 20–50% of children identified as having AD/HD will not meet the full diagnostic criteria for it as adolescents (Barkley et al., 1990; Mannuzza & Klein, 1992).

To account for this decline, one must first consider what might be going on at the level of the symptoms themselves. In one of the few longitudinal studies investigating this, Hart and associates (Hart, Lahey, Loeber, Applegate, & Frick, 1995) annually evaluated a sample of 106 clinic-referred boys with AD/HD over a 4-year period. Their results indicated that the frequency of parent- and teacher-reported hyperactive-impulsive symptoms did decline with age, especially during late childhood and early adolescence. Although slight age-related reductions in the frequency of inattention symptoms were also found, they did not reflect any real developmental change. Similar findings have emerged from a recently completed cross-sectional investigation using teacher ratings of a nationwide community sampling of children between 5 and 18 years (DuPaul et al., 1997). In that study, 11–13-year-old children displayed significantly fewer hyperactive-impulsive symptoms as compared with children 5–10 years of age, and those aged 14–18 years exhibited significantly fewer hyperactive-impulsive symptoms relative to children 13 years and younger. As with the Hart et al. study, no significant changes were found in the frequency of inattention symptoms.

Given that children seem to display fewer hyperactive-impulsive symptoms as they get older, it stands to reason that as teenagers, they will be less likely to receive either the Combined subtype or the Hyperactive-Impulsive subtype classification. Coupled with the fact that inattention symptoms remain relatively constant over time, it is easier to understand why the overall prevalence of AD/HD encompassing all subtyping classifications decreases from childhood into adolescence. This may also explain why, if a teenager receives any AD/HD diagnosis at all, it will most likely be the Predominantly Inattentive subtype, consistent with recent cross-sectional findings (DuPaul, Anastopoulos, et al., 1998; DuPaul et al., 1997).

Very little is known about the manner in which AD/HD unfolds from adolescence into adulthood. Some evidence suggests that no more than 30% of those identified as children or adolescents with AD/HD will continue to meet diagnostic criteria for this condition as adults (Gittelman, Mannuzza, Shenker, & Bonagura, 1985; Mannuzza et al., 1997). Up to 50% will continue to exhibit subclinical symptoms that interfere with daily functioning (Weiss & Hechtman, 1993).

On the basis of such longitudinal findings, some investigators speculate that the overall incidence of AD/HD in the adult population is probably less than 1% (Shaffer, 1994). In a more direct examination of this matter, Murphy and Barkley (1996a) found a somewhat higher overall prevalence rate of 4.7% (1.3% for Inattentive; 2.5% for Hyperactive-Impulsive; .9% for Combined), which was derived from self-reported AD/HD ratings obtained from a local community sample of several hundred adults. As with the child findings, the adult estimate was derived primarily from symptom frequency counts rather than from complete *DSM-IV* criteria. Thus, this figure probably represents an upper limit on the actual prevalence of AD/HD among adults. Bearing this in mind, further analyses of these same cross-sectional data yielded prevalence rates of 1.3%, 2.5%, and .9% for the Predominantly Inattentive, Predominantly Hyperactive-Impulsive, and Combined subtypes, respectively. Of additional interest is that overall symptom frequency declined across the entire adult age span, not only for hyperactive-impulsive symptoms but for inattention symptoms as well. The reasons for the difference between the adult findings and previously reported child results are not clear. Although it is possible that developmental trends are at work, methodological variations (e.g., ratings based on self-report versus other-report) may provide a more parsimonious explanation.

One additional point bears mentioning: The developmental changes assume that the same *DSM-IV* symptom listing is appropriate for individuals of all ages. In fact, the content of the *DSM-IV* items was derived largely from what is known about elementary school children with AD/HD. Few modifications were made for preschoolers, adolescents, and adults, thus many of the *DSM-IV* items are developmentally inappropriate for them. What this means for adolescents and adults is a lower ceiling on the number of possible symptoms they might endorse. For example, instead of there being 9 symptoms per list to consider, there may be only 7 or 8 that realistically could occur, which artificially reduces the overall number of symptoms that adolescents or adults report and thus creates the illusion of a downward developmental trend. Research is obviously needed to clarify the situation. In particular, systematic research comparing the predictive validity of the existing *DSM-IV* items against new items that are more developmentally appropriate for preschoolers, adolescents, and adults should be pursued, not only for diagnostic reasons but also to resolve the ongoing debate regarding AD/HD symptom onset.

Summary

Current findings suggest that most individuals with AD/HD begin to display their symptoms in early childhood, with hyperactive-impulsive difficulties typically preceding inattention problems. Most often such symptoms appear around 3–4 years, but they can surface during infancy or upon school entrance as well. The question of whether AD/HD symptoms can have an onset after age 7 is currently being debated (Barkley & Biederman, 1997). To resolve the debate, researchers must clearly define symptom onset, recognizing that there may be an important distinction between the time when symptoms first appear versus the time when they begin to cause clinically significant impairment.

Upon reaching late childhood and early adolescence, many children with AD/HD begin to display substantially fewer hyperactive-impulsive symptoms. Some also show a reduction in their overall level of inattention, but to a much lesser degree. Little is known about the course that AD/HD symptoms follow from adolescence into adulthood. Potentially complicating this situation is that childhood estimates are based on parent and teacher reports, whereas adult estimates come from self-report. Available evidence shows that adults display fewer AD/HD symptoms than do children or adolescents, and the overall frequency of AD/HD symptoms seems to decline gradually across adulthood. For adults, the declines are evident in both hyperactive-impulsive and inattention symptoms.

PSYCHOSOCIAL IMPACT AND COMORBIDITY

Having AD/HD does not automatically lead to psychosocial difficulties. Having AD/HD does, however, place a person at higher risk for such problems.

The "goodness of fit" concept provides a useful framework for understanding how this disorder can disrupt normal functioning. According to this model, when there is a poor match between the challenges of a particular developmental period and a person's ability to meet those challenges, psychosocial difficulties arise. Thus, it is not just having AD/HD that determines the type of problems one might experience, it is the manner in which AD/HD makes it difficult to do what is expected at a given age.

Unfortunately, most research on the psychosocial impact of AD/HD has not taken developmental expectations into account. Much of it is merely descriptive, with little regard for how AD/HD limits a person's capacity for meeting the demands of a particular developmental period. Also, researchers have focused their attention almost exclusively on elementary school children; essentially no research has been done with preschool AD/HD populations, and very little has been reported for adolescents. Even less exists for adults. Still, it is possible to speculate about AD/HD's impact by considering how this disorder might make it difficult to meet specific developmental challenges.

Early Childhood

If one word can sum up developmental challenges for preschool, it is *readiness*: readiness for school, readiness to explore the world and become more independent from parents, and readiness to interact with others in a positive way.

Academic Functioning

There is a virtual explosion of language, cognitive, and motor skills during the preschool years. Preschoolers develop a rich vocabulary, representational thought, an interest in figuring out why things happen, and the ability to affect their environment through climbing, running, and jumping, and more. All these abilities are necessary building blocks for success in elementary school.

Although taking an active approach to learning is normal at this stage of development, preschoolers with AD/HD take it to an extreme. Research has shown that they engage in more transitional behavior and are less attentive and cooperative during group activities (Alessandri, 1992; McIntosh & Cole-Love, 1996). They also seem to have greater difficulty with motor control and persistence during tasks that require working memory (Mariani & Barkley, 1997). Because of their difficulty sitting still while looking at a book or patiently learning to manipulate crayons, many preschoolers with AD/HD seem immature and do not perform well in preschool or kindergarten settings. Those who do not acquire readiness skills from their early educational experiences have an increased risk of more-serious academic difficulties in later grades.

Family Functioning

Rapidly developing cognitive, language, and motor skills are also put into service as the preschooler becomes focused on initiating activities, making things happen, and being able to say "I can do it!" Initiating activities allows the child to meet another developmental challenge: becoming an individual by separating from parents and primary caretakers. Doing things independently, such as dressing and eating, becomes almost more important than doing them successfully. Increased ability to plan, increased private speech to guide the planning, and improved motor skills to carry out these plans result in independent projects, which form the groundwork for the child's growing sense of self.

For many parents of preschool children with AD/HD, this typical striving for independence becomes an intense battle for control. Daily self-care activities are a test of wills because these children combine a lack of patience for completing such tasks independently with the activity level and impulsivity to fuel long chases around the house. In response to their preschooler's frequent displays of negative and noncompliant behavior (Campbell, 1995; Mash & Johnston, 1982), many parents resort to aversive, coercive, and controlling strategies to keep things in check (Campbell, Breaux, Ewing, & Szumoski, 1986; Lee & Bates, 1985; Mash & Johnston, 1982; Pisterman, Firestone, McGrath, Goodman, Webster, & Mallory, 1992). Over time, such battles very likely contribute to the increased parenting stress and martial discord often found in these families (Barkley et al., 1996; Shelton et al., 1998).

Social Functioning

Another important preschool challenge is entering into the world of peers. During early childhood, children increase the time that they spend in the company of others. Because peer relationships are characterized by a more equal power status, the skills learned in this social context are important for future social relations. Although aggression increases during the preschool years as the children's individual needs for assertion and independence clash with each other, there is also an increase in problem-solving abilities and in using language to settle these disputes. Children's earliest friendships begin as well. Initially based on proximity, these friendships form the basis for learning to take the perspective of others and for developing empathy. Play at this age becomes, as Piaget says, "the child's work." It is a forum for working out problems, fears, and social roles, and for encountering the rules and expectations of family and society, which serves to enhance self-awareness, social knowledge, and self-control.

For many preschoolers with AD/HD, shifting from settling disputes with behavior to settling them with words is delayed. Using language requires foregoing behavior that is likely to be more initially rewarding (e.g., getting a toy) in favor of a problem-solving strategy that takes longer and has delayed results. Thus preschoolers at risk for AD/HD behave more aggressively toward their peers (Campbell, 1990; Campbell & Cluss, 1982; Schleifer et al., 1975). Disrupted friendships may not be as evident initially because they are largely based on proximity (i.e., who lives next to you, who attends the same day care), but some of these children are not learning the play and social skills they will need later when friendships depend more on sharing, perspective-taking, and common interests. Such difficulties may explain why preschoolers at risk for AD/HD so often disrupt the play of others and frequently shift from one activity to another (Campbell, 1995): Their negative interactions lead to peer rejection, and therefore such children find themselves engaged in solitary play more often than they might like (Alessandri, 1992). They may also begin to acquire negative reputations, which can be long-lasting and can set the stage for more-serious social difficulties in the next developmental period.

Middle Childhood

As children progress to elementary school, competence becomes the theme: Competence in controlling their behavior, in school work, in handling family responsibilities, and in interacting with peers.

Behavioral Functioning

A major challenge in the elementary school years is learning and following basic rules. At home this might mean getting ready for school, cleaning one's room, setting the table, taking out the trash, and coming home at designated times. School responsibilities often include keeping a neat and organized desk, transporting endless communiques between parents and teachers, getting to and from lunch and recess, and negotiating the bus. Such tasks can be tedious and boring, and repetition is usually necessary to ensure that the child demonstrates not only knowledge of these skills but also the automaticity necessary for their consistent use.

Inattention and impulsivity render many children with AD/HD unable to consistently follow rules and comply with requests. This may at times seem deliberately defiant or noncompliant, but such behavior is usually unintentional. This is not to say that children with AD/HD do not exhibit defiance or noncompliance. Indeed, they commonly display secondary features of aggression as well as comorbid diagnoses of Oppositional-Defiant Disorder and Conduct Disorder (Jensen, Martin, & Cantwell, 1997). In clinic-referred samples of children with AD/HD, up to 60% will meet criteria for a secondary diagnosis of Oppositional-Defiant Disorder, with another 25% meeting criteria for Conduct Disorder (Barkley, 1990; Pelham, Gnagy, Greenslade, & Milich, 1992). Lower rates have been noted in community samples, with Oppositional-Defiant Disorder (ODD) and Conduct Disorder (CD) occurring up to 32% and 12% of the time, respectively (August, Realmuto, MacDonald, Nugent, & Crosby, 1996).

Although applicable to the AD/HD population as a whole, these comorbidity rates are subject to the influence of demographics and subtyping. As recently noted by Gaub and Carlson (1997b), girls with AD/HD tend to show less aggression than do boys with the same condition. Age may come into play as well. Because AD/HD typically emerges around 3–4 years, some investigators suggest that it may be a risk factor for the later development of ODD, whose peak onset is approximately 6 years; ODD may in turn be a risk factor for the later emergence of CD, whose peak onset is around 9 years (Loeber & Keenan, 1994). The risk for secondary externalizing problems seems greater when hyperactive-impulsive features are prominent, as shown recently in a study that found ODD in 48% of the children with a Combined type AD/HD diagnosis versus 19% of those with a Predominantly Inattentive subtyping classification (Eiraldi, Power, & Nezu, 1997). In that same study, comorbid CD was detected in 44% of those with the Combined type, whereas this occurred in none of those with a Predominantly Inattentive presentation. Higher rates of ODD and CD have also been reported for children with a Predominantly Hyperactive-Impulsive subtyping classification versus those with a Predominantly Inattentive diagnosis (Gaub & Carlson, 1997a).

In view of the high rate of overlap between AD/HD and these two externalizing disorders, some have questioned the degree to which these conditions represent distinct entities (Paternite, Loney, & Roberts, 1995). Empirical findings (Burns, Walsh, Owen, & Snell, 1997; Schachar & Tannock, 1995), as well as literature reviews (Hinshaw, 1987; Waldman & Lilenfeld, 1991), have generally shown that although there *is* substantial overlap, there is enough evidence to support their existence as separate diagnostic entities.

Academic Functioning

During the early elementary years, children must learn to memorize the basic building blocks of learning, such as letter, word, and number recognition, decoding skills, reading for comprehension, basic math computations, numerical reasoning, and forming letters and printing. As children progress into the middle elementary years, expectations shift, and competence is defined by how well they can apply these building blocks to new situations (e.g., using addition and subtraction to solve word problems). There are also increased demands for sustaining attention to task in both desk work and homework. When all goes well, the child enters adolescence with an understanding of how to apply the basics to more-advanced problems and to other subject matter.

Due to difficulty in sustaining attention (Hooks, Milich, & Lorch, 1994), children with AD/HD often fail to finish assigned tasks. Over time this takes its toll, limiting the practice opportunities that are essential for learning. Though most children with AD/HD do not show deficits in their storage and recall of simple information (Cahn & Marcotte, 1995), many have significant difficulties when asked to memorize complex information, especially when it requires organization and deliberate rehearsal strategies (Douglas & Benezra, 1990).

Not surprisingly then, many children with AD/HD have trouble in school. Depending on the exact definition that is used, anywhere from 18–53% of the population will be academic underachievers, performing significantly below the level of their intelligence (Barkley, 1990; Frick et al., 1991). Although younger children with AD/HD can also display significant academic under-achievement, many do not because they have not been in school long enough for this type of problem to develop. They may, however, show deficiencies in the *amount* of work that they produce, a red flag for later academic underachievement (DuPaul & Stoner, 1994). Along with age, subtyping considerations may affect academic achievement, with problems occurring more often among children with either a Combined or a Predominantly Inattentive classification versus those with a Predominantly Hyperactive-Impulsive presentation (Gaub & Carlson, 1997a).

Some children with AD/HD have comorbid learning disorders as well. The reported incidence of such difficulties within the AD/HD population is 10–50%, depending on the learning disorder and how it is defined (August & Garfinkel, 1990; Barkley, 1990; Frick et al., 1991; Tannock & Schachar, 1996). Of the various comorbid learning problems that can arise, reading disorders occur most often (August & Garfinkel, 1990). Other language-based disabilities have also been found fairly consistently, surfacing most often as pragmatic deficits—that is, deficits in organizing, monitoring, and using language—rather than as deficits in speech production, semantics, or syntax (Tannock & Schachar, 1996). There are also reports that children with AD/HD may be at increased risk for central auditory processing disorders (Riccio, Hynd, Cohen, Hall, & Molt, 1994), as well as for deficits in their visual-motor functioning (Barkley, 1998).

As a group, children with AD/HD score slightly lower on standardized intelligence tests than do controls (McGee, Williams, Moffitt, & Anderson, 1989). Whether this represents differences in intellectual functioning, in achievement, or merely in test-taking behavior is unknown. What is known is that AD/HD can be found across all levels of intelligence (Barkley, 1990), with slightly higher rates (i.e., 9–18%) reported for children with developmental delay (Epstein, Cullinan, & Polloway, 1986).

Family Functioning

During middle childhood, children spend less time with their family and more time with their peers, but families continue to play a critical role in the child's overall development. Especially important is the guidance that families provide, interpreting and teaching societal rules. Families also serve as a supportive testing ground for developing new skills, whether they be related to chores, academics, athletics, or the arts.

Inattention and impulsivity make it hard for children with AD/HD to follow through on parental instructions, thus they violate household rules. As depicted in Figure 2.2., this inability to regulate behavior can have a spillover effect, significantly impacting the psychosocial functioning of parents and siblings. As was true for the parents of preschoolers with AD/HD, parents of school-age children with AD/HD may become overly directive and negative in their parenting style (Cunningham & Barkley, 1979). Being unable to control their child's behavior can lead parents to conclude that they are less skilled and less knowledgeable in their parenting roles than they actually are (Mash & Johnston, 1990). They may also experience considerable stress in their parenting roles, especially when their child has comorbid oppositional-defiant symptoms (Anastopoulos, Guevremont, Shelton, & DuPaul, 1992; Johnston, 1996). Of additional clinical concern is that many parents of children with AD/HD become depressed, abuse alcohol, and experience marital difficulties (Cunningham, Benness, & Siegel, 1988; Lahey et al., 1988; Pelham & Lange, 1993). It has been generally assumed that such problems were the direct result of raising a child with AD/HD. Re-

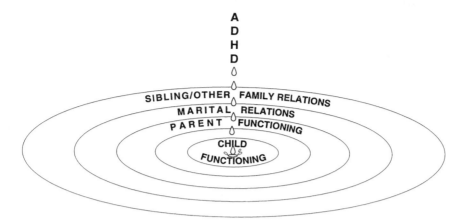

FIGURE 2.2. Impact of AD/HD on family functioning.

cently, however, it has become clear that not all of the blame should fall on the child's shoulders, because these difficulties could also stem from the parents themselves having AD/HD (Murphy & Barkley, 1996b).

Social Functioning

Middle childhood is a developmental period in which interactions with peers increase. In contrast with the preschool years, middle childhood friendships are based less on physical proximity and more on similarities with the friend. Reputations of popularity or unpopularity are developed and reinforced at this time. Thus, empathy, sharing, resolving conflict in a nonaggressive way, waiting one's turn in conversation, and having varied interests are important components of social competence.

Many children with AD/HD jump impulsively into conversations, are unable to take turns, and quit play activities prematurely due to boredom (Pelham & Bender, 1982). This inability to control behavior in social situations complicates the process of making new friends (Grenell, Glass, & Katz, 1987). Often, these behaviors also alienate existing friends, who respond with rejection or avoidance (Cunningham & Siegel, 1987).

Such problems occur more often among children with a Combined classification versus those with a Predominantly Inattentive presentation (Lahey, Carlson, & Frick, 1997). Due to the absence of systematic research in this area, little is known about the manner in which age, gender, and other demographics affect the social relations of children with AD/HD.

Emotional Functioning

Elementary school children begin to define themselves in terms of such areas as physical appearance, academics, sports, and social relations. Much of the basis for this self-evaluation comes from an increasing awareness of how their skills stack up against those of others. To the extent that children perceive themselves as competent relative to their peers, they tend to feel good about themselves. Competence provides a foundation for healthy emotional functioning.

As noted, children with AD/HD are at increased risk for various behavioral and academic problems as well as for difficulties in peer and family relations. Thus, they often have fewer success opportunities and receive more negative feedback than do most other children. This may in part be why as many as 13–51% have emotional disorders (Jensen et al., 1997). In both clinic-referred and community samples, up to 30% had a mood disorder, with Major Depression and Dysthymic Disorder occurring most often (August et al., 1996; Biederman, Newcorn, & Sprich, 1991). Secondary anxiety disorders are common as well, affecting as many as 34% of the AD/HD population (August et al. 1996). There are also reports, albeit controversial, that up to 11% of children with AD/HD have Bipolar Disorder (Biederman et al., 1996).

Little is known about the influence of age, gender, and other demographics on these rates (Russo & Beidel, 1994). Recent findings indicate that subtyping considerations and the presence of other externalizing problems play a moderating role. One study found depression in 19% of children with a Predominantly Inattentive classification versus 7% of those with a Combined diagnosis (Eiraldi et al., 1997). Although this difference is not statistically significant, it is consistent with earlier reports of higher rates of internalizing problems among children primarily displaying inattention (Lahey et al., 1997). Of additional clinical interest is that mood and anxiety disorders are not likely to be present when they are the only comorbid diagnoses. Among children with AD/HD who have just one other diagnosis, only 3% had a mood disorder and another 6% had anxiety problems (August et al., 1996). Rates of depression and anxiety rose to 30% and 34%, respectively, among children with AD/HD who were also diagnosed with CD or ODD (August et al., 1996). Thus, the presence of a secondary externalizing disorder seems to increase the risk for developing an additional internalizing disorder.

Besides reduced opportunities for success and higher rates of negative feedback, other factors often place children with AD/HD at risk for developing emotional problems. From a theoretical point of view (Barkley, 1998), deficiencies in their capacity for behavioral inhibition make it harder to pause and think before reacting emotionally, or to regulate an ongoing emotional reaction. Evidence also suggests that children with AD/HD are less likely to persist in tasks when confronted with failure (Milich & Okazaki, 1991). Moreover, they tend to make more external attributions for both failure and success (Lufi & Parish-Plass, 1995), so they may not even take credit for their accomplishments. Such misperceptions occurring repeatedly over time may seriously interfere with the development of self-esteem and other aspects of healthy emotional functioning.

Adolescence

Striving for independence is a major developmental challenge facing adolescents. It influences not only personal functioning, but also school performance, family interactions, and peer relations.

Behavioral Functioning

The push for independence puts adolescents on a collision course with parents, teachers, and others who have rules and expectations for their behavior. Teenagers are likely to test limits more often and be more rebellious than when they were younger, knowing full well that there may be negative consequences for their actions. Over time, most teenagers learn how and when to exert their new found independence, so as to avoid or reduce such consequences.

For the adolescent with AD/HD, this lesson does not come easy, because it requires pausing and contemplating consequences. Teens with AD/HD, lacking this capacity, are more inclined to display extreme forms of defiance and non-compliance, often warranting a secondary diagnosis of ODD (Barkley, Anastopoulos, Guevremont, & Fletcher, 1991). For similar reasons, teens with AD/HD are also more inclined to engage in theft and to exhibit other features of CD (Barkley et al., 1991).

Academic Functioning

Unlike elementary students, middle and high school students move from one class to another, which increases the demand for self-regulation, such as remembering what to bring to each class, getting to classes in a timely fashion, avoiding the temptation of talking to classmates in the hallways, and so forth. In the classroom, there is an increased emphasis on working independently. Homework takes on increased importance as well, with most assignments requiring systematic planning, organization, and sustained effort. For college-bound students, there is the additional challenge of college board examinations and other standardized tests, all of which require rapid processing, attention to detail, and sustained attention to task.

Because so many of these academic expectations emphasize independence and self-regulation, many adolescents with AD/HD experience significant difficulties in school, such as lower grades and greater use of special-education services (Barkley, Guevremont, Anastopoulos, & Fletcher, 1992). Teens with AD/HD are also more likely to repeat a grade, to be suspended from school, to drop out of high school, and to become employed directly from high school rather than continuing their education (Klein & Mannuzza, 1991).

Family Functioning

Striving for, struggling with, and accepting responsibility for independence become the major focus of teens' relationships with their family. Adolescence is a time when one tries on different roles. Many theorists believe that the attainment of a cohesive adult identity depends on the active exploration of roles in adolescence. This process brings with it a certain amount of conflict with parents. Decisions about friends, curfews, driving, dress, and chores become the proving ground as the adolescent considers "what I choose to be and what I choose not to be."

Although difficult for any adolescent, these challenges are especially hard for teens with AD/HD, whose impulsivity can lead to saying and doing things that get them into trouble. Teens with AD/HD are much more likely to encounter problems in their family relations, such as more frequent and more intense conflicts with parents (Barkley, Anastopoulos, Guevremont, & Fletcher, 1992). Perhaps as a consequence of such conflict, their parents are more likely to be psychologically distressed and dissatisfied in their marriages, especially when comorbid oppositional-defiant features are present (Barkley, Anastopoulos et al., 1992).

Social Functioning

Another major developmental change that takes place during adolescence is that the influence of friends outweighs that of family. Friendships continue to be based on psychological attributes, including loyalty, ability to keep secrets, respect for each other's independence, and how much each reinforces the other's current chosen role. Relationships with same-sex, as well as opposite-sex, peers become more important as the adolescent sorts out what sexuality means for him or her. Additional issues of freedom and independence arise when teens encounter alcohol and drugs, acquire a driver's license, and take on part-time jobs.

Meeting such challenges successfully requires skills and abilities that many adolescents with AD/HD lack, particularly reflection and self-control, taking the perspective of others, and thinking ahead. Thus, their social adjustment is often impaired (Taylor, Chadwick, Heptinstall, & Danckaerts, 1996) in that they have fewer friends and engage in fewer social activities (Barkley et al., 1991). Although some studies have not found increased rates of substance abuse or cigarette smoking (Biederman et al., 1997; Taylor et al., 1996), others have (Barkley et al., 1990; Klein & Mannuzza, 1991; Milberger, Biederman, Faraone, & Jones, 1997). Furthermore, teens with AD/HD are definitely at increased risk for automobile accidents and traffic violations, especially speeding (Barkley et al., 1993; Nada-Raja et al., 1997).

Emotional Functioning

Adolescence also brings many physical changes, including major disruptions in hormonal functioning, which can lead to new emotional experiences, or at least intensify previously learned emotional reactions. Keeping these emotions in check is a challenge for any teen, but especially for those with AD/HD, who lack the capacity for regulating their emotional responses.

Although teens with AD/HD seldom report higher rates of internalizing problems, ratings completed by their parents and teachers often suggest that they are at risk for them (Barkley et al., 1991). This risk is even greater for adolescents with a history of learning difficulties that required special-education assistance (Barkley et al., 1990). Implicit in this finding is the possibility that the emotional problems experienced by adolescents with AD/HD are not entirely due to their diminished capacity for regulating emotions. At least in part, such problems may be the result of long-standing histories of repeated failure and frustration, not only in academics, but also in social and family functioning.

Adulthood

Whereas striving for independence was the driving force in adolescence, knowing what to do with this independence is the central theme for adults. Among the many developmental challenges adults face are merging into society, preparing for and selecting a career, establishing and maintaining a primary relationship or marriage, and maintaining satisfactory relationships with friends and others in the community.

Behavioral Functioning

Upon reaching young adulthood, most people have attained as much independence as they want or need. Defiance and rebellion take a back seat to societal rules and moral and religious beliefs.

Due to their inattention and impulsivity, many adults with AD/HD inadvertently fail to comply with societal rules and expectations. They might miss a payment on a bill, forget to attend an important meeting, or skip work to do something fun. Although the problems of most adults with AD/HD do not go beyond this level, up to 25% exhibit more-serious behavioral difficulties, including Antisocial Personality Disorder (Klein & Mannuzza, 1991; Murphy & Barkley, 1996b). When AD/HD is accompanied by Antisocial Personality Disorder, the risk for arrest and incarceration increases dramatically (Satterfield & Shell, 1997), as does the risk for substance abuse (Gittelman et al., 1985). Drug abuse seems to be particularly problematic (Klein & Mannuzza, 1991; Murphy & Barkley, 1996b); marijuana or cocaine is most often the drug of choice (Mannuzza et al., 1997). Alcohol abuse may also be associated with adult AD/HD, but this finding is less consistent (Murphy & Barkley, 1996b).

Educational Functioning

In contrast to childhood and adolescence, in adulthood the changes in cognitive functioning are far more subtle and gradual. Improvements are usually in the domain of crystallized intelligence, or the base of practical knowledge built up over a lifetime of experience.

Although research has yet to bear this out, clinical experience suggests that many adults with AD/HD lack practical knowledge, because they apparently profit less from their educational experiences. Moreover, adults with AD/HD average 2 to 3 years less overall schooling (Mannuzza, Klein, Bessler, Mallory, & Hynes, 1997). As many as 23% will not complete high school, versus 2% of controls (Mannuzza et al., 1997). Approximately 12% will complete college (Mannuzza et al., 1997), but only 3% of them will go on to receive a graduate degree, versus 16% of controls (Mannuzza et al., 1997).

Occupational Functioning

Educational training provides the preparation necessary for choosing a career. This involves several occupational stages: experimentation, settling on a choice of jobs, a more intense period of work involvement, and then a gradual phasing out, followed by retirement (Atchley, 1975). In this context, early adulthood is a time when psychological processes are organized and mobilized to achieve competence in productive work, and middle adulthood is when the person redefines this work and begins to think about his or her legacy.

Because adults with AD/HD often lack optimal educational preparation, they frequently end up in lower-paying or nonprofessional jobs (Mannuzza et al., 1993). Such positions typically involve a great deal of repetition and tedium, so adults with AD/HD quickly lose interest and thus change jobs more often, either by choice or through being fired (Murphy & Barkley, 1996b). Although prone to numerous job changes, adults with AD/HD generally do not have higher rates of unemployment; they are also more likely to own their own business (Mannuzza et al., 1997). This suggests that many adults with AD/HD may have a prolonged period of occupational experimentation, followed by fewer years and less depth in their career field.

Family Functioning

One of the most important developmental tasks of adulthood is choosing and maintaining a primary relationship, usually defined as marriage. Many things enter into the selection of a partner, including having similar interests and activities, being able to communicate easily, and sharing goals and responsibilities. In the context of this relationship, another major developmental task often emerges: parenting. Whether planned or not, this begins the transition. Once the child is born, couples face many other adjustments requiring numerous negotiations both in their individual roles and in their relationship with each other. How well couples negotiate these adjustments seems to determine whether the transition to parenthood is perceived positively or negatively.

Adults with AD/HD are often inattentive to what others are saying or doing, impulsively interrupting them in midsentence, or forgetting to follow through on commitments. This creates tension in their relationships and obstacles to fulfilling their marital and parenting roles. Although little research has addressed these matters, preliminary findings indicate that adults with AD/HD are more likely to experience marital discord, to separate or divorce, and to report difficulties in their relationships with their children (Murphy & Barkley, 1996b).

Social Functioning

As they did in their youth, adults tend to choose friends who are similar to themselves in personal attributes and who enjoy similar interests and activities. Psychological characteristics such as communication skills, ease of getting along, and perceived social support become even more important. Unlike friendships in youth, adult friendships are characterized by increasing demands on one's time and more variations in the circles in which one lives. Thus, maintaining, as well as initiating, friendships becomes more challenging.

Researchers have yet to examine the social relations of adults with AD/HD. However, for the same reasons that adults with AD/HD would have problems in a primary relationship, they would have problems with friends and other adults. This is, in fact, commonly reported in clinical practice.

Emotional Functioning

To the extent that adults meet the above developmental challenges successfully, they are likely to have a healthy self-esteem and to be satisfied with life. For those who do not meet them well, the end result may be self-doubt, dissatisfaction, and a sadness over lost opportunities.

Thus adults with AD/HD might be prone to emotional difficulties. Support for this contention has been mixed, however. Some researchers report exceedingly high (43–52%) lifetime rates of depression and anxiety (Biederman et al., 1993). Others have found more moderate rates (18–32%; Murphy & Barkley, 1996b). In at least two additional studies, there were no differences in the rates of depression and anxiety experienced by adults with AD/HD versus those of controls (Klein & Mannuzza, 1991; Mannuzza et al., 1997). Such inconsistencies preclude making any definitive statements about the emotional well-being of adults with AD/HD.

Summary

Having AD/HD puts individuals at risk for psychosocial difficulties across the life span, the particulars being determined largely by what is considered typical or normal at a given stage of development. Preschoolers with AD/HD place increased caretaking demands on their parents and frequently display aggression with siblings and peers. Difficulties acquiring academic readiness skills may be evident as well, but these tend to be of less clinical concern than are the family or peer problems that preschoolers present. As children with AD/HD move into elementary school, academic problems are increasingly important. Together with their ongoing family and peer relationship problems, school-based difficulties set the stage for the development of low self-esteem and other emotional problems, which persist into adolescence, but more intensely. New problems may develop as well (e.g., traffic violations, alcohol and drug experimentation), stemming from the increased developmental need for independence, self-regulation, and self-control. Having AD/HD can also make the transition into adulthood difficult; particularly noteworthy are the obstacles it poses to establishing and maintaining a family and career.

Individuals with AD/HD are also at increased risk for having secondary, or comorbid, diagnoses. Preschoolers and children with AD/HD frequently display Oppositional-Defiant Disorder. Among adolescents with AD/HD, Conduct Disorder is common. Antisocial Personality Disorder, Major Depression, and substance abuse are just a few of the possible comorbidities among adults. Such comorbid conditions often increase the severity of overall psychosocial impairment, making the prognosis for such individuals even less favorable.

Relatively little research has taken developmental expectations into account when examining the psychosocial impact of AD/HD. Nor has much empirical attention been directed to the moderating influence of comorbidity. Researchers would be well advised to take these matters into consideration in the future.

CONCLUSION

Attention-Deficit/Hyperactivity Disorder is a chronic and pervasive condition characterized by developmentally inappropriate levels of inattention, hyperactivity-impulsivity, or both. Contrary to popular belief, AD/HD symptoms are highly subject to situational variability, occurring most often under low- and delayed-feedback conditions that are boring, repetitive, or familiar. Although the exact details of what causes AD/HD are not well understood, a recent convergence of theory and empirical findings points to a combination of genetic, neurochemical, and other neurobiological factors. Due to the variable manner in which epidemiological research has been conducted, the exact prevalence of AD/HD is difficult to determine. What is clear is that AD/HD occurs most often among boys and younger children. AD/HD symptoms typically arise in early childhood and persist across the life span, though hyperactivity-impulsivity symptoms diminish somewhat over time. At least in clinic-referred populations, AD/HD is often accompanied by secondary behavioral, academic, social, emotional, and family complications, which increase the severity of psychosocial impairment and the risk for negative outcomes.

3

Implications for Assessment

"Why do you need to ask me so many questions?"

The manner in which *DSM-IV* defines AD/HD has numerous implications for the assessment process. So too does our understanding of how AD/HD presents itself across the life span. This chapter examines these matters more fully and provides the rationale for using a multimethod assessment approach, in which clinical interviews and rating scales play a central role.

IMPACT OF *DSM-IV* CRITERIA ON ASSESSMENT

As noted in the introduction, there is still a great deal of variability in the way that AD/HD is assessed, in part due to the variation in how faithfully child health-care professionals and educators adhere to the *DSM-IV* criteria. Often, some, but not all, of its guidelines are used. Perhaps the best example of this is when clinicians rely on symptom frequency counts as the sole basis for establishing an AD/HD diagnosis. Although this practice offers ease and convenience, it also carries an increased risk of identifying someone as having AD/HD when in fact they do not. Such short cuts should be avoided.

Greater adherence to the *DSM-IV* criteria in their entirety would reduce this variability among practitioners. It would not entirely eliminate it, because *DSM-IV* does not specify which procedures to use to making a diagnosis. This decision rests entirely with the evaluator and is therefore subject to interpretation.

Complicating this process is that the field is currently saturated with a large number and variety of procedures that purportedly assess AD/HD. Among these are clinical interviews, behavior rating scales, psychological tests, observational assessment techniques, and various medical procedures, each with its own variations. For example, clinical interviews come in three forms: *structured*, *semistructured*, and *unstructured*. Behavior rating scales, of which there are dozens, can be *broad-band*, meaning that they assess a wide range of child psychopathology, or *narrow-band*, designed to assess AD/HD exclusively. Both types often come in parent, teacher, and self-report versions. Psychological tests are still another approach. Generally speaking, clinicians administer psychological tests in either a clinic or school-based setting. Some measure AD/HD symptoms directly, including continuous performance tests and tests borrowed from the neuropsychological assessment literature. Others address AD/HD symptoms indirectly—that is, they were originally developed to measure other psychological constructs, but are thought to have some association with AD/HD symptomatology as well. The Freedom from Distractibility factor from the Third Edition of the Wechsler Intelligence Scale for Children is a good example of this. Projective measures also fall into this category. Less commonly used are observational assessment procedures, which allow for a more direct examination of AD/HD. These can be conducted in one of two ways. In naturalistic observations, an evaluator unobtrusively watches a child at home, in school, or wherever the child functions during the day (e.g., day care). Analog observations typically occur in clinics, with evaluators watching through a one-way mirror as the child plays, interacts with a parent, or performs assigned tasks. Pediatricians, child psychiatrists, and others with appropriate medical training have additional options, such as standard pediatric examinations, neurodevelopmental exams, neuroimaging studies, and other neurologically related procedures. Although not usually thought of as an assessment procedure, reviews of medical, psychological, or school records can be an additional source of diagnostically relevant information.

Deciding which procedures to use is a rather formidable task, especially for beginning or inexperienced clinicians. Although it may seem obvious, an often overlooked starting point is to ask the following question: Which procedures do the best job of addressing the *DSM-IV* criteria for AD/HD? We begin to answer this question by looking at each criteria separately.

Criterion A

> *Either (1) or (2):*
> *(1) Inattention: six (or more) of the following symptoms of inattention have persisted for at least 6 months to a degree that is maladaptive and inconsistent with developmental level.*
> *(2) Hyperactivity-Impulsivity: six (or more) of the following symptoms of hyperactivity-impulsivity have persisted for at least 6 months to a degree that is maladaptive and inconsistent with developmental level.*

Inherent in Criterion A are three important diagnostic elements. First, a certain *frequency* of either inattention or hyperactive-impulsive symptoms (i.e., 6 or more from either list) is required. Criterion A also stipulates that these symptoms must have a *duration* of at least 6 months and be *inconsistent with developmental level*.

To meet the frequency requirement, an assessment procedure must allow for direct comparison with the two symptom lists. The more that a given procedure deviates from the content of these lists, the harder it is to make a frequency determination. Most clinical interviews address this requirement, as do most narrow-band scales. Broad-band scales typically do not map exactly onto either list, though they may allow comparisons with some of the symptoms. The same is true for psychological tests, whose data typically do not allow for direct comparison with either list in its entirety. Naturalistic observations can shed light on symptom frequency, but only when they are long enough, are conducted on more than one occasion across multiple settings, and include a formal coding system for tallying behavior. Analog observations seldom allow a complete sampling of AD/HD symptoms, but they may provide documentation for at least some symptoms. Because they typically provide opportunities for informal observation, medical examinations can uncover the existence of some AD/HD symptoms that arise in the office. Other components of the medical evaluation, including standard pediatric examinations, neurodevelopmental examinations, and neuroimaging studies generally do not. Although school and medical records often contain symptom-related information, reviewing them seldom allows a complete assessment of all 18 *DSM-IV* symptoms.

Documenting that AD/HD symptoms have lasted at least 6 months is relatively straightforward. Nearly all interviews and most rating scales address this. When records are available, they too often contain information that allows an assessment of the recent history of these symptoms. Psychological tests, unless administered on repeated occasions spanning a 6-month period, are of little value in making this determination. The same goes for observations and medical tests.

Criterion A also states that AD/HD symptoms must be inconsistent with the child's developmental level. In other words, the degree to which AD/HD symptoms occur must deviate significantly from what is expected of a child of the same gender and the same chronological or mental age. Although child health-care professionals and educators have some sense of what constitutes normal behavior, most would admit (if they were being candid) that the norms in their heads are far from precise. Therefore, to address the requirement for *developmental deviance*, clinicians should not rely on their own subjective appraisals. Instead, they should use assessment procedures with well-established norms that allow them to make a more accurate and objective determination of the degree to which symptoms deviate from those norms. Behavior rating scales are especially well suited to this purpose, as are some psychological tests, such as continuous performance tests, at least with respect to symptoms of inattention and impulsivity. The same would not be true for interviews, observational assessments, medical tests, and prior records, all of which lack norms.

Criterion B

Some hyperactive-impulsive or inattentive symptoms that caused impairment were present before age 7 years.

Criterion B states that there must be evidence that AD/HD symptoms were present and causing impairment *prior to 7 years of age*. This requirement is automatically met when children younger than 7 are brought to a clinic for an AD/HD evaluation. For older children, other forms of documentation are necessary. Most interviews include questions that review the history of AD/HD symptoms in sufficient detail to allow this determination. Records, especially school records, very often include such information as well. This type of historical information cannot be reliably obtained from behavior rating scales or psychological tests. Likewise, observational assessments and medical tests do little to address this requirement.

Criterion C

> *Some impairment from the symptoms is present in two or more settings (e.g., at school [or work] and at home).*

Criterion C requires impairment from AD/HD symptoms in two or more settings. To the extent that an evaluator has access to both parents and teachers, interviews can determine this. Rating scales distributed to parents, teachers, and other significant caretakers can also produce data that document *cross-situational pervasiveness*. Although less likely under managed health-care constraints, observing a child in multiple settings can also serve this purpose. When available, records often include information that documents the existence of AD/HD-related problems in multiple settings. Psychological tests do not fully meet this requirement, but they can show evidence of impairment in at least one setting—namely, the clinic or school where the testing is conducted, via informal observation during the testing and through the test results themselves. Observations of symptoms that arise during a medical examination can serve the same function.

Criterion D

> *There must be clear evidence of clinically significant impairment in social, academic, or occupational functioning.*

As with all *DSM-IV* disorders, there must be evidence of *functional impairment*, that is, clinically significant impairment in social, academic, or occupational functioning. This information can be derived from many of the narrow-band rating scales, such as those assessing academic productivity, social skills, or parent–child interactions. Many psychological tests can also serve this purpose, providing valuable information pertaining, among other things, to academic achievement levels, behavioral inhibition, and working memory. Interviews, observational assessments, and record reviews can help to identify the presence of psychosocial impairment, but in a much less objective and precise way than can rating scales and psychological tests, for which there are usually norms. The interview portion of a medical examination serves a similar function, but other aspects of the medical workup do not address functional impairment.

Criterion E

> *The symptoms do not occur exclusively during the course of a Pervasive Developmental Disorder, Schizophrenia, or other Psychotic Disorder and are not better accounted for by another mental disorder (e.g., Mood Disorder, Anxiety Disorder, Dissociative Disorder, or a Personality Disorder).*

Assuming that criteria A–D have been met, Criterion E stipulates that *alternative explanations* for the symptom patterns need to be ruled out before arriving at an AD/HD diagnosis. This means ruling out mental health conditions (e.g., depression, anxiety, child maltreatment) that can produce AD/HD-like symptoms. Such conditions can be reliably detected through most forms of clinical interviewing, and many rating scales also allow assessment of other psychopathologies. On a more limited basis, psychological tests can be of assistance, such as when academic achievement tests and intelligence tests are used to rule out learning disabilities. In addition, medical examinations can rule out various physical problems that may be producing symptoms that are mistaken for AD/HD. Often this includes testing for sensory deficits, such as hearing and visual problems, and occasionally for seizure disorders and other neurological conditions as well. Observational assessments and record reviews occasionally reveal possible exclusionary conditions, but for the most part they do not.

Summary and Recommendations

No one procedure maps perfectly onto all of the *DSM-IV* criteria. To arrive at an AD/HD diagnosis, a combination of assessment procedures—a *multimethod approach*—is necessary. When deciding which procedures to combine, one should remember that some types of assessment procedures do a better job of addressing the *DSM-IV* criteria than others. As may be seen in Table 3.1., clinical

TABLE 3.1. Adequacy of Assessment Procedures in Addressing AD/HD Criteria

	Assessment procedure					
DSM-IV criteria	Interviews	Rating scales	Psychological tests	Observations	Medical tests	Records
A. Symptom						
Frequency	Yes	Yes	No	Yes	No	No
Duration	Yes	Yes	No	No	No	Yes
Developmental deviance	No	Yes	Yes	No	No	No
B. Onset	Yes	No	No	No	No	Yes
C. Settings	Yes	Yes	No	Yes	No	Yes
D. Impairment	Yes	Yes	Yes	Yes	No	Yes
E. Exclusions	Yes	Yes	Yes	Yes	Yes	Yes

Note: AD/HD = Attention-deficit/hyperactivity disorder; *DSM-IV* = *Diagnostic and Statistical Manual, Fourth Edition*.

interviews and rating scales provide the most comprehensive coverage, meeting all but one of the criteria. Clinical interviews lack the means to address developmental deviance. Rating scales lack the capacity for documenting symptom onset. When used together, what's missing from one is covered by the other. Thus, using clinical interviews and rating scales in combination is an excellent way to address the AD/HD criteria in their entirety.

Multimethod assessments are not limited to clinical interviews and rating scales. Adding other assessment procedures can refine the diagnostic picture. For example, psychological tests can provide further evidence of developmental deviance. They can also document certain functional impairments (e.g., academic underachievement) and can rule out certain conditions (e.g., learning disabilities) that might better account for the presence of AD/HD symptoms. Observational assessments have the potential to address many of the *DSM-IV* criteria. When time and money permit, clinicians should include some type of observational assessment to get a better feel for a child's clinical presentation. But most clinicians do not have this financial and temporal luxury, so observational assessments are generally precluded. Although medical procedures do little to address the inclusionary criteria for AD/HD, they can play an important role in ruling out medical conditions that may be producing AD/HD-like symptoms. Records can often address many of the AD/HD criteria, but they are frequently unavailable. Therefore clinicians cannot rely on them to establish a diagnosis.

IMPACT OF AD/HD RESEARCH FINDINGS ON ASSESSMENT

Voluminous research on AD/HD has greatly increased our understanding of this disorder, which in turn has led to numerous refinements in the diagnostic criteria. Not all that is known, however, is reflected in the diagnostic guidelines. Some aspects of the *DSM-IV* criteria are vague, leaving them open to idiosyncratic interpretation. For reasons such as these it is important to turn to the research literature for additional guidance on conducting an AD/HD assessment. The next section examines many of the research findings that have bearing on the assessment process.

Clinical Presentation

One major complication in assessing AD/HD is the situational variability of its primary symptoms (Zentall, 1985). As noted earlier, AD/HD symptoms do not occur in an either/or, all-or-none fashion. Sometimes they appear, other times they don't; it depends on the situation. For example, symptoms seldom arise when children are doing something they like. Nor do they surface when children are engaged in one-on-one situations with adults who provide immediate and salient feedback. Conversely, children are much more likely to display AD/HD symptoms in low-feedback situations or in group settings that are highly repetitive and boring. This gives insight into why individuals within the same setting sometimes disagree on whether the symptoms are present.

In clinical practice, such discrepancies arise in any number of ways. For example, a child may exhibit clear-cut AD/HD symptoms in school but not at home. Less frequently, parents may observe such symptoms at home even though teachers do not see them at school. In certain families, a mother might be keenly aware of her child's AD/HD symptomatology, whereas the father might not be. A regular-classroom teacher may report that a student shows a high rate of inattention or hyperactivity-impulsivity, whereas the child's special-education teacher seldom, if ever, sees such symptoms. Even when parents and teachers agree that the symptoms exist, they may be at odds with a child health-care professional whose clinic-based observations and direct testing suggest nothing of the sort.

That such discrepancies may occur—and they quite frequently do—has tremendous implications for the assessment process. First, because AD/HD symptoms can vary from one setting to the next, clinicians must employ measures that sample a child's behavior in as many settings as possible, being sure to target settings in which the symptoms are most likely to occur. For instance, preference would be given to procedures that sample behavior from a group setting rather than from a one-to-one interaction. Another important point to bear in mind is that AD/HD symptoms can also vary within the *same* setting. For any given setting, therefore, multiple assessment methods, informants, or both should be used to capture the symptoms as completely as possible. To cover all bases within a school setting, two or more teachers, for example, could be asked for their perceptions of the child's behavior. Having both parents serve as informants is also an excellent way to obtain a more complete picture of the child's behavior at home.

A cost-effective way of obtaining such information is to have parents, teachers, and other caretakers complete rating scales, especially narrow-band questionnaires that focus exclusively on AD/HD symptoms. Although more time-consuming, interviews with these same informants will also yield such data. Although observational procedures also do this, they are often too costly and time-consuming to be practical. Assessment data from rating scales, interviews, and observations will usually address the pervasiveness of symptoms across settings, but occasionally they may produce clear evidence in only the home setting or only the school setting, not in both. If this happens, clinic-based observations and psychological tests suggestive of AD/HD can document symptom existence in a second setting. Reviews of prior records often do this too.

Etiological Considerations

Emerging from the earlier etiological discussion is the idea that neurobiological factors play a major role. Of what clinical significance is this? Unfortunately, very little. Although neurochemical, neuroanatomical, and neurophysiological differences have been found between AD/HD and non-AD/HD comparison groups (Castellanos et al., 1996; Pliszka et al., 1996; Zametkin et al., 1993), such differences are inconsistent from one study to the next. Therefore, there is no neurobiological template for determining the presence of AD/HD. Further, what we do know about AD/HD neurobiology comes from comparisons of group averages. As a group, children with AD/HD may have a neurobiological profile that differs from that of a group of non-AD/HD children, but this does not mean that all children with AD/HD have that profile. What applies to the group may not apply to an individual within the group. Thus, results from group studies may have little bearing on a clinical assessment, which deals with an individual. For this reason, there is little justification for using CT scans, MRIs, PET scans, blood tests, or other such medical procedures to assess AD/HD. Should a more precise neurobiological template emerge in the future, there may be some merit in using such procedures. However, cost will still need to be considered before incorporating them routinely.

Another etiological finding is that genetic and prenatal factors apparently alter neurobiology in a way that mediates AD/HD expression (Cook et al., 1995; Edelbrock, Rende, Plomin, & Thompson, 1995; Streissguth et al., 1995). Again, such studies are plagued by some of the same limitations noted above, including an overreliance on group averages. Not all children with AD/HD have a family history of it, a genetic marker for it, or any evidence of pregnancy complications. Thus there is little reason to include chromosomal analyses or other such tests in the assessment. This is not to say that such information is of no diagnostic value; even though it cannot be used to diagnose AD/HD, knowing that a child has a family history of it or a history of pregnancy risk factors can add detail to the diagnostic picture emerging from other assessment procedures. Thus, clinicians should consider incorporating this type of information into their assessments, which can be done through interviews, through parental completion of developmental history and health history questionnaires, or through reviewing any medical records that may be available.

Based upon what we know about the neurobiology of AD/HD, Barkley (1998), Quay (1997), and others have recently theorized that it results from a core deficit in behavioral inhibition. Barkley takes this one step further, speculating that the inhibition deficits disrupt four major areas of executive functioning, which sets the stage for AD/HD problems to occur. If valid, this concept has numerous implications for the assessment process. Foremost among these is the need for documenting a deficit in behavioral inhibition. The most precise way to do this is via psychological tests that measure behavioral inhibition. Barkley's theory also creates a need to address the four major areas of executive functioning that are presumably disrupted. Psychological tests are the only method that assesses these four areas, which are: (1) working memory, (2) emotion regulation, (3) internalization of language, and (4) the processes of reconstitution and synthesis. Although assertions of a core deficit in behavioral inhibition have a great deal of intuitive appeal, they are theoretical models, and new ones at that. Whether to include such psychological testing procedures in an assessment battery depends largely on one's confidence in these models.

Epidemiological Considerations

One of the most important points to emerge from a consideration of the epidemiology of AD/HD is that its apparent prevalence is influenced by many factors. Teachers tend to report higher rates of AD/HD symptoms than do parents, and higher rates are reported for younger children versus older children and for boys versus girls. Ethnic diversity also exerts an influence; higher rates of AD/HD symptoms are reported for African American versus Caucasian children.

Awareness of epidemiological variation is of diagnostic value. Assume for a moment that a preschooler's assessment suggests the presence of AD/HD, Predominantly Hyperactive-Impulsive type. Although this conclusion may be wrong, it is consistent with the research on subtype variations across development—namely, that very young children are more likely to display the Predominantly Hyperactive-Impulsive subtype, which adds confidence to the diagnostic conclusion. Conversely, if a teenager is evaluated as having AD/HD, Predominantly Hyperactive-Impulsive type, it may signal a diagnostic error. This is not to say that teenagers cannot have this diagnosis. They certainly can, but because most do not, it is even more important to consider the possibility that another condition may be producing the symptoms.

Clinicians would also be well advised to pay close attention to ethnic diversity. As noted, several studies have recently shown that both parents and teachers rate African American children as having higher rates of AD/HD symptoms than Caucasian children (DuPaul et al., 1997; DuPaul, Anastopoulos, et al., 1998). Cultural bias in the *DSM-IV* criteria, racial bias across informants, and other unknown factors may artificially elevate AD/HD rates within African American populations. If in fact these rates are higher than they should be, currently available assessment procedures may be faulty in some way, leading to overidentification. Clinicians should thus exercise caution when evaluating African American children. In particular, it seems necessary for clinicians to build an especially strong case before arriving at this diagnosis. Practically speaking, clinicians need to incorporate more procedures into their assessments in order to gather as much assessment information as possible. They must also make every effort to use procedures that included minority youth in their development and standardization to reduce potential bias in their administration and in their norms.

Developmental Considerations

Research shows that the onset and course of AD/HD symptoms can be highly variable. With respect to onset, a debate is now in progress over the 7-year cutoff criteria (Barkley & Biederman, 1997). At the heart of the debate is a distinction between when AD/HD symptoms were first noticed and when they first caused problems. According to Applegate et al. (1997), nearly all children with AD/HD display inattention and hyperactivity-impulsivity before age 7. Most also exhibit symptoms associated with psychosocial problems before this age. A substantial minority, however, do not. Clinicians need to be aware of this distinction when conducting evaluations, particularly in the context of parent interviews.

Another developmental finding of clinical importance is that AD/HD symptoms seem to change their expression across the life span (Hart et al., 1995).

Because the *DSM-IV* criteria were developed primarily using elementary school children, they are less applicable to preschoolers, adolescents, and young adults. Thus clinicians should also look at other developmentally appropriate manifestations of AD/HD. This information can be gathered easily through interviews with parents and teachers, and possibly with children and adolescents themselves.

The fact that AD/HD symptoms vary across the life span also has implications for meeting the developmental deviance requirement. In general, rating scales and psychological tests are an excellent way to meet this particular criteria, but some do it better than others, largely as a function of the adequacy of their norms. Quality norms for rating scales and psychological tests are generally derived from large numbers of individuals across the full age spectrum. Clinicians need to take this into account when choosing which rating scales and psychological tests to use.

Psychosocial Impact and Comorbidity

Having AD/HD places individuals at risk for lifelong difficulties in multiple psychosocial domains. In addition to being affected by the disorder itself, individuals with AD/HD are also at increased risk for a variety of comorbid conditions. For clinicians who simply wish to screen for the presence of AD/HD, such circumstances are of little concern. For those conducting a more comprehensive evaluation, however, comorbidity takes on tremendous clinical importance. Knowing the extent to which AD/HD is affecting a child and being aware of which comorbid conditions might be present sheds light on the overall severity of the child's difficulties, which can help clinicians plan appropriate interventions.

School Functioning

Academic functioning is particularly sensitive to the effects of AD/HD (DuPaul & Stoner, 1994). Nearly all young people with this disorder have trouble producing satisfactory amounts of school work, and this diminished productivity can eventually interfere with learning, causing a child to fall behind. Research has also shown that children with AD/HD are at slightly higher risk for reading disorders and other learning disabilities (Tannock & Schachar, 1996).

Not uncommonly, children referred to child health care professionals for AD/HD evaluations have already undergone school-based testing that serves to clarify their level of intelligence, academic achievement, and for the presence or absence of learning disorders. If such data are unavailable, the clinician must gather it. This can be done using IQ and psychoeducational tests, which are used exclusively for this purpose. School records frequently document retentions, special services, and other classroom accommodations that have arisen as a result of AD/HD symptomatology. Another way to gather information on school performance is through classroom observations or teacher completion of rating scales that assess academic productivity and other facets of school functioning.

Although less cost effective, teacher interviews can also serve this purpose. In contrast, medical tests play no role in documenting functional impairment in school performance.

Behavioral Functioning

Having AD/HD places a child at risk for developing secondary behavioral complications. Anywhere from 40–60% of the AD/HD population exhibits Oppositional-Defiant Disorder or Conduct Disorder (August et al., 1996; Barkley, 1998). Such conditions are serious clinical referral problems in themselves and they warrant intensive intervention. Therefore, determining whether they exist is essential. Interviews and rating scales are especially well suited to addressing comorbid conditions, and clinical interviews in particular allow direct determination of whether the *DSM-IV* criteria for ODD and CD are met. Observational assessments may reveal the existence of some, but not all, features of comorbid conditions, as can various records, which may contain information on school suspensions or expulsions, criminal activities, or other manifestations of ODD or CD. Data drawn from psychological and medical tests have little bearing on these concerns.

Emotional Functioning

Children and adolescents with AD/HD experience a great deal of failure and frustration, and they frequently receive negative feedback from parents and others with whom they come into contact. As a result, many have emotional difficulties. Although there is some disagreement about actual rates, there is little argument over the fact that such children and adolescents are at increased risk for clinical depression and anxiety disorders (August et al., 1996; Biederman, Newcorn, & Sprich, 1991). Some researchers have also raised the possibility, albeit a controversial one, that these children are at increased risk for Bipolar Disorder (Biederman et al., 1996). Each of these emotional conditions is itself a serious mental health problem with potentially debilitating or even life-threatening consequences. Therefore, clinicians must incorporate procedures that screen for their presence. Again, clinical interviews are well suited for this. Although rating scales typically do not lend themselves to generating actual diagnoses, they can reveal the existence and severity of emotional symptoms, as can observational assessments and certain types of psychological testing, such as projective techniques. At times a child's records may contain evidence of emotional disorders. Medical tests are of limited value in making these sorts of diagnostic determinations.

Social Functioning

Up to 50% of those with AD/HD have peer relationship difficulties (Barkley, 1998). Although this can involve problems making friends, these difficulties usually center around maintaining established relationships. Just as parents and teachers find the behavior of children with AD/HD unpleasant and aversive, so too do other children. As a result, many face constant ridicule, teasing, and rejection from their peers, which leads to frequent shifting from one group to the next. Because research has shown that peer relationship problems are predictive of many negative outcomes, the value of detecting them cannot be overstated. It is critical for any AD/HD evaluation to include procedures that assess social functioning. Although costly and time-consuming, an especially effective way to do this is through naturalistic observations, particularly at school. Indirect evidence can also be gathered fairly reliably through clinical interviews and rating scales. Psychological tests shed little light on social functioning, nor do records and medical procedures.

When the referral involves an adolescent, additional social areas must be addressed, including involvement in school organizations, dating history, possible experimentation with alcohol and drugs, driving record if they're licensed, and their job performance, if they have an employment history. Clinical interviews and questionnaires are the best way to assess these areas.

Family Functioning

Parents of children with AD/HD often have psychosocial difficulties themselves, which commonly include low parenting self-esteem and high parenting stress (Anastopoulos et al., 1992; Shelton et al., 1998). They may also manifest symptoms of adult AD/HD, depression, anxiety, or other psychopathology (Cunningham et al., 1988). Moreover, marital relations may be strained. Siblings are also at increased risk for displaying AD/HD and other behavioral problems. Even when they are unaffected, brothers and sisters very often resent a sibling with AD/HD because the sibling's behavior demands and controls so much of the family's time, attention, and energy. How many of these family complications are a direct consequence of living with a child who has AD/HD is an interesting matter requiring further research. Even without such research, this remains a clinically relevant issue with bearing on the assessment process.

Certain family problems (e.g., marital discord) can exacerbate a pre-existing AD/HD condition or lead to other child difficulties of diagnostic significance. Working from the assumption that a child's behavior might have a "ripple effect," the clinician should learn whether other family members are experiencing problems that warrant treatment for themselves. Regardless of their source, such family problems need to be addressed, not only to benefit the affected family member but to facilitate family efforts to implement treatment strategies on behalf of the child with AD/HD.

From a systems point of view then, some portion of the assessment battery should focus on the family context in which the child with AD/HD functions. Failure to do so can lead to incomplete diagnostic formulations and ineffective interventions or to far less effective interventions, at least. Clinical interviews offer insight into many areas of family functioning. So too do most rating scales, particularly parent self-report scales. Observing family interactions can also reveal a lot about the functioning of its various subsystems as well as of its individual members. Records may contain relevant information about the family and should be reviewed when available. Psychological tests do not address these areas, nor do medical procedures.

Summary and Recommendations

What research has taught us over the years has enormous implications for the assessment of AD/HD, implications that go well beyond the boundaries of the *DSM-IV* criteria. For example, because the symptoms are subject to situational variability, it is necessary to include assessment procedures that provide a comprehensive sampling of this disorder from multiple settings. This can often be achieved through some combination of clinical interviews, rating scales, and observational procedures. Knowing that a child has a family history of AD/HD or a history of pregnancy risk factors does not confirm an AD/HD diagnosis but can add to the diagnostic picture. Such information is often available through records, clinical interviewing, and parent-completed developmental and health history questionnaires. Based on recent theories, some clinicians may also wish to include procedures that assess a child's capacity for behavioral inhibition and the integrity of his or her executive functions, which are thought to be involved in the expression of AD/HD. At present, psychological testing is the only reliable and valid way of measuring these cognitive domains.

Because the psychosocial impact of AD/HD is far reaching and because the risk for comorbidity is high, clinicians also need to incorporate procedures that address these areas. As noted in Table 3.2., a combination of clinical interviews, rating scales, and observational procedures can assess functional impairment in all of the pertinent psychosocial domains. Clinical interviews offer the unique advantage of determining whether the *DSM-IV* criteria for various behavioral and emotional disorders have been met. A particular strength of rating scales is that they offer insight into parent and family functioning. Observational assessments are especially well suited to addressing deficits in social relations. Psychological testing procedures are the primary method for gathering information on academic achievement levels and learning disorders. Records can occasionally document psychosocial impairment, but their uncertain availability

TABLE 3.2.   Adequacy of Assessment Procedures
in Addressing Psychological Effect and Comorbidity

Functional domain	Assessment tool					
	Interviews	Rating scales	Psychological tests	Observations	Medical tests	Records
Academic	Yes	Yes	Yes	Yes	No	Yes
Behavioral	Yes	Yes	No	Yes	No	Yes
Emotional	Yes	Yes	Yes	Yes	No	Yes
Social	Yes	Yes	No	Yes	No	No
Family	Yes	Yes	No	Yes	No	Yes

limits their usefulness. Although valuable for other reasons, medical tests contribute little to the assessment of psychosocial impact or comorbidity.

CONCLUSION

No procedure by itself can provide all the assessment data needed to address the complete *DSM-IV* criteria for AD/HD. Neither can any single procedure assess all major domains of psychosocial functioning and possible comorbid conditions. Such circumstances dictate that a multimethod assessment approach be used. Given the depth and breadth that they provide, clinical interviews and rating scales should serve as the foundation of the assessment battery. Upon this foundation, other assessment procedures can be added, depending on the nature of the referral question and on any practical and financial constraints that may exist.

4

Assessment Procedures

"Isn't there a blood test for this?"

Thus far, we have presented our rationale for using a multimethod approach in the assessment of AD/HD and given our reasons for making clinical interviews and rating scales the foundation of this approach. In this chapter we describe specific assessment procedures that clinicians might use when conducting evaluations. Given the large number and variety of assessment procedures on the market, some guidance is in order, thus, we examine many of the interviews and rating scales, as well as psychological tests and observational procedures, that can be incorporated into AD/HD assessments. For each we provide a general description of its purpose, format, and content. We also review each measure's psychometric properties and discuss its utility in the assessment process.

INTERVIEWS

As noted in the preceding chapter, clinical interviews are the foundation of the multimethod assessment. These interviews vary with respect to their purpose. Some are for diagnostic purposes, others are for gathering background information, and still others attempt to do both. Clinical interviews also vary in how they are conducted. They range from structured to semistructured to unstructured formats. Clinical interviews are usually conducted with parents and other caretakers, but they can also be administered to children, adolescents, and teachers.

Structured Interviews

DSM-III gave clinicians and researchers their first real opportunity to use well-defined diagnostic guidelines. The new criteria created a need for valid and reliable assessment tools that could generate childhood diagnoses compatible with *DSM-III*. This was the impetus for the development of structured interviews.

Generally speaking, structured interviews are comprehensive, encompassing most childhood diagnostic conditions. Structured interviews require clinicians to read questions exactly as written and in the order that they are presented. Informants typically respond to questions categorically—that is, either *yes* or *no*. Presenting questions in this way increases the uniformity of administration and makes it possible for those with relatively little clinical training to administer them. These structured interviews are very useful for both clinical practice and research, where a high degree of diagnostic consistency is desired.

Two structured interviews have dominated the field for the past 20 years. Both are reviewed below.

Diagnostic Interview Schedule for Children-IV

The original version of the Diagnostic Interview Schedule for Children-IV (DISC-IV; NIMH, 1997) was developed in 1983 by the National Institutes of Mental Health for use in its epidemiological studies of childhood behavior disorders. The DISC has undergone numerous revisions, prompted primarily by the changes in the *DSM*. The current version, known as the DISC-IV, parallels *DSM-IV* criteria and is compatible with *ICD-10*.

The DISC-IV is organized into six major sections: Anxiety Disorders, Mood Disorders, Disruptive Disorders, Substance Use Disorders, Schizophrenia, and Miscellaneous Disorders (e.g., eating, elimination). These sections contain 24 diagnostic modules, from which more than 30 *DSM-IV* diagnoses may be generated. Using a graded question format, information is gathered about symptom onset, duration, and severity. Some are stem questions, which are broad and address the most salient aspect of a symptom; they are asked of every respondent. The rest are contingent questions, asked only if a stem or previous contingent question is answered positively. Informants respond to these questions primarily with *yes* or *no*.

The DISC-IV is usually administered to parents of children 6–17 years old (DISC-P). A youth version is also available for administration to children and adolescents 9–17 years old (DISC-Y). Both take about 45–90 minutes to administer, depending on the number of diagnostic modules included, the number of symptoms endorsed, and the informant's response pace. A teacher version of the DISC-P, limited to disorders seen in a school setting (e.g., disruptive disorders, certain internalizing symptoms), is currently being developed. Also under development is a version for parents of preschool children.

The structured nature of the DISC-IV questioning permits a reliable and valid interview even when administered by lay—that is to say, clinically inexperienced—interviewers. In contrast to earlier versions that used a rather cumbersome paper-and-pencil approach, the DISC-IV is now administered via computer, using Windows-compatible software. Clinicians read the questions from the monitor and enter the informant's responses directly into the computer. Once the DISC-IV is completed, clinicians can use the scoring feature to generate several different types of reports to summarize the diagnostic findings. The DISC-IV also includes an optional module that covers lifetime diagnoses.

Psychometric Properties. Results of initial psychometric studies using the DISC-IV show test-retest reliabilities similar to those in previous versions (Fisher et al., 1997). They are highest for simple phobias (.90s) and AD/HD (.79) and the lowest for conduct disorder (.43). Because the DISC-IV revision is relatively new, most of the information about its psychometric properties is inferred from earlier studies using *DSM-III* and *DSM-III-R* criteria. Results from the Methods for the Epidemiology of Child and Adolescent Mental Disorders study (MECA; Shaffer et al., 1996) show satisfactory reliability for symptom and criteria counts in both the parent and the child forms. Previous versions also possessed satisfactory interrater reliability (Anderson, Williams, McGee, & Silva, 1987). Test-retest reliability improves as the child gets older (Edelbrock, Costello, Dulcan, Kalas, & Conover, 1985). In terms of validity, research shows that the DISC discriminates between psychiatrically referred and control groups (Breslau, 1987; Costello & Edelbrock, 1985; Costello, Edelbrock, & Costello, 1985). Using the DISC alone, however, is inadvisable because it can result in an overestimation of psychiatric symptoms (Cohen, Velez, Kohn, Schawb-Stone, & Johnson, 1987). Parent–child agreement is low to moderate (Edelbrock, Costello, Dulcan, Conover, & Kalas, 1986), similar to parent–child concordance for rating scales. Agreement is greater for older children and adolescents versus younger children, and higher for externalizing versus internalizing disorders.

Advantages and Disadvantages. The reliability and validity of the DISC-IV are more than adequate. Because of its direct relationship to the *DSM-IV* criteria, the DISC-IV has several assessment advantages. Data are systematically gathered about the frequency, severity, onset, and duration of not only AD/HD symptoms but also symptoms of various comorbid conditions. Although the administration order of the diagnostic modules is fixed, clinicians do not have to use all modules. They may select a subset of them, which can be changed from client to client. Computer administration of the DISC-IV simplifies the process of posing questions; the computer guides the clinician from one question to the next. Another advantage is that the DISC-IV uses a scoring program based on computer algorithms that directly correspond to *DSM-IV* criteria for both parent and child versions. Completed interviews can be reviewed by clinical supervisors as necessary, and data can be imported into various statistical programs for further analysis.

Because of its comprehensiveness, administering the DISC-IV can be time-consuming. For a child with multiple difficulties, the time can extend beyond 1.5 hours. Using the DISC-IV also requires a Windows based computer and the DISC-IV software which can cost several hundred dollars. As with all structured interviews, increased reliability must be weighed against restricted flexibility. Some clinicians and researchers may also find the repetitive structure of the questions tedious, thereby tempting them to stray from standard administration of the procedure.

Diagnostic Interview for Children and Adolescents-IV

The Diagnostic Interview for Children and Adolescents-IV (DICA-IV; Reich, Welner, Herjanic, & MHS Staff, 1996), developed in 1969, was patterned after the Renard Diagnostic Interview (Helzer, Robins, Croughan, & Welner, 1981) assessing symptomatology according to the modified International Classification Criteria and the Feighner criteria (Feighner et al., 1972). It was revised in 1981 to assess symptomatology according to the *DSM-III* criteria (Welner, Reich, Herjanic, & Jung, 1987) and revised again in 1988 to incorporate the *DSM-III-R* criteria (i.e., DICA-R). The most recent version, DICA-IV addresses all major child and adolescent diagnoses in the *DSM-IV*.

The DICA-IV's primary purpose is to screen children and adolescents for psychiatric disorders. Just like the DISC-IV, the DICA-IV gathers clinically relevant information through a combination of stem and contingent questions presented via computer, using Windows-based software. Responses are entered directly into the computer, which then guides the clinician to the next question. The DICA-IV can be administered either to parents of children and adolescents 6–17 years old, or directly to children and adolescents themselves. The parent version has the same categories as the child and adolescent versions have, with the exception of two additional categories that provide data on pregnancy, birth, and the child's early development. Parallel forms of the child and the adolescent versions are available for children ages 6–12 and for adolescents ages 13–17. Each of the DICA-IV's 28 diagnostic categories takes 5–20 minutes to complete. In addition to the *DSM-IV* categories, the DICA-IV includes a listing of critical items tapping six high-risk areas: conduct disorder, alcohol use, street-drug use, marijuana use, major depressive disorders, and posttraumatic stress disorder.

Psychometric Properties.   The psychometric properties of the DICA-IV are largely inferred from its earlier versions. In one such study (Reich, Cottler, McCallum, Corwin, & VanEedewegh, 1995), test-retest reliability for the computerized version of the DICA-R was satisfactory for most diagnoses. Kappas were higher for adolescents than for younger children, and reliability increased when assessing only agreement on symptom presence. Values went down when age of onset and duration criteria were added, suggesting that many children have difficulty with these concepts. This was particularly true of conduct disorder. In several other studies, the DICA displayed good reliability and moderate to good validity (Welner et al., 1987) across all diagnostic categories.

Advantages and Disadvantages.   The DICA-IV shares many advantages and disadvantages with the DISC-IV. Its psychometric properties are satisfactory. It is directly related to the *DSM-IV* criteria for AD/HD and all other disorders. The automatic branching of its computerized questions reduces clinician error, and clinicians have the option of administering some, rather than all, of its diagnostic categories. Unique to DICA-IV is the inclusion of a critical-items list that provides a quick screen for high-risk behaviors (e.g., suicidal behavior) that may need to be addressed before the diagnostic process is completed. Other unique features include the availability of pregnancy, birth, and early development sections in the parent version, as well as two youth versions that can accommodate developmental differences in responding between children and adolescents. The DICA-IV also allows for probing beyond the simple *yes/no* format characteristic of structured interviews, thereby yielding more comprehensive information. But this also requires greater clinical skill and expertise, and is therefore more challenging for inexperienced personnel. Allowing probing may also lengthen the interview. As with the DISC-IV, the DICA-IV requires a computer on which to run DICA-IV software; the cost may be prohibitive to some.

Semistructured Interviews

For clinicians who have reservations about structured interviews, semistructured interviews may be a more palatable alternative. The format allows more freedom to probe certain areas and more flexibility in follow-up questioning, particularly helpful when interviewing very young children. Another difference is that most semistructured interviews elicit responses about symptom severity as opposed to mere presence. But such advantages must be weighed against the need for increased clinical training and familiarity with the *DSM* criteria, without which one could not benefit from this format's flexibility.

Like structured interviews, semistructured interviews developed closely on the heels of *DSM-III*. Since then, numerous versions have made their way into the field, with varying degrees of success. Several are reviewed below.

Schedule for Affective Disorders and Schizophrenia for School-Age Children

The Schedule for Affective Disorders and Schizophrenia for School-Age Children (K-SADS; Puig-Antich & Chambers, 1978) is a semistructured interview originally developed for researchers to examine childhood depression. Modeled after the adult Schedule for Affective Disorders and Schizophrenia (Endicott & Spitzer, 1978), the original K-SADS content emphasized symptoms of depression. Five versions of this interview have been developed: a present episode version (K-SADS-P; Chambers et al., 1985), a lifetime version (K-SADS-L; Klein, 1993), a IV-R version (K-SADS-IVR; Ambrosini & Dixon, 1996), an epidemiologic version (K-SADS-E; Orvaschel, 1994), and a present and lifetime version (K-SADS-PL; Kaufman et al., 1997). The K-SADS-PL is the most current version and the one most useful for assessing AD/HD.

The K-SADS-PL is designed for children and adolescents 6–17 years. It contains a number of major sections, including introductory, screening, and checklist completion sections, plus the Children's Global Assessment Scale (C-GAS) ratings.

The Unstructured Introductory Interview covers demographics, health, presenting complaints, prior psychiatric treatment, school functioning, hobbies, and peer and family relations. Its purpose is to develop rapport and to elicit information for treatment planning. The Screening Interview consists of 82 symptoms divided into 20 diagnostic areas. Screening questions are surveyed first, and skip-out options are available within each diagnostic area. Respondents rate symptomatology with regard to current (C) and most severe past (MSP) symptoms simultaneously. The diagnostic areas can be surveyed in any order and can follow priorities expressed in the previous interview. Similarly, the probes do not have to be stated verbatim but can be adjusted to the child's developmental level. All sections must be completed, however. The Supplement Completion Checklist helps the interviewer determine which of the five diagnostic supplements to administer based on skip-out criteria in the Screening Interview. The diagnostic supplements comprise Affective, Psychotic, Anxiety, Behavioral, and Substance Abuse and Other Disorders. Supplement administration order parallels the chronological unfolding of these difficulties. Information gathered from the supplements allows the interviewer to generate current and lifetime estimates of *DSM-III-R* and *DSM-IV* diagnoses, including AD/HD.

The K-SADS-PL is typically administered first to parents, then to the child or adolescent, and takes 30–90 minutes, depending on the informant and the scope and severity of reported difficulties. Diagnoses are based on both child and parent data. When there are discrepancies, interviewing the parent and child together is recommended to try to resolve them. If disagreements persist, greater weight is generally given to parent input on externalizing behaviors and child input concerning subjective experiences and internalizing problems. Ultimately, the interviewer must decide the weighting, which necessitates considerable training.

Psychometric Properties.   Initial psychometric ratings, based on a relatively small sample, are moderate overall. Interrater reliability across the 20 diagnostic screening areas is excellent (mean = 99.7%; range = 93–100%). Test-retest reliabilities regarding assigning diagnoses over 1–5 weeks are excellent for major depression, anxiety, conduct disorder, and oppositional-defiant disorder. Reliabilities are good for AD/HD (.63 for present diagnosis, .55 for lifetime diagnosis), only slightly less than those for structured interviews. Test-retest reliability for the skip-out criteria is only fair to good. Concurrent validity is good for depression, anxiety, and AD/HD.

Advantages and Disadvantages.   The K-SADS-PL is psychometrically sound. It permits diagnosis-specific impairment ratings, has skip-out criteria to shorten administration time, and samples current as well as lifetime occurrence, which can help to determine onset and duration. It is especially good at identifying depression and anxiety. Another advantage is that it includes sections addressing relevant background and history information. A major disadvantage is that its administration requires substantial clinical training and expertise. Also problematic is the absence of guidelines for resolving informant discrepancies, leaving this up to the interviewer's subjective judgement. Also, although by no means unacceptable, its reliability for AD/HD is slightly less than that reported for structured interviews.

Semistructured Clinical Interview for Children and Adolescents

Developed in 1989, the Semistructured Clinical Interview for Children and Adolescents (SCICA; McConaughy & Achenbach, 1994) has been recently revised. The SCICA can be administered to children and adolescents 6–18 years of age. There is a protocol of questions and probes, as well as a self-report and an observation form for rating what the child or adolescent says and does during the interview. Administration takes approximately 60–90 minutes and the data can be hand-scored or computer-scored. Scoring profiles, available only for 6–12 year olds, yield information for eight syndrome scales: Aggressive Behavior, Anxious, Anxious/Depressed, Attention Problems, Family Problems, Resistant, Strange, and Withdrawn. There are also several global indices: Internalizing, Externalizing, and separate Total Problem scales for the Observational and Self-report items. The structure closely parallels that of other Achenbach scales. A training videotape is available that includes segments of child and adolescent interviews for practice scoring.

Psychometric Properties. Interrater reliability for the syndrome scales is good overall, except for the Anxious (.45) and Attention Problems (.57) scales. Test-retest reliabilities range from good to very good for the global indices (McConaughy & Achenbach, 1994).

Advantages and Disadvantages. The SCICA is part of the Achenbach System of Empirically Based Assessment (ASEBA), which covers a wide age range as well as multiple informants. Its empirical basis makes it well suited to dimensional analyses, thus permitting examination of developmental deviance. This same characteristic, however, makes comparison with the *DSM-IV* categories difficult, especially on the Attention Problems scale, which, besides having low interrater reliability, does not map closely onto the *DSM-IV* criteria, particularly for the hyperactive-impulsive subtype. This lack of *DSM-IV* correspondence renders the SCICA less than ideal for most clinical practice settings, because arriving at a *DSM-IV* diagnosis is essential (e.g., for managed care reimbursement). As such, its utility in a multimethod assessment battery for AD/HD is limited.

Other Semistructured Interviews

The Interview Schedule for Children (ISC; Kovacs, 1982) and the Child Assessment Schedule (CAS; Hodges, McKnew, Cytryn, Stern, & Kline, 1982) are two additional semistructured interviews that have been used in research and clinical practice. The ISC is similar to the K-SADS in that most of its items assess depression. Information about "attention deficit disorder" is based on *DSM-III* and *DSM-III-R* criteria. The CAS samples a broader range of behaviors, but its diagnostic categories reflect *DSM-III* conceptualizations. To our knowledge, neither of these interviews has been revised for compatibility with *DSM-IV* criteria.

A relative newcomer to the field is the Child and Adolescent Psychiatric Assessment (CAPA; Angold et al., 1995). Like the ISC and the CAS, the CAPA is a semistructured interview that can be used with children and their parents. The CAPA focuses on many child psychopathology symptoms occurring during the preceding 3 months. The question format is not completely fixed, but one must determine the presence or absence of all items in a section. The CAPA includes a detailed symptom review section that mirrors not only *DSM-IV* but also *ICD-10*. Another interesting aspect of the CAPA is that it generates incapacity ratings. At present the CAPA has not been published and full psychometric data are unavailable, but indications are that it has adequate reliability, with kappas ranging from .55 for conduct disorder to 1.0 for substance abuse/dependence (Angold & Costello, 1995). Little is known about its utility in AD/HD assessments.

Unstructured Interviews

Ease of administration, flexibility, and low cost often make unstructured interviews the interviews of choice among clinicians. As the term implies, the content and format of unstructured interviews are whatever an interviewer wants them to be. They may be limited to a review of AD/HD criteria, they may cover 20 or more diagnostic categories, or they may fall somewhere in between. Although such flexibility can be advantageous, it also carries the potential for serious assessment problems. For one thing, unstructured interviews can be highly unreliable because of their lack of clarity about diagnostic-decision rules, judgment errors, and interviewer bias (Achenbach, 1985; Costello, 1986). Another problem is that administration varies greatly from one clinician to the next, because there is nothing to keep systematic errors or unwanted interviewer bias out of the process. In clinics where many staff conduct assessments, what is identified as AD/HD by some clinicians may be identified as something else by others, sometimes leading to clinical management complications when a treatment referral is made to other staff members (e.g., when a staff psychiatrist receives a request to place a child on stimulants but does not concur with another staff's assessment).

Also, the administration of unstructured interviews can vary greatly from client to client, even when conducted by the same clinician. Without formal guidelines to follow, clinicians may cover certain material one day but not the next, due to forgetfulness or various other distractions. The manner in which the same clinician asks questions about the same content area can also fluctuate, multiplying the chances for diagnostic error, and in turn of inappropriate treatment services, thereby delaying improvements in the child's functioning.

For reasons such as these, clinicians should refrain from using unstructured interviews, especially for the diagnosis portion of the assessment. Given the availability of several structured and semistructured interviews that are psychometrically sound and have documented utility in assessing AD/HD and other conditions, there is little reason to choose an unstructured interview.

That said, many structured and semistructured interviews do not routinely collect background information such as developmental history, health history, school history, family history, and so on. When using a structured or semistructured interview that lacks this capacity, clinicians must find an alternate way to gather the information, and here unstructured interviews can play a role.

To increase the overall accuracy of an unstructured interview, the clinician can impose a modicum of structure on it. Rather than just randomly reviewing background information, one can follow a predetermined outline. Additional structure can be achieved by using a similar response format in all content areas.

In our own clinical work, we have routinely used an unstructured interview to gather background data. The interview begins by asking parents or other caretakers to clarify the nature of the presenting concerns. It then shifts to a discussion of the child's developmental history, with questions about pregnancy, birth, delivery, neonatal course, developmental milestones, and early temperament. A thorough review of the child's current and past health status typically follows. Attention is also directed to the child's language development, intellectual progress, and sensory functioning (e.g., hearing). Further details are then obtained concerning the child's school and social history. Thereafter, efforts are made to gather information about parenting style, recent psychosocial stressors, and current and past functioning of the child's immediate and extended family.

Whenever possible, an unstructured interview with the child's teacher adds a great deal to the diagnostic picture. Teachers can usually provide much needed information about the child's school functioning, particularly the effect of AD/HD on classroom behavior and performance. Information about the child's current academic achievement and social functioning with classmates can also be gathered. Differences in behavior due to subject matter, class size, number of teachers in the classroom, and so on should be described in detail, not only to aid in establishing a diagnosis but to identify strengths and weaknesses for treatment planning.

Unstructured interviews can also be done directly with children and adolescents, which provides an opportunity to gauge their understanding of why they are being evaluated. Further questioning can reveal the child's play and recreational interests, as well as self-perceptions of academic, behavioral, social, emotional, and family functioning. Interviewing children and adolescents also affords an opportunity for observing their appearance, manner, thought processing, language functioning, and interpersonal skills.

Summary

Several empirically validated structured and semistructured interviews are available for assessing AD/HD. Among them, the DISC-IV and the DICA-IV seem best suited for a multimethod battery that assesses AD/HD and its associated features. Although use of these instruments can be time-consuming and expensive, the advantages far outweigh the disadvantages. Advantages include diagnostic accuracy, comprehensive diagnostic coverage well beyond AD/HD, ease of administration for lay interviewers, and empirically derived computer scoring. But none of these instruments provides in-depth coverage of historical information; this must be gathered from other sources. Unstructured interviews can serve this purpose. So too can some of the rating scales considered next.

RATING SCALES

There are many reasons for including rating scales in an assessment of AD/HD. Rating scales address not only the presence of AD/HD symptoms, but also their severity and degree of developmental deviance. Many rating scales also allow a detailed examination of comorbid conditions. In addition to addressing child psychopathology, rating scales can assess functional impairment in many psychosocial domains. Compared with the less-structured interviews, rating scales are better standardized, which decreases subjectivity and thus increases reliability. Rating scales can also be completed by parents or teachers before any face-to-face evaluation. Thus, rating scales are a cost-effective method for gathering information from multiple informants across different settings. As such, they represent a practical alternative to clinical interviews, which take longer and cost more. Rating scales also offer advantages over observational procedures. For example, they provide access to infrequently displayed behaviors likely to be missed by time-limited observations. They can also summarize information across longer time intervals than those usually afforded by observation.

Despite these advantages, there are some important caveats. Rating scales assume that the informant is familiar enough with the child's behavior to inform reliably. The informant must also have access to the information and understand the questions. Another potential problem is that adult psychopathology can distort parent and teacher perceptions of child behavior.

Partly in response to such concerns, there has been a recent surge of interest in the use of *self-report* scales for children and adolescents. Additional factors have also prompted increased interest, particularly a growing recognition of the child's unique position as observer of self and environment. There is also greater emphasis on children's thoughts and feelings as potential targets for treatment using cognitive-behavioral interventions. At the same time the field has become more aware of the existence of childhood depression and other internalizing disorders, for which self-report is especially revealing. Greater sensitivity to developmental issues has yielded more-flexible formats in self-report, leading to increased availability of psychometrically sound self-report instruments. The primary argument against self-reports is that children and adolescents may not reflect on and report their behavior accurately. Younger children especially may have difficulty accessing and describing their feelings. Even when access to thoughts and feelings is available, it may not translate into accurate reporting due to the powerful need of some children to present themselves in a positive light.

In sum, many parent- and teacher-completed rating scales, as well as child self-report rating scales, are now available to assess not only AD/HD but also other types of psychopathology and functional impairment. Although a complete discussion of all rating scales is beyond the scope of this text, we review those that we believe are used most often in research and clinical practice.

Broad-Band Rating Scales

As their name implies, broad-band rating scales sample a wide range of behaviors. Most broad-band rating scales include some type of composite score for internalizing, externalizing, and total problems, as well as specific subscale scores (e.g., depression, aggression). A few include indices of adaptive functioning and behavioral competence. Most have norms that allow comparison of the child's behavior with that of same-age and same-gender peers, and thus, objective assessment of developmental deviance.

Behavior Assessment System for Children

The Behavior Assessment System for Children (BASC; Reynolds & Kamphaus, 1992) is a relatively new family of instruments. It is a multimethod, multiinformant, and multidimensional system designed to assess adaptive as well as maladaptive behaviors for children 2.5–18 years of age. There are three core instruments: Teacher Rating Scales (TRS), Parent Rating Scales (PRS), and Self-Report of Personality (ages 8–11 and 12–18). In addition, there is the Student Observation System (SOS; described later in this chapter) and the Structured Developmental History form.

Both the parent and teacher scales contain a preschool, child, and adolescent version. For low-level readers there is an audiotaped administration. There is a Spanish version as well. The 130-item scales, encompassing a wide range of child psychopathology, take approximately 10–20 minutes to complete. Respondents rate the frequency of each item on a 4-point scale from *never* to *almost always*. Five composite scores can be derived: Behavioral Symptoms, Externalizing Problems, Internalizing Problems, School Problems, and Adaptive Skills. Within these five domains are 14 specific assessment areas: Adaptability, Aggression, Anxiety, Attention Problems, Atypicality, Conduct Problems, Depression, Hyperactivity, Leadership, Learning Problems, Social Skills, Somatization, Study Skills, and Withdrawal.

The BASC also has a self-report form comprising 170 *true/false* questions. There is one version for children ages 8–11 and another for adolescents 12–18. Each takes approximately 30 minutes. As with the parent version, there is an audiotaped administration for low-level readers or nonreaders. Four composite scales can be derived: School Maladjustment, Clinical Maladjustment, Personal Adjustment, and the Emotional Symptoms Index. Fourteen specific areas of functioning are also assessed: Anxiety, Attitude toward School, Attitude toward Teachers, Atypicality, Depression, Interpersonal Relations, Locus of Control, Relations with Parents, Self-esteem, Self-reliance, Sensation Seeking, Sense of Inadequacy, Social Stress, and Somatization.

All versions of the BASC can be hand-scored, but most often they are computer-scored, either from on-line administration or keyed in from a protocol. Scored data are presented in a number of ways, including raw scores, *T* scores, and percentile rankings. Scores can be interpreted with reference to either community-based national norms or clinic-referred norms, presented separately for each gender as well as collapsed across gender.

The 12-page Structured Developmental History form can be completed in questionnaire or interview format. Included in this survey are questions relating to social and family history; birth and developmental history; health history; and speech, hearing, vision, and language functioning.

Psychometric Properties.   All three rating scales were nationally standardized on large community samples (PRS, $n = 1,088$; TRS, $n = 763$; SRP, $n = 4,423$) and clinical samples (PRS, $n = 401$; TRS, $n = 693$; SRP, $n = 411$), that reflect United States socioeconomic, ethnic, and geographic distributions. The scales were refined through item-level covariance structure analysis, with each item contributing to only a single scale. The authors report high internal consistency for the composites (.80s–.90s) and for the scales (.70s–.90s), along with moderate to high test-retest reliabilities. The least reliable scales are Somatization and Anxiety at the younger ages on the teacher form, and Atypicality and Conduct Problems on the parent rating scale. Interrater consistency is similar to that of other multisource assessment systems, where moderate discrepancies across informants are common.

Construct validity was established through factor analysis. The TRS scales correlate highly with corresponding scores on Achenbach's Teacher Report Form (TRF), the Revised Behavior Problem Checklist, and Burks' Behavior Ratings Scales, but they do not correlate significantly with the Conners' Teacher Rating Scale-39. For the PRS, there is a high correlation with the CBCL and with the externalizing scale of the Conners' Parent Rating Scale-93. Correlations with the revised Personality Inventory for Children (Lachar, 1982) and Behavior Rating Profile are moderate.

In terms of differentiating children with AD/HD from those without, Ostrander, Weinfurt, Yarnold, and August (1998) found the BASC was more parsimonious and more predictive than the CBCL. Of additional clinical interest is that 88% of their sample was correctly identified as having AD/HD using a clinical cutoff on the Attention subscale.

Studies on the self-report form found that scores were strongly related to similar personality dimensions on the MMPI, the Youth Self-report of the CBCL, the Behavior Rating Profile, and the Children's Personality Questionnaire. Group profiles for specific diagnoses had good discriminant validity for teacher and parent ratings. Although the self-report profiles for conduct disorder, behavior disorder, and depression were distinct, less sensitivity was found for self-report on AD/HD and learning problems.

Advantages and Disadvantages.   Although relatively new, the BASC offers several advantages in assessing AD/HD. Separate ratings are obtained for both attention problems *and* hyperactivity on all forms, essential when using *DSM-IV* subtyping criteria. Similar to other broad-band rating scales, the BASC taps 14 domains of child psychopathology and adaptive functioning, thus permitting assessment of not only AD/HD but of comorbid conditions as well. The BASC covers a wide age range, which allows for repeated assessments across development. Domains for both parent and teacher scales are the same, which facilitates assessment of cross-situational symptom pervasiveness, as well as cross-informant comparisons.

Another BASC advantage is its sampling of adaptive skills, which includes not only social competence but strengths, such as leadership and self-reliance, unlike many rating scales that sample only problem behaviors. This makes the BASC particularly helpful in strength-based assessments. The composite score in the adaptive domain addresses AD/HD impairment criteria very well. Validity checks and a developmental history form are additional advantages.

In the self-report versions, the domains sampled and the scoring may be less helpful in establishing the presence of inattention or hyperactivity-impulsivity. Self-report can be useful, however, when examining the child's or adolescent's view of the impact of AD/HD on various areas of functioning.

The psychometric characteristics of the BASC are quite good, equaling or exceeding the standardization levels of similar instruments (Adams & Drabman, 1994; Hoza, 1994). The recent revision of this measure for preschoolers has not only extended the age range from 4 down to 2.5 years, but has also addressed certain previous psychometric limitations inherent in other preschool measures.

The BASC has few disadvantages, but because it is relatively new, it does not have the background of research of several other rating scales. Also unclear is how well certain BASC components, specifically Classroom Observation and Developmental History, work together with other BASC components to yield a comprehensive clinical picture. Given that many other rating scales lack interview or observational components, this shortcoming is not a major disadvantage.

In summary, the BASC offers a comprehensive, psychometrically sound multi-informant approach to assessing child behavior that closely parallels the *DSM-IV* criteria. Thus it is well suited for inclusion in multimethod AD/HD assessments.

Conners' Rating Scales

Without question, the Conners' Rating Scales are one of the most commonly used rating scales for evaluating AD/HD symptomatology. Recently revised (Conners, 1997), the new parent and teacher versions are the result of 30 years of research. There are English, Spanish, and French-Canadian versions, computer scoring programs, treatment progress plot forms, feedback forms, and general teacher information forms for collecting additional information on children 3–17 years of age. In addition, a self-report version has recently been developed for use with adolescents 12–17.

Both a long form (CPRS-R;L) and a short form (CPRS-R;S) of the Revised Conners' Parent Rating Scale have been developed. The long version contains 80 items encompassing many child problems. Parents indicate on a 4-point scale the degree to which certain items characterize their child, which takes approximately 15–20 minutes. This long form yields subscale scores for the following: Oppositional, Cognitive Problems/Inattention, Hyperactivity, Anxious-Shy, Perfectionism, Social Problems, Psychosomatic, *DSM-IV* symptom subscales, an ADHD Index, and a Conners' Global Index. Norms for children 3–17 years are available, with separate norms for boys and for girls provided in 3-year intervals. The 27-item short form takes only 5–10 minutes and yields scores on fewer subscales: Oppositional, Cognitive Problems/Inattention, Hyperactivity, and the ADHD Index.

The new ADHD Index contains the 12 items that most reliably distinguish children with AD/HD from those without it. This index is combined with the *DSM-IV* criteria to form several shorter scales known as the Conners' ADHD/*DSM-IV* Scales (CADS), with parent (CADS-P), teacher (CADS-T) and adolescent (CADS-A) versions available.

The Conners' Global Index (CGI), which can be used alone or as part of the longer parent and teacher scales, was once termed the "Hyperactivity Index" of the Abbreviated Symptoms Questionnaire. The new name more accurately reflects the 10-item scale's purpose, which is to provide a concise measure of general psychopathology. There are also global indices for restless-impulsive behaviors and emotional lability.

The teacher versions of the Conners' scales have also been revised. The current long form of the Revised Conners' Teacher Rating Scale (CTRS-R;L) consists of 59 items, uses the same format as the parent version, and includes the same subscales as the long parent version across the same age range. The short form (CTRS-R;S) consists of 28 items and specifically taps AD/HD as well as ODD symptoms.

A new addition is the Conners–Wells Adolescent Self-Report Scale, in both a long (CASS;L) and a short (CASS;S) form. Both are available for adolescents 12–17 years and sample a broad range of problem behaviors. The 87-item CASS;L includes the following subscales: Family Problems, Conduct Problems, Anger Control Problems, Emotional Problems, Cognitive Problems/Inattention, Hyperactivity, ADHD Index, and *DSM-IV* Symptom Subscales. The 27-item short form taps areas similar to the parent and teacher short forms: Conduct Problems, Hyperactivity, Cognitive Problems/Inattention, and ADHD Index.

Psychometric Properties.   Norms for the parent scale were drawn from over 200 data collection sites, using ratings from more than 2,000 parents (Conners, Sitarenios, Parker, & Epstein, 1998a). As with the previous versions, this new parent scale has excellent psychometric characteristics. Internal reliability coefficients average .80, the Inattention subscales are above .90 across the age range, and the Hyperactivity-Impulsivity subscales range from .75 for adolescent females to above .90 for younger children. Test-retest reliability is generally strong; the Inattention and Hyperactivity-Impulsivity subscales are above .70. Moderate reliabilities are reported for the Anxious-Shy subscale (.47) and the Emotional Lability Global Index (.54). Factor analyses support the validity of the subscales. Further attesting to its validity is that the Conners' scales reliably distinguish between children with AD/HD and those without AD/HD, with an overall correct classification rate of more than 90%.

With excellent normative data from over 2,000 teachers, the revised teacher versions demonstrate the same strong psychometric characteristics (Conners, Sitarenios, Parker, & Epstein, 1998b). Internal reliability estimates parallel the parent version, ranging from .73–.95 for the Inattentive/Cognitive Problems subscale to .80s–.90s for the Hyperactivity-Impulsivity subscale. Test-retest reliability for the Hyperactivity-Impulsivity subscale is good (.72), but it is only moderate for the Inattention/Cognitive Problems subscale (.47). Discriminant validity is strong, with an overall correct classification rate of over 80%. The standardization sample for the self-report version is also comprehensive, and it has separate age and gender profiling.

Advantages and Disadvantages.   The current versions replace myriad earlier Conners' scales. There were two parent scales and numerous teacher scales (e.g., Iowa Conners), as well as the Hyperactivity Index and the Abbreviated Symptom Questionnaire. Although these measures had strong psychometric characteristics and reflected the prevailing conceptualizing of AD/HD, the many versions caused variability in clinical practice and research. The new versions provide much-needed uniformity while building upon the strong research base of the earlier versions. Additional improvements include the compatibility with the *DSM-IV* criteria. Subscales can be scored by counting the number of items in each category as well as by comparing the results with normative data— the latter very helpful when addressing the *DSM-IV* criterion for developmental deviance. The new scales also cover behavioral difficulties more comprehensively, thus permitting examination of possible comorbid conditions. In contrast to the original normative sample, which was small and not geographically or culturally diverse, the current sample is broad and better reflects the United States population.

Another advantage is the availability of compatible parent and teacher versions, essential for establishing the presence of impairment in multiple settings, as *DSM-IV* criteria require. Furthermore, the new ADHD Index contains the 12 items that most reliably distinguish children with AD/HD from those without, and it is a good screening tool for detecting children who need a more comprehensive evaluation. In addition, the short parent and teacher forms can screen for behavioral difficulties beyond AD/HD.

One advantage of the Conners' system versus the BASC is that the subscale structure of its self-report is comparable to its parent and teacher scales. In addition, the CASS contains separate subscales for inattention and hyperactivity that facilitate AD/HD diagnosis. The BASC does not. In contrast to the BASC self-report, the content of the CASS focuses somewhat more on disruptive behaviors and somewhat less on the internalizing symptoms for which youth self-report is so valuable. One limitation of the Conners' relative to the BASC and the Achenbach scales (described next) is the lack of a way to assess adaptive functioning. Although one can consider the absence of problems to be strengths, a more direct assessment of social and adaptive competence is helpful for strength-based assessment and treatment planning, as well as for impairment evaluation.

In summary, the revised Conners' Scales address most of the major limitations of previous Conners' scales, and they maintain the same psychometric strength and applicability to AD/HD. Thus, this family of questionnaires can be used with confidence in comprehensive AD/HD assessments.

Achenbach System of Empirically-Based Assessment

Another comprehensive system of broad-band rating scales is the Achenbach System of Empirically-Based Assessment (ASEBA). Like the BASC and Conners' scales, the ASEBA includes parent, teacher, and self-report versions. All rating scales within this system use a similar response format in which the respondent indicates on a 3-point scale the degree to which a particular behavior is true (*not true, sometimes true, very* or *often true*). Depending on which scale is used, time frames differ, ranging from the past 6 months for parent and self-report to the past 2 months for teacher and parent report on the CBCL/1½–5. Similar to the BASC, a direct observation form is available. Unique to the ASEBA is the availability of a semistructured interview for children and adolescents (the SCICA, reviewed earlier).

There are three parent rating scales. Perhaps the best known is the Child Behavior Checklist and Profile for parents of children ages 4–18 (CBCL/4–18; Achenbach, 1991a). The 118 items and two open-ended questions cover a wide range of behavioral and emotional difficulties, which parents rate on a 3-point scale according to their frequency over the past 6 months. The CBCL/4–18 yields *T* scores and percentiles for eight cross-informant syndromes, as well as Internalizing, Externalizing, and Total Problem scales. The eight cross-informant areas are Aggressive Behavior, Anxious/Depressed, Attention Problems, Delinquent Behavior, Social Problems, Somatic Complaints, Thought Problems, and Withdrawn. An additional 20 items estimate specific competencies with regard to Child Activities, Social Relationships, and School Performance, along with a Total Competence score.

To assess parents' perceptions of their toddler, one option had been the Child Behavior Checklist/2–3 (CBCL/2–3; Achenbach, 1992). This has been replaced with the recently developed 99-item CBCL/1½–5 (Achenbach & Rescorla, 2000) for use with parents as well as day care providers and preschool teachers. Using a new national normative sample and larger clinical samples, the following cross-informant syndromes are available on both the parent and teacher forms: Emotionally Reactive, Anxious/Depressed, Somatic Complaints, Withdrawn, Attention Problems, and Aggressive Behavior. There is also the Sleep Problems subscale that was available on the CBCL/2–3. In addition, Internalizing, Externalizing, and Total Problems scales are scored from both forms. Unlike the CBCL/4–18, there is no competence scale.

In response to the criticism that the Achenbach scales did not easily map onto *DSM-IV* criteria, the CBCL/1½–5 includes a profile of *DSM*-oriented scales.

These scales were developed from items on the parent and teacher scales that experienced psychiatrists and psychologists from ten cultures rated as being very consistent with *DSM* diagnostic categories. The *DSM*-oriented scales are: Affective Problems, Anxiety Problems, Pervasive Developmental Problems, Oppositional Defiant Problems, and one devoted specifically to Attention-Deficit/ Hyperactivity Problems.

In addition, the CBCL/1½–5 now includes the Language Development Survey (LDS). The LDS uses parents' reports of vocabulary and word combinations to identify language delays in children at ages 18–35 months. It can be completed independently by a parent in about 10 minutes and requires only fifth grade reading skills. All forms are available in Spanish and have computer scoring and cross informant comparisons.

A relatively new addition to the parent rating scales, representing an upward extension of the CBCL, is the Young Adult Behavior Checklist (YABCL; Achenbach, 1997a) for ages 18–30. This checklist is designed for parents, but it also can be completed by others, such as spouses, close friends, or supervisors. Like the Young Adult Self-Report (YASR), the YABCL samples adaptive functioning via 113 items and two open-ended questions in the areas of friends, work, family, spouse, education, and mean adaptive functioning. The remaining 107 items and two open-ended questions yield eight syndrome scales: Aggressive Behavior, Anxious/Depressed, Attention Problems, Delinquent Behavior, Intrusive, Somatic Complaints, Thought Problems, and Withdrawn, as well as global Internalizing, Externalizing, and Total Problem scores. A substance use scale taps tobacco, alcohol, drug, and overall substance use.

Two teacher rating forms are available. The first is the Teacher Report Form and Profile for Ages 5–18 (TRF; Achenbach, 1991b). The TRF includes 118 items, 93 of which are the same as the parent-completed CBCL. Additional items sample behaviors seen only in school, such as "disturbs other pupils" and "disrupts class discipline." Scales from the TRF include Academic Performance, Adaptive Characteristics, and the same eight cross-informant syndromes and global indices as in the parent scale. Recently two additional profiles were added, tapping the two AD/HD factors of inattention and hyperactive-impulsive behavior. Teachers also rate the child's academic performance in terms of grade level for each subject area on a 5-point scale, ranging from *far below* to *far above*. Adaptive functioning is rated on a 7-point scale pertaining to how hard the child is working, how much the child is learning, how appropriate the child's behavior is, how much the child is learning, and how happy the child seems to be.

Until recently, the Achenbach scales could only sample teacher reports for children down to 5 years of age. In 1997, the Caregiver–Teacher Report Form and Profile (Achenbach, 1997b) was developed to capture the preschool period. As mentioned earlier, this form has now been replaced with the CBCL/1½–5. As with the CBCL/4–18, both parents and teachers review the same items which facilitates cross informant comparisons. Another advantage is that the CBCL/ 1½–5 is one of the few measures that can be used to assess behavior across both the toddler and preschool years.

There are two self-report measures that together cover adolescents and adults 11–30 years old. The Youth Self-Report and Profile for Ages 11–18 (YSR; Achenbach, 1991c) is a counterpart to the Child Behavior Checklist. This 112-item questionnaire, which shares 102 items with the CBCL/4–18, requires a minimum fifth grade reading level, but it can be administered orally. There are two competence scales that sample across family, friends, hobbies, and work; the same eight cross-informant syndromes used in the parent and teacher versions; and Internalizing, Externalizing, and Total Problems composite scores. Four open-ended questions examine physical problems, concerns, and strengths.

An upward extension of the Youth Self-Report is the Young Adult Self-Report Form (YASR: Achenbach, 1997). The YASR can be completed by 18–30-year-olds to describe their adaptive functioning in five areas: Friends, Education, Job, Family, Spouse, and Overall Functioning. Scores for eight problem areas are produced as well: Aggressive Behavior, Anxious/Depressed, Attention Problems, Delinquent Behavior, Intrusive, Somatic Complaints, Thought Problems, and Withdrawn. This scale also includes three open-ended questions about tobacco, marijuana, and alcohol use. These scores, as well as the composite scores for Internalizing, Externalizing, Total Problems, and Substance Use, can be compared with ratings obtained from others on the companion Young Adult Behavior Checklist. Although both the YSR and YASR can be used with 18-year-olds, the authors suggest using the YSR for those still living at home and the YASR for those living independently (for example, in college).

Psychometric Properties.   Thorough reviews of the psychometric qualities of the various Achenbach measures are found in the manuals for the individual measures. In addition, a bibliography of published studies using the Achenbach scales is updated yearly and available for purchase (Vignoe & Achenbach, 1999). Psychometric data are generally strongest for scales sampling ages 4–18, and is weaker or less-available for the preschool and young-adult versions. Psychometric data for the composite scores are stronger than for the subscales, and both are stronger than any of the competence sections. A brief sampling of the comprehensive psychometric data for the various scales is presented below.

The CBCL/4–18 scales were derived from parent ratings of 4,455 clinically referred children and normed on 2,368 nonreferred children in the United States. The 1991 revision improves on the original sample by addressing some earlier criticisms of nonapplicability to culturally diverse groups. For the behavior problem portion, test-retest reliability is good for the subscales (.80s) and excellent for the composite scores (high .80s to .90s). Similar findings are reported for interparent reliability and internal consistency on all cross-informant subscales except Thought Problems, possibly reflecting the subjective nature of the questions and the fact that some parents interpret the items differently from the original intent. The Competence Scale is also less solid psychometrically. Internal consistency is around .5 and most children score fairly high, so it may be better at distinguishing difficulties than at identifying strengths *per se*. The questions tend to pull for more-subjective responses, leading to less reliable data.

With regard to validity, the CBCL/4–18 has often been the gold standard against which other measures determine their own validity. In one study comparing the BASC and the CBCL, the BASC seemed more parsimonious and accurate in distinguishing AD/HD from non-AD/HD students and for identifying the AD/HD-combined type (Ostrander et al., 1998). In the same study, however, the CBCL had a slight edge in identifying primarily inattentive students, probably because of the CBCL's empirically based structure, which yields a separate Attention Problems subscale but no hyperactive-impulsive score. Other validity studies found high concurrent correlations with related instruments, such as the older Conners' Parent Rating Scale and the Quay Problem Behavior Checklist.

The CBCL/1½–5 is based on a new U.S. national sample of ratings of 1,728 children and normed on 700 children. The reliability and validity are strong as with the other Achenbach scales. In the past, the CBCL/2–3 differentiated children referred for mental health services from nonreferred children (Achenbach, Edelbrock, & Howell, 1987). It would appear that the new form would be equally helpful but with the additional advantages of encompassing a wider age range, permitting cross-informant comparisons across all subscales, addressing *DSM-IV* criteria, and permitting a more direct examination of AD/HD behaviors.

The YABCL scales are based on ratings by 1,455 clinic-referred young adults and 1,532 parents, as well as ratings from 1,058 nonreferred young adults and 1,074 parents. Internal consistency is similar to the other scales, with test-retest reliabilities in the upper .80s and interparent reliability in the low .60s. Because it is relatively new, there is little validity data beyond that reported in the initial development of the measure.

The TRF Scales were based upon on 2,815 students referred to clinics and normed on 1,391 nonreferred students. Reliability and validity are similar to those of the parent version, with test–rest reliability in the low .90s and interteacher agreement in low .60s. Little is known about the inattention and hyperactive-impulsive profiles because they have only recently been published and researchers have not yet examined them.

The YSR and YASR have somewhat limited psychometric data because they too were recently published. The YSR was developed on 1,272 clinic-referred teens and normed on 1,1315 nonreferred teens. Test-retest reliability is in the high .70s, with good internal consistency overall. The YASR was developed on a clinic-referred sample of 1,455 young adults and normed on 1,058 individuals. Test-retest reliability is higher than for the YSR, falling into the upper .80s.

Advantages and Disadvantages.   The Achenbach scales are perhaps the most frequently used broad-band measures in research, with at least 1,700 published studies using some version of them. Such popularity stems directly from the many advantages inherent in the Achenbach system. Many have praised its empirically based approach as being a purer measure of what is really occurring in child behavior as opposed to merely reflecting the changing nature of diagnostic systems. It takes a continuous, rather than categorical, approach to examining behavior disorders. There is similarity across the measures, with parallel parent, teacher, and self-report measures permitting a determination of symptom pervasiveness, as well as ease in longitudinal assessments. All versions have machine-readable and direct-client-entry formats as well as computer scoring via a Windows-based Assessment Data Manager, which is user-friendly

and permits a variety of scoring and report options. The cross-informant program for the parent, teacher, and youth self-report forms is another strength,
indicating the degree of agreement between informants and then comparing the
correlations with reference samples. Also, many of the Achenbach's scales have
been translated into 50 different languages.

The new CBCL/1½–5 is one of the few broad-band rating scales in this age
range. With the exception of some temperament scales, and now the BASC's
extension down to 2.5 years, few scales are appropriate for toddlers. Although
it is unlikely that sufficient evidence would exist for making a AD/HD diagnosis
in a toddler, there are instances when some type of diagnosis is warranted; the
CBCL/1½–5 can be helpful in documenting the developmental deviance of a
toddler's behavior. Similarly, with the exception of the BASC, the CBCL/1½–5 is
the only instrument in the preschool range that evaluates behavior from other
informants. The self- and other report forms that range into early adulthood are
also helpful when assessing AD/HD in college students and young adults.

The Achenbach's greatest disadvantage arises from one of its strengths—
namely, its empirically derived dimensional nature. Because of this, the scales
did not closely map onto *DSM-IV* in the past, making them particularly problematic with respect to AD/HD. As mentioned earlier, there is an Attention Problems subscale, but hyperactivity and impulsivity are not well represented on
this dimension. To address this, Achenbach has recently added a separate
inattention and hyperactive-impulsive profile to the TRF. Achenbach reports
some nationally normed cut-points that seem to have predictive value, but the
profiles have not been used extensively in diagnostic studies (Achenbach, 1996),
nor is there any companion profile available for parents, which limits cross-
situational comparison. The new preschool version, however, does permit an
assessment of 5 *DSM*-oriented categories while maintaining the cross-informant
comparison of previous scales.

Achenbach and colleagues are to be credited for attempting to measure
adaptive functioning. In a sea of pathology-oriented rating scales, the CBCL was
one of the first behavior rating scales to address this area. Limited internal consistency, however, and the absence of items reflecting actual strengths, have led
some to characterize its competence scale as a measure of social *incompetence*.

Still, the Achenbach scales have many advantages overall and are well-
suited for use in research and in many clinical settings. Although they can be
used in multimethod assessments, the Achenbach scales may be less clinically
helpful in assessing AD/HD than either the BASC or the Conners', primarily
because they do not generate scores paralleling the *DSM-IV* two-factor symptom
structure of AD/HD. The utility of the newer *DSM* scoring will need to be
established.

Devereux Scales of Mental Disorders

The Devereux Scales of Mental Disorders (DSMD; Naglieri, LeBuffe, &
Pfeiffer, 1994) is another broad-band measure of psychopathology in children
and adolescents. Its content is derived primarily from the diagnostic criteria in
DSM-IV. The DSMD includes a 110-item child form for children ages 5–12 and a

111-item form for youth ages 13–18, both of which require a sixth grade reading level. Both can be filled out by parents, teachers, and other caregivers. Raters indicate on a 5-point scale the degree to which specific behaviors were apparent during the previous month.

Scores are obtained on 10 behavioral indices. As with the other broad-band scales, there is a Total Score as well as separate scores for an Externalizing and Internalizing composite. The Externalizing composite encompasses conduct and attention subscales for ages 5–12, and conduct and delinquency subscales for ages 13–18. The Internalizing composite includes anxiety and depression subscales. There is also a Critical Pathology composite composed of the Autism and Acute Problems subscales. The DSMD takes only 15 minutes to complete and 10 minutes to score. A new computerized scoring program scans for items endorsed at a critical level and lists specific *DSM-IV* criteria associated with them.

Psychometric Properties. Adequate levels of internal, test-retest, interrater, and intrarater reliability are reported, along with excellent internal consistency. Because the DSMD used a broad national standardization sample, excellent norms are available, broken down by age, gender, and informant.

Advantages and Disadvantages. The DSMD's strengths include ease of completion and scoring, ability to screen for severe emotional problems, and utility in documenting improvement during treatment, particularly residential treatment. Some weaknesses are that only negative behaviors are identified and the individual subscales comprise only a few items. Of particular concern is that there are only 4 inattention items, 3 impulsivity items, 3 hyperactivity items, and no separate subscales for the two major components of AD/HD. So caution must be taken when using the DSMD in AD/HD evaluations.

Child Symptom Inventory

Another relatively new broad-band measure is the Child Symptom Inventory (CSI; Gadow & Sprafkin, 1995). Its purpose is to provide a checklist for evaluating behavior according to diagnostic criteria. The newest version is a *DSM-IV* updating of the CSI-3R, which was developed for *DSM-III-R*. The 97-item parent checklist taps 17 disorders, and the 77-item teacher checklist taps 13. Both include AD/HD categories. There is also a preliminary 122-item adolescent version, the Adolescent Symptom Inventory (ASI-4), completed by parents, teachers, and other caregivers to screen for 24 *DSM-IV* disorders, including AD/HD. Respondents rate each item on a 4-point frequency scale (*never* to *very often*). The CSI is appropriate for use with children 5–12 years old. It has a Spanish version.

Psychometric Properties. Limited norms are available. As reported in the manual, preliminary findings attest to its content, concurrent, and construct validity. All else concerning its psychometric properties is inferred from previous research with the CSI-3R.

Advantages and Disadvantages.   Because this measure is relatively new, re-search on its utility is limited, but its correspondence to *DSM-IV* is helpful. Although the same information can be obtained from many of the interviews described earlier, the fact that the information can be obtained quickly through a paper-and-pencil measure that goes beyond a *yes/no* format makes it attrac-tive. As a screening instrument, therefore, the CSI seems promising, but more research is needed to demonstrate the tool's sensitivity and specificity in screen-ing children who need a more comprehensive evaluation. It is also unclear to what degree the CSI is useful in a larger multimethod assessment of AD/HD.

Other Broad-Band Scales

Two additional behavior rating scales have frequently been used to assess AD/HD in both research and clinical settings, but because they do not reflect the new *DSM-IV*, they are now of little clinical utility. We describe them briefly, primarily to acknowledge their historical significance.

Revised Behavior Problem Checklist

The Revised Behavior Problem Checklist (RBPC; Quay & Peterson, 1983, 1987) is an expanded version of the original Behavior Problem Checklist (BPC; Quay & Peterson, 1975). The RBPC was one of the most commonly used scales to rate problem behaviors in children and adolescents 5–18 years of age. It contains 89 items, takes 15–20 minutes to complete, requires 10 minutes to score, and yields scores on six factors, including Conduct Disorder, and Attention Problems-Immaturity.

Psychometric Properties.   Norms are available for children K–12. Test-retest reliability and internal consistencies are fair to moderate, depending on the scale. The scale differentiates between those having ADD with and without hyperactivity using *DSM-III* criteria (Aman & Werry, 1984; Lahey et al., 1984.

Advantages and Disadvantages.   When first published, the BPC was one of the premier rating scales, appearing in numerous studies. Its relationship to *DSM-III* set a precedent for the rating scale as a mechanism for quantifying a somewhat subjective diagnostic system, but lack of revision limits its current utility. Primary drawbacks are its lack of representative norms, its relative insen-sitivity to treatment effects, and its lack of correspondence with the *DSM-IV's* two-factor AD/HD conceptualization. Although Attention Problems—Immaturity and Motor Tension—Excess scales somewhat mirror the *DSM-IV* AD/HD fac-tors, they do not specifically address impulsivity.

Personality Inventory for Children

The Personality Inventory for Children (PIC; Wirt, Lachar, Klinedinst, & Seat, 1977) is a broad based instrument for parents and caregivers of children 3–16 years of age. The 420 items tap behavior, affect, and cognitive status. There are three separate administration options. Typically, the parent completes the first 280 items, which takes approximately 25–30 minutes and yields a profile of 20 scales. The clinical scales include intelligence, family relations, hyperactivity, and more. There are four validity-screening scales and four broad-band scales. All 420 items must be administered to obtain the longer item analysis from the computer report. If a brief screening is needed, the first 131 items will yield scores for the Broad-Band Factor and the Lie Scale. The PIC can be hand-scored or computer-scored; computer scoring provides specific diagnostic and placement information. Completion time varies from 20 minutes to 2 hours, depending on the version.

Psychometric Properties.   Test-retest reliability is good. Internal consistency varies considerably. The revised scale differentiates among hyperactive, behavior-disordered, learning-disabled, and normal children using *DSM-III* diagnostic criteria (Breen & Barkley, 1983; Porter & Rourke, 1985) and is sensitive to medication effects (Voelker, Lachar, & Gdowski, 1983).

Advantages and Disadvantages.   Like the Revised Behavior Problem Checklist, the PIC had several advantages during the middle to late 80s, but these are now outweighed by limitations that include its length, its response format, its lack of an inattention subscale, and its lack of a teacher version. Thus it adds little to AD/HD assessment.

Narrow-Band Rating Scales

The increased interest in AD/HD has yielded a plethora of tools specifically designed to assess it. Some also assess other disruptive symptomatology, such as oppositional-defiant behavior and conduct disorder, which often accompany AD/HD.

AD/HD Rating Scale-IV

The AD/HD Rating Scale-IV (DuPaul, Power et al., 1998) is an 18-item parent and teacher rating scale that focuses exclusively on AD/HD. It presents the 9 inattention and 9 hyperactive-impulsive symptoms from *DSM-IV* in an alternating fashion: inattention in odd-numbered positions and hyperactive-impulsive in even-numbered positions. The word *often* is dropped from each symptom description to allow parents and teachers to rate symptom frequency using a 4-point scale, ranging from *not at all* to *very often*. Scores are summed across the odd-numbered items to generate an inattention score, across the even-numbered items to produce a hyperactive-impulsive score, and across all items to yield a total score. Corresponding percentile scores are derived from norms drawn from a large, nationally representative sample of more than 4,000 children ages 5–18 years. For statistical and practical reasons, the norms are broken down according to age, gender, and informant. Another scoring option is to count the number of odd items endorsed as a *2* or a *3* (i.e., *often* or *very often*) to obtain a quick screening for the *DSM-IV* frequency requirement of 6 or more inattention symp-

toms. Similarly, the frequency of hyperactive-impulsive symptoms can be esti-
mated by totalling the even numbers endorsed as *2* or *3*.

Psychometric Properties.   The AD/HD Rating Scale-IV is a psychometrically
sound instrument showing substantial reliability and validity across many peer-
reviewed studies (e.g., DuPaul, Power, McGoey, Ikeda, & Anastopoulos, 1998).
Parent and teacher ratings are internally consistent, stable over a 4-week period,
and significantly correlated with observations of classroom behavior, as well as
with corresponding subscales on the Conners' Parent and Teacher Rating Scales
(DuPaul et al., 1997). Factor analyses reflect a structure that closely parallels
the two-factor structure described in *DSM-IV* (DuPaul, Anastopoulos et al.,
1998). Normative and psychometric data are now being collected for a national
preschool sample, which should be available in 2001.

Advantages and Disadvantages.   Given its direct relationship to the *DSM-IV*
criteria, its ease of use (e.g., administration takes approximately 5 minutes), and
its sound psychometric features, the AD/HD Rating Scale-IV is well-suited for
inclusion in a multimethod AD/HD assessment battery. It also appears promising as an AD/HD screening measure.

The McCarney Evaluation Scales

Over the past decade, McCarney and colleagues have developed a family of
rating scales designed to evaluate and diagnose AD/HD. The original 1989 versions have been revised to correspond to the *DSM-IV* criteria. It comprises the
Attention Deficit Disorders Evaluation Scales (ADDES, home and school versions; McCarney, 1995) for children K–12; the Early Childhood Attention Deficit
Disorders Evaluation Scale (ECADDES, home and school versions; McCarney,
1995) for children ages 2–6; and the Adult Attention Deficit Disorders Evaluation Scale (A-ADDES, self-report, home, and work versions; McCarney, Anderson, & Jackson, 1996) for adults 18–65 years.

The ECADDES was field-tested and standardized on 4,783 children representing national percentages of gender, residence, race, geographic area, and
parental occupation. The home version has 50 items. The school version has 56
items, and it samples behaviors generally appropriate for kindergarten, preschool, and day care settings. The ADDES home version contains 46 items and
the school version has 60 items. It was standardized on 8,210 students, including some with AD/HD, from 4.5–18 years of age. Separate norms are available for
males and females and for older students (ADDES Secondary-Age Student) ages
11.5–18 years. As with the ECADDES, the standardization sample reflects national percentages. The A-ADDES, was standardized on 6,074 ratings of its three
versions, with separate norms for men and women. The self-report version has
58 items; the home version contains 46 items, and should be completed by a
significant other in the home; the work version contains 54 items for a super-
visor or coworker to complete.

All versions share the same response format and take approximately 20
minutes. Respondents answer the items using frequency quantifiers. Each item

is rated on a 5-point scale, from *(0) does not engage in the behavior* to *(4) one to several times per hour.* Four types of scores can be obtained: frequency ratings for each item, which reflect both frequency and severity; subscale raw scores; standard scores for inattentive and hyperactive-impulsive subscales; and a percentile score, which is the global index of behavior in all areas of the total scale. The scales include technical manuals, intervention manuals, and parent guides. They are available in Spanish and have computer scoring packages that identify the items that directly correspond to the *DSM-IV* criteria.

Psychometric Properties. For the ECADDES, internal consistency is quite high (.99 for the total scale), with test-retest reliability exceeding .89 for the two subscales. Interrater reliability is moderate, .64–.66, and its criterion validity is based on comparison with the Conners'. Internal consistency, test-retest reliability, and interrater reliability are also excellent for the ADDES. Its construct validity was established with respect to the Conners' Scales, ACTeRS, and the CBCL. Similar psychometric qualities are reported for the A-ADDES.

Advantages and Disadvantages. The McCarney system of rating scales has several advantages. Comparable parent, teacher, self-report, and other report versions across the age range permit cross-informant comparisons, determination of symptom pervasiveness in multiple settings, and longitudinal assessments— all without substantially changing forms. Psychometric characteristics are strong as well. The frequency-referenced response options are unique and are very specific with regard to the presence of behaviors.

The revised scales mirror the structure of the *DSM-IV* criteria, and the item-comparison analysis permits a specific examination of the 18 symptoms. The intervention manuals contain many useful strategies that translate assessment results into treatment plans, individualized educational plans (IEPs), or 504 Accommodations.

There are few limitations other than the newness of the scales, on which there is a limited published research base, so the success of the scales at identifying AD/HD is still undetermined. Still, they appear to have great potential for making a significant contribution to AD/HD assessment, either as a screening tool or as part of a multimethod battery.

Adolescent Behavior Checklist

The Adolescent Behavior Checklist (ABC; Adams, Kelley, & McCarthy, 1997) is a 44-item self-report measure for assessing AD/HD and associated features in adolescents 11–17 years. The response format is similar to other rating scales: respondents rate each item on a 4-point scale (*not at all* to *very much*), yielding a total score and scores on six factors: Inattention, Impulsivity/ Hyperactivity, Conduct Problems, Poor Work Habits, Emotional Lability, and Social Problems/Competence.

Psychometric Properties. The norming and standardization sample approached 1000, including a broad representation of age and ethnicity but somewhat limited geographic diversity. Separate means and standard deviations are reported for males and females. Internal consistency is high (.90s). Test-retest reliabilities are moderate to good, ranging from a low of .62 for Social Problems/Competence to a high of .81 for Inattention. Initial evidence for convergent and divergent validity is strong, based on the ABC's correlations with the Achenbach scales (YSR, CBCL) and the older Conners' scales (CPRS-48). Research shows that the ABC can differentiate clinical from nonclinical samples and those with AD/HD from psychiatric controls (Adams, Reynolds, Perrez, Powers, & Kelley, 1998).

Advantages and Disadvantages. The ABC reflects a growing appreciation of the need for psychometrically sound and developmentally appropriate measures of AD/HD in the adolescent age group. It is briefer and more easily administered than some of the other measures for adolescents (e.g., YSR). It mirrors the *DSM-IV* criteria and includes sampling of other age-appropriate behaviors, which can help to establish impairment (e.g., Poor Work Habits). Its main limitation is the lack of studies attesting to its utility. Nonetheless, the ABC seems promising for assessing AD/HD in adolescents.

Child Attention Problem Rating Scale

The Child Attention Problem Rating Scale (CAP; Edelbrock, 1991) is a 12-item rating scale comprised of items from the Teacher Report Form of the Achenbach system. A factor analysis of the CAP derived separate factors for Inattention and Overactivity (Edelbrock, 1991). The scale can be used by both parents and teachers and yields Inattention, Overactivity, and Total scores. Norms are available for 1,100 children and adolescents ages 6–16 (Barkley, 1990). Although it was developed prior to the *DSM-IV* criteria, the CAP is still suited to the assessment of AD/HD using *DSM-IV* criteria because it samples the two primary factors. A cutoff score at the 93rd percentile has been used successfully in research with children to differentiate AD/HD from non-AD/HD (Barkley, DuPaul, & McMurray, 1991).

The SNAP/Disruptive Behavior Disorders Rating Scale

Since *DSM-III*, Pelham and colleagues have used the SNAP to assess AD/HD and other disruptive behavior disorders. The SNAP (Atkins, Pelham, & Licht, 1985) was originally published to translate *DSM-III* criteria for ADD with Hyperactivity into a rating scale for teachers. Each criterion was rated as being present *not at all, just a little, pretty much,* or *very much.* The SNAP has appeared in numerous journal articles, and its use has been extended to parents.

To address the changing criteria and to include other disruptive behaviors, the SNAP has undergone periodic revision, first appearing as the SNAP-IV, or the Disruptive Behavior Disorders (DBD) Rating Scale (Pelham, Evans, Gnagy, & Greenslade, 1992; Pelham, Gnagy, Greenslade, & Milich, 1992). The most recent version consists of the *DSM-IV* symptoms of ADHD, ODD, and CD, rated on a 4-point scale (*not at all* to *very much*). Using respondent ratings of *pretty much* or *very much* to indicate the presence of symptoms, one can derive scores for inattention, hyperactivity-impulsivity, oppositionality, and conduct disorder. Means and standard deviations are reported across various research samples. Both scales are widely used, have adequate internal consistency, and are helpful for quick screening and for research purposes (e.g., Washchbusch, Willoughby, & Pelham, 1998). Its advantages are similar to those of the AD/HD Rating Scale-IV because of its shared structure and its use in numerous research endeavors. Norm availability for the AD/HD Rating Scale-IV perhaps gives it an edge over the SNAP in establishing an AD/HD diagnosis, but a clear advantage of the SNAP is its ability to address AD/HD and other disruptive behavior disorders simultaneously.

Eyberg Behavior Inventories

Eyberg and colleagues have developed a short parent and teacher rating scale for disruptive behaviors. The parent version is the Eyberg Child Behavior Inventory (ECBI; Eyberg & Ross, 1978), a 36-item checklist of conduct problems for the parents of children and adolescents between ages 2–17. It takes about 10 minutes to complete, and each item is rated for frequency on a 7-point scale, and on a *yes/no* scale as to whether the behavior is a problem. This in turn yields Total Intensity and Total Problem scores.

The Sutter–Eyberg Student Behavior Inventory (SESBI; Sutter & Eyberg, 1984) is the parallel teacher report. It shares 11 items from the ECBI and has 36 items overall. As with the ECBI, teachers rate the frequency of each behavior on a 7-point scale ranging from *never* to *always* and indicate whether it is a problem by circling *yes* or *no*. The SESBI yields a Total Problem and a Total Intensity score. Factor analyses revealed a four-factor solution encompassing Overt Aggression toward Others, Emotional-Oppositional Behavior, Attentional Difficulties, and Covert Disruptive Behavior (Burns, Sosna, & Ladish, 1992).

Psychometric Properties.   With respect to the ECBI, norms are available on a wide range of children aged 2–12, with a smaller, less-representative sample for adolescents. Test-retest reliabilities and internal consistencies are good (.80s–.90s) with little practice effect. In addition, the scale distinguishes between children with and without significant behavior problems across the age range (Boggs, Eyberg, & Reynolds, 1990; Eyberg & Ross, 1978; Eyberg & Robinson, 1983). The ACBI also seems sensitive to treatment effects, such as parent training (Eisenstadt, Eyberg, McNeil, Newcomb & Funderburk, 1993; Eyberg & Robinson, 1982; Webster-Stratton, 1984).

The Intensity and Problem scores correlate with the Externalizing scores on the Achenbach, which lends criterion validity. Though not assessing the two dimensions of AD/HD specifically, it appears to be a valid screen for conduct problems, especially for children in the late preschool to early elementary school, where its norms are strongest. Test-retest reliability for 1–3 week intervals is approximately .90 (Burns et al., 1992), and .48–.52 over 1 year (Burns, Walsh, & Owen, 1995).

The SESBI teacher report measure has strong internal consistency and test-

retest reliabilities (high .80s–.90s). Scores do not decrease on second administration, a problem with some of the other rating scales. Interrater reliability is
also strong (.85–.95 for Intensity, .84–.87 for Problems). The two subscales are
moderately correlated, indicating that they measure a closely related but not
identical construct. Principal components analyses have identified one primary
factor as accounting for 38–53% of the variance.

Validity was established with the parent and teacher versions (4–18) of the
Achenbach Child Behavior Checklist. Although the Intensity and Problems
scores correlated with the Externalizing score (.87 and .71, respectively), they
did not relate strongly to the Internalizing score (.25). The scale differentiates
between children with disruptive behavior disorders and those with either
internalizing disorders or no difficulties.

Advantages and Disadvantages. The strengths of the scales are brevity, face
validity for behaviors that are most problematic for parents and teachers, separate intensity and frequency scores, and the number of studies that have used
the measure. As a brief screen for disruptive behaviors, these scales accomplish
their purpose.

Difficulties are the more limited standardization samples, particularly for
the older age group scale. Given this limitation, and the lack of correspondence
to the two-factor AD/HD diagnostic conceptualization in *DSM-IV*, the ESBI and
the SESBI are not as helpful as many newer measures in multimethod AD/HD
assessments.

Home and School Situations Questionnaires—Revised

A somewhat similar approach to the Eyberg scales is found in the revised
Home and School Situations Questionnaires (HSQ-R, SSQ-R; Barkley & Edelbrock, 1987; DuPaul & Barkley, 1992). The HSQ-R is completed by parents of
children and adolescents 4–18 years and consists of 16 situations in which
problematic child behaviors can occur. Parents and caregivers rate whether the
problem behavior is present in that setting; if so, they rate its severity on a
9-point scale. The companion SSQ-R samples 12 typical school situations.

Psychometric Properties. Numerous studies support the reliability and validity of these measures (e.g., Breen & Altepeter, 1991; DuPaul & Barkley, 1992).

Advantages and Disadvantages. These scales are particularly helpful in establishing impairment in one or more settings, its pervasiveness, and specific
problematic situations. They are also sensitive to treatment effects (e.g., Wodrich & Kush, 1998). Thus, the HSQ-R and SSQ-R can aid in establishing a
diagnosis, in generating treatment plans, and in evaluating the efficacy of behavioral and pharmacological interventions.

One limitation is the absence of norms. Another problem is that the scales
are not well suited to adolescents. Although adolescents were included in both
the original and the revised scales, some of the behavior problems listed are
not appropriate for this age group (e.g., "while with the babysitter"). In addition,

some important situations (e.g., curfew, driving) are not included. To address this, Adams, McCarthy, and Kelley (1995) modified the HSQ and SSQ, developing three similar forms: the Adolescent HSQ—parent report (AHSQ-PR), Adolescent HSQ—self-report (AHSQ-SR), and the Adolescent SSQ—self-report (ASSQ-SR). The standardization sample included close to 1,000 adolescents ages 11–17. Internal consistency and test-retest reliabilities are good (.80s). Criterion validity with the Achenbach scales seems promising. With additional psychometric data, the adolescent version, along with the HSQ and SSQ, would seem to be a very helpful adjunct to a comprehensive battery.

The ADD-H: Comprehensive Teacher Rating Scale

The *ADD-H*: Comprehensive Teacher Rating Scale (ACTeRS; 2nd edition; Ullmann, Sleator, & Sprague, 1985) is a psychometrically sound, 24-item checklist that describes four classroom factors: Attention, Hyperactivity, Social Skills, and Oppositional Behavior. Teachers rate the child on each item using a 5-point scale ranging from *almost never* to *almost always*. Scores can be translated into percentiles, and the 1991 norm revision and expansion project yielded norms and profiles by gender for children K–8. The checklist can be hand- or computer-scored. However, because it was developed during the *DSM-III* era and is unrevised, the *ADD-H* is primarily of historical significance and adds little to the assessment of AD/HD as currently defined.

Attention Deficit Disorder Behavior Rating Scales

The Attention Deficit Disorder Behavior Rating Scales (ADDBRS; Owens & Owens, 1993) is a 50-item checklist originally designed in 1982 to screen for AD/HD in children ages 6–16. Revised in 1993, this measure rates items on a 5-point scale according to frequency, and it examines 10 behaviors. Three relate specifically to the tripartite conceptualization of AD/HD (i.e., inattention, impulsivity, and hyperactivity); 7 are based on the authors' observations of clinically relevant behaviors (e.g., anger control, academics, and more). Data are limited on reliability and validity, and its normative sample is small (e.g., 200 for the 1993 scale) and contains little information about the gender, ethnicity, and geographic or SES distribution. Items were generated from clinical experience exclusively with no subsequent factor analyses. Although scoring is simple and straightforward, the absence of psychometric data severely limits the utility of this measure.

Ratings of Functional Impairment

In addition to assessing AD/HD and other types of child psychopathology, rating scales can address various domains of psychosocial functioning as well. This capability further highlights the role that rating scales can play in assessing AD/HD, partly because *DSM-IV* requires evidence of functional impairment, and partly because of the influence that this type of information can have on treatment planning.

As noted in Chapter 2, AD/HD can affect multiple domains of psychosocial functioning. School performance is particularly sensitive to its effects. Social functioning is another frequently impaired area. Disruptions in family functioning are also common. Although rating scales are not the only way to assess impairment in these areas, they can nevertheless shed much light on them. Thus, clinicians are well advised to consider including them in their assessment. With this in mind, we now turn to a discussion of many functional impairment measures.

Academic Functioning

Psychological testing and classroom observations generate the lion's share of functional impairment evidence pertaining to a child's performance in school, but when such procedures are not feasible, the door is opened for rating scales to address this impairment.

One especially well-suited tool for this is the Academic Performance Rating Scale (APRS; DuPaul, Rapport, & Perriello, 1991), developed to obtain teacher ratings of academic skills deficits in students with disruptive behavior difficulties. The APRS produces a Total Score and two subscale scores, Academic Success and Academic Productivity. These scores provide estimates of school functioning that differ from those that clinicians and educators usually employ in assessing academic impairment—namely, discrepancies between predicted and actual achievement. The Academic Productivity subscale can identify low rates of school productivity, which set the stage for later underachievement. Although based on a small number of studies, the APRS appears psychometrically sound. It has adequate test-retest reliability and good criterion validity based on comparisons with other measures of children's academic achievement, including weekly classroom performance. The APRS can also differentiate between children with and without behavior problems and is sensitive to treatment effects (Barkley, 1998; Danforth & DuPaul, 1996).

Social Functioning

Because AD/HD can disrupt social relations, it can interfere with the development of stable, positive friendships. Direct observation is an excellent way to gather information about this, but it is time-consuming and therefore cost-ineffective. Some of the broad-band scales described earlier (e.g., BASC, CBCL/4–18) include subscales that address social functioning, but their rather general nature gives little actual insight into it.

To gain such insight, clinicians can use any one of several rating scales developed specifically for assessing social relations. Among these are the Social Skills Rating System (SSRS; Gresham & Elliott, 1990), the Matson Evaluation of Social Skills with Youngsters (MESSY; Matson, Rotatori, & Helsel, 1983), and the Taxonomy of Problem Social Situations for Children (TOPS; Dodge, McClaskey, & Fledman, 1985). Because the SSRS is often used, we now describe it in greater detail.

The SSRS is a standardized, norm-referenced instrument that can be completed by parents, teachers, and students themselves. The parent and teacher versions are further subdivided into three developmental levels: preschool and grades K–6 and 7–12. Two student forms are available for children in grades 3–6 and 7–12. The parent form yields four subscale scores: Cooperation, Assertion, Responsibility, and Self-Control, as well as a Total Social Skills score. Scores for Externalizing and Internalizing problem behaviors and a Total Problem Behavior score are also produced. The teacher form generates all but the Responsibility score. The standardization sample is fairly broad, and there is strong evidence of construct validity, internal consistency, and test-retest reliability. The Assessment-Intervention Record (AIR), which integrates information obtained from all informants, provides a nice analysis of student strengths and weaknesses that can serve as a link from assessment to intervention.

Family Functioning

Children with AD/HD can place a tremendous strain on family functioning, such as greatly increased caretaking demands on their parents that can disrupt parent–child relations and cause changes in parenting style. Such strains may have a ripple effect, disrupting sibling relations as well as marital relations and personal parental functioning. Although the child's AD/HD may not actually cause these problems, research shows that families who have a child with AD/HD also have higher rates of marital discord, parental depression, and various other psychiatric difficulties. Regardless of their source, these circumstances have bearing on a child's prognosis, because parents and other caregivers are usually the primary agents for implementing treatment, whether it is ongoing parent training or adherence to daily medication regimens. For reasons such as these, information about family functioning should be gathered as part of the assessment process. Ease of administration and convenience make rating scales a cost-effective way of doing so. Many of these scales are reviewed below.

Parenting Style

Two scales seem particularly well suited to assessing parenting style. The first is the Parenting Scale (PS; Arnold, O'Leary, Wolff, & Acker, 1993), a 30-item instrument that examines dysfunctional discipline practices in parents of preschoolers. The PS generates three indices of parenting style: Laxness, Overreactivity, and Verbosity. It has been used with nonreferred elementary-age children and also in many research studies on children with AD/HD. Adequate internal consistency and test-retest reliability have been reported. Factor scores are related to observations of ineffective parenting and of child misbehavior, as well as maternal ratings of child behavioral difficulties and marital discord. Another scale of this sort is the Parenting Practices Scale (PPS; Strayhorn & Weidman, 1988), a 34-item scale used to assess the extent to which parents use parenting practices that are commonly taught in behavioral parent training programs.

Parenting Stress and Efficacy

One of the possible consequences of raising a demanding child is that it can be stressful day in and day out, which in turn can fuel doubts about one's competence as a parent. Four empirically derived rating scales used frequently in AD/HD research are available for assessing these aspects of parenting.

The best known of these is the Parenting Stress Index (PSI; Abidin, 1995), which specifically examines stress levels in the parent–child system. Two forms are available for parents of children ages 1–12. The long form consists of 120 items that address the degree and source of the stress via global domain scores and a life-events subscale. Individual subscales can also be examined within these larger domains, permitting a more refined examination of areas such as parental perceptions of the child's temperament, the parent's sense of competence, the informant's relationship with a spouse, and how reinforcing the child is to the parent. The PSI has excellent reliability and validity and has been used extensively to examine parenting stress and response to parent training among parents of children with AD/HD (Anastopoulos et al., 1992; Anastopoulos, Shelton, DuPaul, & Guevremont, 1993). In addition to the long form, there is also a short form version (PSI-SF), consisting of 36 items that take about 10 minutes to complete. Scores on four parallel scales are obtained: Total Stress, Parental Distress, Parent–Child Dysfunctional Interaction, and Difficult Child. The PSI-SF also includes a subscale for detecting excessive bias in responding. Correlations with the long form are high (.80–.90). The Stress Index for Parents of Adolescents (SIPA; Sheras & Abidin, 1998) is a recent upward extension of the PSI for parents of adolescents ages 11–19 years. The 112 items require a fifth grade reading level, take approximately 20 minutes, and examine the relationship of parenting stress to four areas: Adolescent Characteristics, Parent Characteristics, Adolescent–Parent Interactions, and Stressful Life Circumstances. Adolescent characteristics include moodiness and emotional lability, social isolation and withdrawal, delinquency and antisocial behavior, and failure to achieve or persevere. The SIPA has good initial reliability and validity, with norms on both community and clinical samples.

A useful instrument for directly addressing parenting efficacy is the Parenting Sense of Competence Scale (PSCS; Johnston & Mash, 1989), a self-report scale examining two domains, degree of self-perceived competence and overall satisfaction as a parent. The PSCS produces separate raw scores for each. Norms are based on nearly 300 parents of children ages 4–9. Principal components analyses confirm the two factors (Johnston & Mash, 1989; Lovejoy, Verda, & Hays, 1997).

Parental Psychopathology

Many parents of children with AD/HD have personal difficulties. Whether these arise from the stress of raising a child with AD/HD or from factors independent of the child may vary from family to family, but either way, these parents are at increased risk for depression, anxiety, adult AD/HD, and other psychopathology, which can exacerbate pre-existing child problems and complicate the process of implementing home-based treatment. Thus, there is good reason to screen for these factors.

The Symptom Checklist-90-Revised (SCL-90-R; Derogatis, 1983) is an especially cost-effective way to screen for parental psychopathology. As its title suggests, the SCL-90-R®* requires respondents to indicate on a 5-point Likert scale how much discomfort each of 90 problems has caused over a specified period of time. Scores are obtained on nine factors: Somatization, Obsessive-Compulsive, Interpersonal Sensitivity, Depression, Anxiety, Hostility, Phobic Anxiety, Paranoid Ideation, and Psychoticism. Three global scores are also obtained: Global Severity Index, Positive Symptom Total (number of items rated higher than zero) and Positive Symptom Distress Index (average rating of items rated higher than zero). Norms allow conversion from raw scores to *T* scores, using gender-based norms referenced for psychiatric outpatients, psychiatric inpatients, adult nonpatients, and adolescent nonpatients.

Despite its brevity, the scale has good reliability, with internal consistency ratings of .70–.90 (Derogatis & Cleary, 1977a, 1977b). There is some concern about the independence of the subscales due to the overlap of Depression and Anxiety in validity studies (Gotlib, 1984), but the Global Severity Index seems to be a good measure of the overall degree of psychological distress, and it is an excellent screen for psychological difficulties among the child's caregivers.

If one is particularly interested in depression or anxiety, there are measures specifically designed to tap these conditions. Two scales authored by Aaron Beck are particularly useful in this regard. The Beck Depression Inventory-II (BDI-II; Beck, Steer, & Brown, 1996) is a widely used self-report inventory that measures the overall severity of depression in adults. The revised (from 1961) version contains 21 symptoms rated on a 4-point severity scale. The items correspond reasonably well with the depression symptoms listed in *DSM-IV* and cover the cognitive, affective, somatic, and vegetative dimensions of depression. The BDI-II is quick to complete, easy to score, psychometrically sound, and has been used in more than 3,000 studies over 30 years.

The Beck Anxiety Inventory (BAI; Beck & Steer, 1993) follows a format similar to the BDI. Twenty-one anxiety symptoms are rated on a 4-point Likert scale for presence during the past week. The BAI is brief and has good reliability, although there are few reliability studies (e.g., Hewitt & Norton, 1993). One criticism is the amount of overlap between the BAI and the BDI, with correlations averaging in the .50s. Nevertheless, it is a quick, helpful way to screen for anxiety symptoms among adults.

Another possible type of parental psychopathology is adult AD/HD. Parents who have AD/HD themselves are likewise at increased risk for many of the above mentioned personal problems. Adult AD/HD symptoms may also affect parenting skills and the parents' ability to implement treatment recommendations for their child. Thus, there is reason to screen for this problem when conducting child AD/HD evaluations. This may be accomplished by having one or both parents complete the *DSM-IV* AD/HD Symptom Rating Scale (Barkley & Murphy, 1998), an upward extension of the AD/HD Rating Scale-IV that parents and teachers complete on children. Separate norms are available for males and females 18 years and up (Barkley & Murphy, 1998).

---

*"SCL-90-R" is a registered trademark of Leonard R. Derogatis, Ph.D.

Marital Relationship

Parents of children with AD/HD are at increased risk for marital difficulties, which can affect both the child's daily functioning and the parents' ability to implement treatment on behalf of their child. Thus, one should assess the marital relationship. Several measures are available, including the Martial Satisfaction Inventory (Snyder, 1981), the Dyadic Adjustment Scale (Spanier, 1989), and the Locke–Wallace Marital Adjustment Scale (Locke & Wallace, 1959). All are useful for both research and clinical purposes. Another aspect of the marital relationship that can have an impact on child functioning is the degree to which both parents agree on their parenting approach. Hypothetically, two parents might be poorly matched on many marital dimensions, may score poorly on a marital satisfaction questionnaire, and yet may be very allied in regard to parenting. The 20-item Parenting Alliance Inventory (PAI; Abidin & Brunner, 1995) questionnaire examines parents' perspectives on how cooperative, communicative, and mutually respectful they are with regard to caring for their child. Each item is rated using a 5-point scale. The PAI is quick to complete, requires only a third grade reading level, and has separate norms (*T* scores and percentiles) for both fathers and mothers, as well as norms for community and clinical samples of children with AD/HD and other behavior disorders.

Summary

Due to their many practical and psychometric advantages, rating scales are an extremely popular method for assessing AD/HD in children and adolescents. Table 4.1. shows that of the many available broad-band measures, the BASC, the Conners', and the Achenbach scales seem best suited for inclusion in a multi-method AD/HD assessment. Because of their excellent norms, the AD/HD Rating Scale-IV and the McCarney ADDES scales should also be considered. Other narrow-band rating scales that can make a significant contribution to AD/HD assessment are the SNAP, the CAP, the Home and School Situations Questionnaires and their adolescent adaptations.

In addition to addressing AD/HD and other child psychopathology, rating scales can assess functional impairment in a variety of domains, including school, social, and family functioning. The actual measures that one selects to measure these will vary depending on the referral question, the child's home circumstances, and so on. Some of the rating scales that address functional impairment appear in Table 4.2.

PSYCHOLOGICAL TESTS

Neuropsychological measures of sustained attention are widely used in clinical practice. One reason for their popularity stems from concerns that interviews and rating scales are not objective, are not pure measures of attention, and do not permit a component analysis of the construct of attention.

TABLE 4.1. Utility of Rating Scales in Multimethod Assessment of AD/HD

Assessment measure	DSM-IV criteria	Comorbid conditions	Impairment indices	Parallel forms	Age range	Psychometric properties
Broad-band measure						
Behavior Assessment System for Children	A-dd C, D, E	Internalizing Externalizing	Social Academic Adaptive	Parent Teacher Self-report	2½–18	R/V: Excellent Norms: National
Conners' Scales	A-f/dd C, D, E	Internalizing Externalizing	Social	Parent Teacher Self-report	3–17	R/V: Excellent Norms: National
Achenbach System of Empirically Based Assessment	C, D, E	Internalizing Externalizing	Social Academic	Parent Teacher Self-report	1½–30	R/V: Excellent Norms: National
Devereux Scales of Mental Disorder	C, D, E	Internalizing Externalizing	Social	Parent Teacher	5–18	R/V: Excellent Norms: National
Child Symptom Inventory	A-f C, E	Internalizing Externalizing	None	Parent Teacher	5–12	R/V: Satisfactory Norms: Limited
Narrow-band measures						
AD/HD Rating Scale-IV	A-f/dd C	None	None	Parent Teacher Self-report	5–18	R/V: Excellent Norms: National
Attention Deficit Disorder Evaluation Scales	A-f/dd C	None	None	Parent Teacher Self-report	3–65	R/V: Excellent Norms: National
Adolescent Behavior Checklist	A-dd D	Externalizing	Social	Self-report	11–17	R/V: Satisfactory Norms: National
Child Attention Problem Rating Scale	A-dd C	None	None	Parent Teacher	6–16	R/V: Excellent Norms: National
SNAP	A-f C	Externalizing	None	Parent Teacher	5–17	R/V: Satisfactory Norms: Limited
Home and School Situations Questionnaires	C, D	None	Home School	Parent Teacher	4–18	R/V: Satisfactory Norms: Limited

Note: AD/HD = Attention-deficit/hyperactivity disorder; *DSM-IV = Diagnostic and Statistical Manual, Fourth Edition*; A-f = Frequency aspects of criterion A; A-dd, Developmental deviance aspect of criterion A; B = Onset criterion; C = 2+ Settings criterion; D = Impairment criterion; E = Exclusionary criterion; R/V = Reliability/validity. Rating scale authors are cited within the text.

TABLE 4.2. Rating Scales for Assessing Functional Impairment

Rating scale	Area of functioning assessed	Psychometric properties
Academic Performance Rating Scale	Academic success and academic productivity via teacher report	Satisfactory
Social Skills Rating System	Social skills via parent, teacher, and self-report	Very good
Parenting Scale	Dysfunctional parental disciplinary practices	Satisfactory
Parenting Practices Scale	Parenting style	Satisfactory
Parenting Stress Index	Source and degree of stress in parent–child system	Excellent
Parenting Sense of Competence Scale	Perceived competence or efficacy and overall satisfaction in parenting role	Satisfactory
Symptom Checklist-90-Revised	Global and specific types of psychological distress and psychopathology in parents	Very good
Beck Depression Inventory II	Frequency and severity of depression symptoms in parents	Excellent
Beck Anxiety Inventory	Frequency and severity of anxiety symptoms in parents	Satisfactory
Adult AD/HD Rating Scale-IV	Frequency and severity of AD/HD symptoms in parents	Satisfactory
Marital Satisfaction Inventory-Revised; Dyadic Adjustment Scale; Locke-Wallace Marital Adjustment Scale	Overall marital satisfaction	Satisfactory
Parenting Alliance Inventory	Degree to which parents work together in parenting roles	Excellent

Note: Test authors are cited in the text.

Although neuropsychological measures of AD/HD are less affected by these concerns, they are by no means free of them, nor are they as objective as some contend. Performance on these measures can be confounded by other psychological abilities, such as memory, intelligence, language abilities, and so on. In addition, they have low to moderate ecological validity and may be less accurate in predicting attention problems in school and other naturalistic settings (Barkley, 1991). Many also lack the normative data that are so essential for diagnostic purposes.

But psychological tests can serve other important purposes, such as assessing intelligence, academic achievement levels, speech and language problems, learning disorders, working memory, and other types of executive and neuropsychological functioning.

A complete discussion of all psychological tests might be used in AD/HD assessments is beyond the scope of this text. Instead, we now provide a detailed discussion of those most frequently used.

Vigilance and Sustained Attention

One very popular instrument for assessing vigilance is the continuous performance test (CPT). This term was first coined in the 1950s by Rosvold and colleagues (Rosvold, Mirsky, Sarason, Bransome, & Beck, 1956) to describe a procedure that assessed attention lapses in individuals with petit mal epilepsy. Contemporary CPTs are designed to detect momentary lapses of attention primarily via omission errors, but commission errors also occur, which many view as an indicator of impulsivity (Sostek, Buchsbaum, & Rapoport, 1980).

There is no one CPT, but rather a number of them that share certain characteristics. Three primary models are described in the literature (Rapport, 1993). The *X version* involves having the child watch for a particular target throughout the entire test. The child responds each time he or she observes the designated target. The more difficult *AX version* has the child respond to a particular letter, number, or other target only when it is immediately preceded by a different letter, number, or target. This version requires that the child not only respond to the appropriate target but be exceptionally vigilant as well. The most difficult type of CPT is the *double letter version* (Friedman, Vaughan, & Erlenmeyer-Kimling, 1978), which requires a response to any letter, number, or target that is repeated. In this version, any number or letter is a potential target.

Conners' Continuous Performance Test

The Conners' Continuous Performance Test (CPT; Conners, 1994) is a computer-assisted procedure that assesses attention and impulsivity in research and clinical settings. In the standard administration of the Conners' CPT, the child or adolescent is asked to respond to any letter *except* for letter X over a duration of 14 minutes (the reverse of the X and AX CPT versions). In this sense, the Conners' CPT is truly a test of *continuous* performance. The 6 trial blocks each have 3 subblocks containing 20 trials. The interstimulus interval is 1, 2, or 4 seconds. The standard administration paradigm can be changed to the traditional X and AX version by varying the target letters, presentation time, interstimulus response time, number of blocks, and number of trials and targets per block. The computer program generates many output variables, including total number of stimuli, number correct, omission errors, commission errors, and various reaction times, expressed as raw scores, T scores, and percentiles.

Psychometric Properties. There are normative data for both the general population and for children ages 4–18 who have been diagnosed with AD/HD. More-detailed norms for preschoolers are being developed. Error rates are low; false positives and false negatives average 10–15% or lower. Practice effects are minimal, and several studies show sensitivity to changes in behavior related to drug treatment (Conners, March, Fiore, & Butcher, 1993; Conners, 1994; Solanto & Conners, 1982).

Advantages and Disadvantages. The standard administration attempts to avoid some of the problems inherent in the other CPT versions. For example, many *X* or *AX* CPTs have a "floor effect" due to the infrequency with which targets are presented. As a result, only the most inattentive or youngest individuals may be identified as having difficulties. The Conners' CPT also provides more useful reaction time measures because of the greater number of responses required. The chance of impulsive target errors is maximized because the child or adolescent is continuously responding. In this regard, the Conners' CPT places a premium on response inhibition, consistent with current theoretical conceptualizations of AD/HD (Barkley, 1998). Because children with AD/HD have more difficulty with temporal uncertainty (Sergeant & Scholten, 1985; Zahn, Kruesi, & Rapoport, 1991), variable administration increases the likelihood of distinguishing children with AD/HD from those without it. These advantages seem borne out by the discriminant validity of the measure. Despite such supportive data, Conners cautions that the CPT should not be used alone; he recommends using it in the context of a comprehensive battery.

Test of Variables of Attention

The Test of Variables of Attention (TOVA; Greenberg & Waldman, 1993) is a standardized visual continuous performance test. The authors suggest that it has several uses, including screening for attentional difficulties, being part of a multimethod complete evaluation, and evaluating and monitoring medication response in children and adults with attention deficit disorders. Its format has several advantages for tapping the two major components (attention and impulsivity) and for separating them from some common learning difficulties. This is accomplished by using geometric as opposed to alphanumeric stimuli, thus requiring neither recognition of numerals and letters nor right–left discrimination, commonly difficult for children with learning disorders.

The task consists of two easily discriminated visual stimuli (a square containing a small square adjacent to its top or bottom edge) that are presented for 100 milliseconds at 2-second intervals. The stimulus within the inner square adjacent to the top edge is the designated target. There is a 2.25 minute practice test followed by two 11-minute test conditions for clients over age 5. Children 4 and 5 years old take a shorter version that lasts 11 minutes. The first half of the task presents the target infrequently (target-to-nontarget ratio of 1:3.5). This rate is designed to elicit boredom and thus measures the child's ability to sustain attention. The second half presents the target frequently (target-to-nontarget ration of 3.5:1) and is designed to measure impulsivity. Scores on 7 variables are calculated: errors of omission, errors of commission, mean correct response time, standard deviation response time, anticipatory responses (guesses), postcommission mean correct response times (average number of correct responses immediately following a commission error), and multiple responses (more than one response per stimulus).

Psychometric Properties.   Normative data are available on 1590 normal children and adults (4–80), by gender, in 2-year intervals for ages 4–19 and in 10-year intervals thereafter. The authors report that the TOVA has good sensitivity in distinguishing children with AD/HD from those without (Greenberg &

Crosby, 1992) and can also discriminate among AD/HD, CD, and undifferenti-ated ADD (Greenberg & Waldman, 1993). The authors also note that the TOVA is sensitive to medication effects as well (Greenberg, 1987), although the number of subjects studied was small.

Advantages and Disadvantages.   The TOVA's primary advantage is in measur-ing pharmacotherapy outcome. One component of the TOVA is the challenge test, which assesses peak drug effects 1.5 hours after a baseline "no-medication" test is completed. This more objective measure of responsiveness seems to have an advantage over behavior rating scales, which can be subject to bias. In contrast, the face validity of improvement on the TOVA and its potentially limited ability to generalize to "real world" behaviors such as completing work must be considered. At this point, the TOVA's utility for the diagnostic process is not well documented.

Gordon Diagnostic System

The Gordon Diagnostic System (GDS; Gordon, 1983) is a portable, freestand-ing electronic device about the size of a bread box. Three tasks are available: Vigilance, Distractibility, and Delay. The Vigilance Task is the classic *AX* format; the child is told to press a button every time a *1* is followed by a *9*. The number of correct responses, omission errors, and commission errors are tabulated. A parallel *AX* version using a *5-3* combination is also available. For preschool children, there is an *X* format where the child is asked to press the button every time a *1* (or *0* for the parallel format) appears.

The Distractibility Task is similar to the Vigilance Task except that random numbers flash at random intervals on either side of the target. The Delay Task requires the child to refrain from responding for at least 6 seconds. When the child does this, a light flashes and the child is rewarded with points. The Delay Task yields three scores: the number of responses, the number of correct re-sponses (the number of times the child delays for the specified interval), and the percentage of correct responses (or Efficiency Ratio).

Psychometric Properties.   Norms are based on an extensive standardization sample of over 1,600 children and adults, but they are not broken down by gen-der. Though the author indicates that this is because gender is not related to performance, studies indicate that variability does relate to gender (e.g., TOVA).

Test-retest reliability is moderate over 2–45 days ($r = .60$s) and stable over a 1-year period ($r = .52$; Gordon & Mettelman, 1988). Some studies show discrimi-nant validity, distinguishing between children with hyperactivity versus those without, as well as among children classified as having ADD and those with learning disabilities, overanxious tendencies, and normal behavior. Other studies, however, have found more limited discriminant validity, particularly with regard to false negative rates that approach 50% (DuPaul, Anastopoulos, Shelton, Guevremont, & Metevia, 1992). The Vigilance Task commission score is sensitive to the effects of stimulant medication, especially at higher doses (Barkley, DuPaul, & McMurray, 1991).

Advantages and Disadvantages.   One advantage of the GDS over other systems is its portability, making it more attractive when cost or space prohibit CPTs that require computer equipment and software. A disadvantage is that its assessment utility varies. Gordon (1995) notes that part of this variability is due to the absence of a reliable gold standard in the assessment of AD/HD. That is, the rate of false negatives with the GDS varies from 43–73%, depending on the child's age and whether one uses parent ratings, teacher ratings, or both to make an AD/HD diagnosis (Gordon & Mettelman, 1988). If a 93rd percentile cutoff is used for just one of the scores, the false negative rate is high, averaging 50% (DuPaul, Anastopoulos et al., 1992). If abnormality on any one of the three GDS tasks is used, both false positive and false negatives drop to 25% (Gordon, 1995) as compared with teacher-based classifications of AD/HD. Although this is an improvement, it is still relatively high, as Gordon (1995) acknowledges, but he suggests that the disagreement between the GDS scores and clinical diagnoses may yield important information about the child. Gordon and colleagues report that children who are diagnosed with AD/HD but who have normal GDS scores tend to be brighter, older, have less-severe symptomatology, and be half as likely to respond to medication as children with AD/HD have abnormal GDS scores (Fischer, Newly, & Gordon, 1995). Conversely, children who have abnormal GDS scores but are not identified as having AD/HD by teacher report also have significantly higher levels of internalizing problems, such as anxiety and depression, and higher levels of noncompliance (Fischer et al., 1993). Though there is no gold standard in the diagnosis of AD/HD, the psychometric data reported by Gordon and colleagues tend to be based on children identified primarily by teachers. It is not clear whether the GDS might show less clinical utility if one included the *DSM-IV* requirement of cross-situational pervasiveness.

Auditory Continuous Performance Test

The Auditory Continuous Performance Test (ACPT; Keith, 1994) was designed to identify children ages 6 to 11 who have auditory attention disorders as well as those who have AD/HD. It is individually administered by audio cassette. The child listens to a man speaking rapidly, in a monotone but with good articulation. He repeats a 96-word list of 20 monosyllabic words six times. Total administration time is about 15 minutes. The child is instructed to listen for the word "dog" which appears 20 times per 96-word trial. The child indicates that the word is heard by raising a thumb.

The scoring approach is similar to the GDS in that the children can make either errors of inattention (not giving a "thumbs up" to the right word) or impulsivity (giving a "thumbs up" to a wrong word). In addition, the child receives a Total Error score, which is the sum of the first two scores. Examiners also compute a Vigilance Decrement score for each child consisting of the number correct on Trial 1 minus the number of correct on Trial 6.

Psychometric Properties.   The standardization sample is small ($n = 510$) but well stratified. Reliability data are weak (5-day test-retest .67–.74). There is limited but promising evidence for construct validity. In one study, the ACPT did reliably distinguish a group of children with AD/HD from a group without it on the Total Error scores and Vigilance Decrement scores; the false positive rate for children with AD/HD was 18–29%, and it was 2–8% for those without the diagnosis.

Advantages and Disadvantages. The primary advantage of this CPT is that it is auditory rather than visual. Unfortunately, the ACPT's disadvantages outweigh its promising format. Its scoring is difficult; the examiner must be especially careful to notice the child's thumb movements during the rapid word presentation. Recording of response latency would be difficult as well, and the age range is also somewhat restricted. Thus, despite the ACPT's advantage of tapping auditory attention, its limitations and scoring difficulties make other CPTs more efficacious with respect to AD/HD. Even for measuring auditory attention specifically, other measures, such as the Intermediate Visual and Auditory Continuous Performance Test (IVA: Sandford & Turner, 1994), may be more effective.

Other Tests of AD/HD Symptoms

Several research procedures have been used to assess impulsivity in children with AD/HD. The best known is the Matching Familiar Figures Test (MFFT: Kagan, 1966). Although some studies indicate that the MFFT has distinguished children with AD/HD from those without (Campbell, Douglas, & Morgenstern, 1971), it has not done so reliably across studies and has been criticized as being heavily confounded by IQ (Milich & Kramer, 1984). Its sensitivity to stimulant drug effects is also unreliable (Barkley, 1977).

Impulsivity has more recently been assessed by using a direct reinforcement of latency task (DRL; Gordon, 1979, 1983). Many studies have also used the Porteus Mazes Task to evaluate planning and impulse control in children with AD/HD (Douglas, 1983). A major problem with all of these instruments is their low intercorrelation, implying that each measures a different facet of impulsivity (Milich & Kramer, 1984). In view of this, there is little reason to consider them in clinical practice.

Numerous measures of activity level have also been employed in AD/HD research. They span many activities, including locomotion, total body movement, and motion of arms, legs, and trunk (Tryon, 1984). Their lack of normative data, low intercorrelation, low reliability in some cases, low inter-correlation, and poor relationship to parent and teacher activity level ratings argue against their use in clinical practice. The inability of these instruments to take situational influences into account also makes them less likely to contribute to treatment planning.

Psychological Tests of Functional Impairment

Intellectual and Academic Functioning. Because of the relatively high incidence of learning disabilities among children with AD/HD, it is often necessary to expand the assessment protocol to include well-standardized tests of intelligence and academic achievement. In the case of complex, mixed, or unusual learning disorders, neuropsychological testing may also be needed to gain a clearer picture of the child's cognitive strengths and deficits. At the very least, one should screen for achievement problems, because it may not be apparent from other sources whether poor school performance is the result of AD/HD or of a learning disability. Tests such as the third editions of the Wechsler Intelligence Scale for Children (WISC-III; Wechsler, 1991) and the Woodcock–Johnson Psychoeducational Assessment Battery (WJ-III; Woodcock, McGraw, & Mather, 2000) provide adequate coverage of the three major domains of general mental development (verbal, performance, and perceptual-motor). For academic achievement, and more specifically for predicting achievement from intellectual ability, tests such as the Wechsler Individual Achievement Tests (WIAT; Wechsler, 1991) and the third edition of the Woodcock–Johnson Psychoeducational Battery (WJ-III; Woodcock et al., 2000) can be helpful.

Factor analyses of the revised Wechsler Intelligence Scale for Children (WISC-R; Wechsler, 1974) and the WISC-III have consistently yielded three factors, including a "freedom from distractibility" factor (FD). Some investigators contend that the FD factor is of diagnostic significance because it can distinguish groups of children with AD/HD from nonreferred samples, but there is little empirical justification for using the FD factor for this purpose in clinical practice. In general, poor scores on this factor are not reliable indicators of AD/HD (Cohen, Becker, & Campbell, 1990), primarily because so many additional factors can affect performance on these subtests (Ownby & Matthews, 1985; Wielkiewicz, 1990). Moreover, though they may distinguish *groups* of children with AD/HD from groups of nonreferred children, such results do not apply to all individuals within the group, given that rates of false negatives approaching 50% have been found (Anastopoulos, Spisto, & Maher, 1994; Reinecke, Beebe, & Stein, 1999). Thus, the WISC-III results are useful for assessing intelligence and for predicting academic performance, but they contribute little to the process of diagnosing AD/HD.

Neuropsychological Functioning. Assuming a neurobiological basis for AD/HD, it seems reasonable that neuropsychological tests would enhance the diagnostic validity of a test battery. In fact, many neuropsychological tests, including the Wisconsin Card Sort Test (WCST; Heaton, Chelune, Talley, Kay, & Curtiss-Glenn, 1993), have been used both clinically and for research purposes with regard to AD/HD. Unfortunately, most of the research examined group differences and did not include diagnostic "hit rates" for individual children. In three studies that did look at diagnostic utility (e.g., Barkley & Grodzinsky, 1994; Grodzinsky & Barkley, 1996; Matier-Sharma, Perachio, Newcorn, Sharma, & Halperin, 1995), neuropsychological measures did not add much to the process. False negative rates were unacceptably high, and although abnormal scores on these measures were likely to reflect the presence of *some* disorder, it was not necessarily AD/HD as defined by *DSM-IV* criteria. Thus, most of these measures seem to tap executive functioning processes rather than AD/HD symptoms *per se*.

Summary

Continuous performance tests are a commonly used method for assessing AD/HD in clinic settings. Among them, the Conners' CPT seems best suited for inclusion in a multimethod assessment battery. It has strong psychometric characteristics, excellent norms, and emphasizes behavioral inhibition, which is consistent with current AD/HD theory. Regardless of which CPT is selected, all yield a direct, relatively objective clinical assessment of AD/HD that lends itself to examining the developmental deviance of inattention and impulsivity. Therein lies a problem, however, in using this approach—namely, it taps into just 2 of the 3 core symptoms, omitting hyperactivity, which may partly explain why the results of CPTs do not always correspond well with parent and teacher input, which includes perceptions of hyperactive behavior.

Tests of intelligence and academic achievement also play a role in AD/HD assessments, primarily by identifying comorbid learning conditions and degree of academic impairment. On a more limited basis, so can tests measuring executive functioning and other neuropsychological processes.

DIRECT OBSERVATIONAL PROCEDURES

In school assessments, observation can be an extremely informative evaluation component, for several reasons. First, observations in the classroom are better than observations in analog settings at distinguishing children with AD/HD from those without it. Children and adolescents with AD/HD have higher rates of off-task behavior, gross motor activity, and negative vocalizations than do children without AD/HD. This has been documented using some of the early classroom observation systems developed for this purpose, including the systems used by Abikoff and colleagues (Abikoff, Gittelman-Klein, & Klein, 1977) and by O'Leary and colleagues (Jacob, O'Leary, & Rosenblad, 1978). A potential drawback is that many of the these systems do not have extensive normative data. However, if one conducts concurrent observations of the target child's classmates, specific "norms" can be obtained. At least one, and preferably several, observations of the child performing independent academic work should be made to corroborate the existence of problems with attention, impulsivity, and restlessness reported by parents and teachers.

When a direct observation in a school or other natural setting is not possible, observations in analog settings can sometimes provide information unavailable from rating scales or interviews. Routh and Schroeder (1976) were among the first to use this type of observation to distinguish children with and without hyperactivity. Since then, many protocols have been developed, such as the Restricted Academic Playroom Situation (Roberts, Ray, & Roberts, 1984; Roberts, 1990), which assess activity and attentional variables during three instructional sets: free play, restricted play, and a restricted academic task. The academic task is particularly helpful in differentiating among children with and without AD/HD, and it is sensitive to stimulant drug effects as well (e.g., Barkley, Fischer, Newby, & Breen, 1988; Roberts, 1990). Although analog observations are more convenient that naturalistic ones, there are constraints. Most require that the clinic be equipped with a one-way mirror and audio–video recording capabilities. (If the behavioral codes are complicated, a computer coding system can be used.) Apart from this, analog observations can be a useful adjunct to the assessment process.

Two recently developed school-based systems and one clinic-based (analog) system are described below.

Direct Observation Form and Profile

The Direct Observation Form and Profile for Ages 5–14 (DOF; McConaughy & Achenbach, 1994) is part of the Achenbach system. It provides a great deal of information via direct observation of the child's behavior in group or classroom settings. There are 96 items scored on 4-point rating scales over 10-minute periods. It is recommended that children be observed on three or more occasions to obtain the most representative sample of the child's behavior. There is a section for scoring on-task behavior at 1-minute intervals, as well as a section for the observer to write a narrative description of the behavior. After the observation, the observer rates the problems observed during that period. The form should be completed for the target child and also for two other children in the classroom. On-Task, Internalizing, Externalizing, and Total Problems scores can be averaged for up to six observation sessions. The computer-scored profiles include six additional scales: Withdrawn-Inattentive, Nervous-Obsessive, Depressed, Hyperactive, Attention-Demanding, and Aggressive.

Norms are available for children ages 5–14, based on observations of 287 children in classroom settings. There are many advantages of this particular system. Although it was developed before publication of the *DSM-IV*, the computer-scored subscales document either inattention or hyperactivity. Not only does this address the presence of these behaviors, it also addresses the degree to which they are out of line with what would be expected for other children of the same age. The items correspond to those of the CBCL, allowing consideration of cross-situational pervasiveness. Another advantage is that this system examines not only AD/HD behaviors, but a broad range of internalizing and externalizing behaviors as well.

The BASC Student Observational System

The BASC Student Observational System (SOS; Kamphaus & Reynolds, 1992) allows coding of directly observed adaptive and maladaptive classroom behaviors. During and following a 15-minute observation period, the observer completes three sections. Part A is a frequency checklist of 65 behaviors in 13 categories. Four are adaptive and nine are maladaptive. The observer notes not only whether the behavior occurred but also if it disrupted the class. Part B records behaviors during thirty 3-second observations across a 15-minute total observation period. Part C is for any additional observations, such as the teacher's response to the child's behavior or teacher–child proximity.

The SOS format is well-suited to being part of an initial assessment, as well being a good tool for evaluating the effectiveness of classroom interventions. The SOS taps both adaptive and maladaptive behaviors and is helpful in rating the degree to which certain maladaptive behaviors are disruptive. Its teacher–child observation is particularly helpful in measuring the effectiveness of classroom interventions. A potential limitation is the very brief time-sampling procedure. It may be hard to identify consistent patterns of interaction between the child's behavior and classroom contingencies during 3-second observations. In addition, no norms are available, and the manual's description of the psychometric properties of the SOS is limited.

AD/HD Behavior Coding System

In the AD/HD Behavior Coding System (Barkley, 1990), a child or adolescent is observed while completing an independent academic task, usually a set of math problems. The child is instructed to complete as many problems as possible, to stay seated, and to not touch any of the toys or objects that are placed in the room as potential distractors. The key is to select math problems that are not too difficult (i.e., well within the child's academic ability) yet not too easy. The child's behavior is coded for 15 minutes, either at the time or later from a videotape. Five categories are coded: off-task, fidgeting, leaving the seat, vocalizing, and playing with the toys and objects. Every 30 seconds the coder checks to see whether any of the five behaviors are present. The occurrence percentage of each behavior and a total occurrence for all behaviors are calculated, as are the number of task problems completed and those completed accurately. This same system can be used to code behavior during other tasks, such as continuous performance tasks (Barkley, DuPaul, & McMurray, 1991).

Intercoder agreement is good, ranging from .77–.85 in previous studies. Children with AD/HD tend to exhibit more difficulties in these categories than do children without AD/HD (Breen, 1989). The coding system is sensitive to drug and dose effects of stimulant medication (Barkley et al., 1988; Barkley, DuPaul, & McMurray, 1991). The categories provide a glimpse of the particular difficulties a child has when asked to complete work independently in class, or even at home (homework). Lack of norms limits this procedure's contribution to the diagnostic process, but it is still helpful in identifying targets for intervention and in evaluating medication responsiveness.

Summary

Direct observational assessments can yield information that may be unavailable through other assessment modalities. Not only can observation document the existence of AD/HD problems reported by parents and teachers, it can also be invaluable in treatment planning and outcome. Furthermore, direct observation is less susceptible to any inherent biases of other adults completing various measures. Still, the lack of norms makes it difficult to determine how far a child's behavior deviates from that of peers. Moreover, observation is time-intensive and therefore cost-ineffective, a serious drawback in the age of managed care. Thus, although highly desirable, observations are not well-suited for routine inclusion in multimethod AD/HD assessments.

MEDICAL EVALUATIONS

Often, the first person parents consult when they have concerns about their child is a pediatrician. Coupled with a belief that AD/HD is biologically based, this leads many to assume that some type of medical evaluation or laboratory tests will detect AD/HD or confirm an AD/HD diagnosis. Many pediatricians, especially those with training in developmental and behavioral pediatrics, as well as pediatric neurologists, are knowledgeable about developmental and behavioral screening measures. Standardized neurological exams (David, 1989), mental status exams, neuromaturational batteries such as the Pediatric Examination of Educational Readiness (PEER; Levine, 1985), more-extensive developmental examinations such as the Denver Developmental (Frankenburg et al., 1990), EEGs (electroencephalograms) and CT scans are just a few of the approaches that may be considered. Can they reliably identify children with AD/HD? Unfortunately, there is no one approach that can be used by physicians, or anyone else for that matter, that is definitive. That aside, typical neurodevelopmental evaluations are not by themselves sufficient to rule a diagnosis of AD/HD in or out with any certainty.

Children with AD/HD often display more neurological "soft signs," minor physical anomalies, and abnormal findings on brief mental status examinations than children without AD/HD, but abnormalities are also found in children with learning disabilities, developmental disabilities, pervasive developmental disorders, and even in children with no behavioral or developmental problems at all. Thus, abnormal neurological exams do not necessarily indicate AD/HD, anymore than having normal exams rule it out (Reeves & Werry, 1987).

This is not to say that physical examinations and developmental evaluations are not useful. Routine and thorough pediatric physicals are definitely important, because it *is* possible that physical difficulties are causing the AD/HD symptoms. Though rare, children with seizure disorders may have AD/HD-like symptoms exacerbated by phenobarbital (Wolf & Forsythe, 1978), or AD/HD may have developed following head trauma or infection of the central nervous system. The child may have AD/HD as a result of lead poisoning, which needs medical intervention, or may have a condition in addition to AD/HD (e.g., enuresis, learning disabilities) that warrants intervention in its own right. A thorough physical examination is also necessary before initiating drug treatment as well as for its subsequent monitoring.

In summary, there is a place for medical evaluations in the assessment process. Although they cannot establish an AD/HD diagnosis, medical procedures are important for ruling out physical causes of any symptoms, for targeting and treating conditions that may mimic or accompany AD/HD, and for ensuring that drug therapy is medically indicated and proceeding smoothly.

CONCLUSION

There are numerous procedures for assessing AD/HD. Among them are clinical interviews, rating scales, psychological tests, observational approaches, and to a limited extent, medical procedures. Clinical interviews and rating scales are especially well suited for a multimethod assessment battery. Structured interviews such as DISC-IV and DICA-IV provide the most accurate and comprehensive diagnostic picture. The BASC, Conners', and Achenbach rating scales are among the best broad-band measures available, shedding light not only on AD/HD but also on exclusionary and comorbid conditions. Several narrow-band measures, such as the AD/HD Rating Scale-IV and the McCarney family of rating scales, do an excellent job of assessing AD/HD symptoms in even greater detail. Numerous other rating scales can determine the presence or absence of functional impairment in various psychosocial domains, including academic, social, and family. In combination with interviews and rating scales, psychological tests can add a great deal to the battery's overall comprehensiveness. Continuous performance tests such as the Conners' shed light on the existence and developmental deviance of AD/HD symptoms in a clinic setting. Intelligence tests, academic tests, and other testing procedures can illuminate comorbid conditions or impairments in the cognitive domain. Although desirable and clinically useful, observations are less likely to be included in multimethod assessments because they are more time- and labor-intensive and therefore cost-ineffective. Though medical procedures cannot diagnose AD/HD, they are often necessary to rule out exclusionary conditions and to determine the appropriateness of starting and maintaining a child on a medication.

5

Establishing a Diagnosis

"He's just being a boy ... he'll grow out of it."

The first step in conducting an AD/HD evaluation is to select the procedures that will be incorporated into a multimethod assessment battery. The next step is to administer these procedures in a reliable, valid, and cost-effective way. Once the assessment data have been collected, the clinician determines whether the *DSM-IV* criteria for AD/HD have been met, and also assesses whether any comorbid conditions are present. Having arrived at a diagnosis, the clinician puts together a treatment plan tailored to the individual needs of the child or adolescent. Feedback about diagnostic conclusions and treatment recommendations is then communicated to parents and other interested parties, after which the clinician begins implementing treatment. Once started, treatment must be evaluated to determine whether it is working.

The above sequence of events may sound familiar to many clinicians. What may not be so evident is exactly how each step is put into practice. The remainder of this text discusses these clinical management issues. This chapter kicks off the discussion by describing the first part of this process, beginning with a description of what we believe is a comprehensive yet cost-effective multimethod assessment approach. Next is a review of the factors that influence the final selection of assessment procedures. Also covered are several issues that have bearing on how assessment data are collected. Against this background, we then detail the many steps that need to be taken to establish an AD/HD diagnosis. In the context of this discussion, we also provide suggestions for diagnosing comorbid conditions.

SELECTING ASSESSMENT PROCEDURES

Because no procedure alone can address everything that needs to be addressed in an AD/HD evaluation, clinicians must use a multimethod approach. As noted in Chapter 3, clinical interviews and rating scales provide a good

foundation for this approach. Psychological testing and various other procedures are often added to this foundation. Which specific interviews, rating
scales, and psychological tests should be included? Having just reviewed many
of them in the preceding chapter, we now are in a position to begin answering
this question.

Assembling a Comprehensive Assessment Battery

To illustrate the process of assembling a comprehensive multimethod assessment battery, assume that you have been asked to evaluate the prototypical
AD/HD referral—an 8-year-old third grade boy, whose behavior and performance concern his parents and teacher. Further assume that this boy has never
undergone any formal assessment of his difficulties and therefore carries no
prior diagnoses. In short, you have been asked to conduct a comprehensive
assessment that will allow you to determine whether AD/HD, or some other
condition, is responsible for the boy's difficulties.

Because of the important role that interviews play in multimethod assessments, clinicians must first decide which interview to use. Ideally, the interview
selected should possess high levels of reliability and validity to increase the
accuracy of its information. We favor structured diagnostic interviews due to
their superior reliability and validity. We recognize that structured interviews
can be time-consuming, inflexible, and tedious, but they yield the most accurate
diagnostic information and do the best job of mapping onto the *DSM-IV* criteria.
Structured interviews also reduce unwanted variability across interviewers, an
especially attractive feature when consistency across evaluators is desired, as
is the case in many clinics where multiple staff conduct AD/HD assessments.

The DISC-IV and the DICA-IV stand out for their excellent psychometric
properties, comprehensiveness, and ability to differentiate AD/HD from other
conditions. Either would be an excellent selection for any child or adolescent.
In our clinic we have a slight preference for using the DISC-IV, for two reasons:
First, we are very familiar with it through various research projects that we have
conducted. Secondly, the DISC-IV requires less clinical training and therefore is
more easily used by our staff of graduate students.

Because the DISC-IV does not directly address the *DSM-IV* requirement for
developmental deviance of AD/HD symptoms, this documentation must come
from other sources. As noted earlier, certain rating scales and psychological tests
serve this role well. Among these are several narrow-band questionnaires, including the AD/HD Rating Scale-IV and the McCarney scales. Given our roles
in the development of the AD/HD Rating Scale-IV and our long experience
with it in both research and clinical practice, our preference is to use this
instrument (Appendix A). If this scale was unavailable, we would not hesitate to
use McCarney's ADDES.

Having a parent complete the AD/HD Rating Scale-IV is usually sufficient
for documenting the developmental deviance of AD/HD symptoms. Sometimes
it's not. This is because AD/HD symptoms in home settings are often milder than
they are in school or other settings. To avoid drawing the wrong conclusion—

that is, concluding that there is no evidence of developmental deviance when in fact there is—additional assessment procedures must be used. One option is to have the child's teacher complete the school version of the AD/HD Rating Scale-IV. Using a parallel version of the AD/HD Rating Scale-IV allows for direct cross-informant comparison, thereby facilitating interpretation of the results. Like the parent version of this scale, the teacher version possesses excellent psychometric qualities, and its norms were drawn from a nationally representative sample that allows analyses by age and gender, making it an excellent choice for addressing developmental deviance in a school setting. Moreover, the information can be used to document symptom pervasiveness across settings.

The parent- and teacher-completed versions of the AD/HD Rating Scale-IV usually yield enough data for clinicians to determine developmental deviance, but sometimes their results fall into a "gray" area, the *subclinical* or *borderline clinically significant* range. Although ambiguity is the exception rather than the rule, it nevertheless occurs frequently enough that clinicians should have additional assessment procedures in place to address it. Useful information can often be acquired through psychological tests, such as continuous performance tests, that can be administered in clinical settings under the careful eye of the clinician. Many CPTs are available, but the Conners' CPT seems especially appropriate for inclusion in a multimethod battery. We use the Conners' for several reasons, not the least of which is that it maps closely onto the construct of behavioral disinhibition, which many see as the core deficit of AD/HD (Barkley, 1998; Quay, 1997). The Conners' CPT also has excellent psychometric properties, superior norms, and lower rates of misclassification than those reported for most CPTs.

Although these procedures—the DISC-IV, the AD/HD Rating Scale-IV, and the Conners' CPT—provide reasonably good coverage of most *DSM-IV* criteria, they do not fully address the functional impairment requirement. The only procedure for gathering any evidence of functional impairment is the DISC-IV, and the type of information this interview provides is less than ideal, because the DISC-IV does not allow quantification of its results. Therefore at best, the DISC-IV identifies the presence or absence of functional impairment, but its utility in assessing the degree to which functioning deviates from developmental expectations is limited.

To achieve greater certainty regarding the presence and severity of functional impairment—information that has bearing on treatment planning—additional measures must be in place. At a minimum, these should include procedures that address school, social, and family functioning.

For many children, school performance is the area most affected by AD/HD. One way to gather information about school matters is through the APRS (Appendix B), which elicits teacher perceptions of the child's academic success and classroom productivity. Although the APRS provides insight into the existence of academic impairment in the classroom, it does not address all areas that would interest a clinician, such as the child's academic achievement in different subject areas. Additional assessment procedures must be used, and school records are an excellent place to begin. Often they contain summaries of intellectual and educational achievement testing results that can be incorporated into the clinician's diagnostic conceptualization and treatment planning. If the records indicate that such testing has never been done, or it hasn't been done for quite some time, the clinician will need to do it at the time of the AD/HD evaluation.

This can be accomplished through any one of several intelligence tests, including the WISC-III. To address achievement, measures such as the WIAT or the WJ-III can be given. Intelligence testing allows clinicians to make predictions about educational achievement. The WIAT or the WJ-III results can then be compared with the WISC-III predictions to determine whether a child is working up to his or her capability. Significant discrepancies between predicted and actual levels of academic achievement may indicate impairment. Such discrepancies can often be traced to the impact that AD/HD has on classroom performance.

Social functioning can also be affected by AD/HD. To determine whether impairment exists in this domain, clinicians can employ observational procedures as well as parent- and teacher-completed rating scales. Due to their ease of administration and convenience, parent and teacher rating scales are often the method of choice. One such scale, which is psychometrically sound and available in parallel parent and teacher versions, is the Social Skills Rating System (SSRS). Given the amount of detailed information that this measure yields, it is particularly well suited when serious concerns about social impairment exist. When these concerns are less prominent but one still wishes to screen for social deficits, such information can be derived from some of the broad-band rating scales discussed earlier, such as the BASC and the CBCL.

Due to the high potential for disruptions at home, clinicians must also gather detailed information about family functioning. Many rating scales are available for this. Among those we find particularly helpful are the Parenting Scale (Appendix C), which gives a detailed description of parenting style, and the short form of the PSI (Appendix D), which estimates the source and magnitude of stress that parents may be experiencing in their parenting roles. We also find it beneficial to have parents complete the Adult AD/HD Rating Scale—Self-Report Version (Appendix E) and the Symptom Checklist-90-Revised (Appendix F) to screen for any parental psychopathology that may be exacerbating child problems or contributing to difficulties in implementing treatment. When working with two-parent families or families with one parent and a significant other, the stability of the adult's relationship needs to be addressed. This can be accomplished through caretaker completion of a number of questionnaires designed for this purpose, such as the revised Dyadic Adjustment Scale (Appendix G), which assesses overall relationship satisfaction. The Parenting Alliance Inventory (Appendix H) can also determine the extent of caretaker agreement on parenting issues.

In addition to addressing impairment, another assessment goal is ruling out diagnostic conditions that better account for the AD/HD symptoms, and determining whether comorbid conditions are present. Of the many procedures in our battery thus far, only the DISC-IV addresses both matters. It has limitations, however. For example, the DISC-IV does not lend itself to dimensional analysis, thereby restricting its utility in assessing the degree to which non-AD/HD symptoms deviate from developmental expectations. Due to its length, it is seldom given to multiple informants. Therein lies a potential problem, because information about exclusionary and comorbid conditions then comes exclusively from one informant, usually a parent. Although parents often know a good deal about their child, they commonly are unaware of symptoms of ODD, CD, depression, and other internalizing disorders that occur in settings other than the home. For this reason it is imperative to gather information about exclusionary and comorbid conditions from additional informants. At the very least this should include teacher input.

How might such information be gathered? One could interview a teacher, but it would have to be done in a semistructured or unstructured format, because structured teacher interviews are not yet available. Even if one is inclined to conduct a teacher interview, doing so may not be viable due to time and cost constraints. An alternative and far more cost-effective approach is to have teachers complete a broad-band rating scale. Along with providing extensive coverage of internalizing and externalizing disorders, broad-band rating scales allow a dimensional analysis of reported symptoms. Thus, they make it possible for clinicians to more accurately appraise developmental deviance. Because the same is true for parent-completed broad-band scales, parents should complete a parallel version of the rating scale for teachers. The clinician can then address the developmental deviance of parent-reported symptoms in a way that goes well beyond the capabilities of the DISC-IV.

Among the various broad-band measures that are available, the BASC, the Conners', and the Achenbach scales are all worthy of consideration. At various times each has appeared in our own assessment batteries. Over the past few years we have used the parent and teacher versions of the BASC (Appendix I). Our preference for the BASC over these other high-quality measures stems from three primary considerations. First, the BASC data are compatible with *DSM-IV*'s two-factor conceptualization of AD/HD; most of the Achenbach scales are not. Second, the BASC yields more information about functional impairment than do the Conners' Scales. Third, the BASC uniquely yields information about a child's strengths, which can aid treatment planning.

Although the above combination of assessment procedures produces an enormous amount of clinical data, there are still aspects of a child's current functioning and life circumstances to address, particularly information pertinent to what prompted the referral. This, of course, can be generally inferred from the nature of the evaluation (e.g., something to do with AD/HD), but specifics are lacking. Is the child being evaluated to establish an initial diagnosis? To look for comorbid conditions? To assess the efficacy of an ongoing treatment plan? Also still needed is information about the child's demographics or family circumstances, including number of siblings, quality of the sibling relationships, parental educational levels, parental occupations, and so on. Moreover, none of the above procedures yields detailed information about the child's history, whether it be school history, family history, health history, or early developmental history.

Because this information is clinically relevant, efforts must be made to collect it. To some extent this can be accomplished through parent or caretaker completion of the child and family information forms, which elicit factual information about demographics and family background (Appendix J). Similar forms can collect information about the child's early development and health history (Appendix K). Another option, used successfully in our clinical work, is a semistructured interview (Appendix L) with parents or other caretakers, which also clarifies the reasons for a child's referral and yields other information as well. In the absence of a more reliable and valid structured interview or rating scale to address these areas, the above mentioned forms and semistructured interview are acceptable methods for gathering such information.

A summary of the multimethod assessment battery assembled thus far appears in Table 5.1. In brief review, this battery includes the DISC-IV, which is administered to parents or other caretakers. Parents also provide input about their child through their responses to the AD/HD Rating Scale-IV and the BASC. Other questionnaires completed by parents include the Parenting Scale, the short form of the PSI (PSI-SF), the adult AD/HD Rating Scale—Self-Report Version, the SCL-90-R, the Revised Dyadic Adjustment Scale, and the PAI. Parents also provide background information through their responses to semi-structured interview questioning and from their completion of demographic, health history, and developmental history forms. Teacher input is obtained from the BASC, the AD/HD Rating Scale-IV, and the APRS. During the clinic visit, children respond to semistructured interview questioning and undergo psycho-

TABLE 5.1.   Components of a Multimethod Assessment Battery

Input		
From	About	Assessment component
Parent	Child	Diagnostic Interview Schedule for Children-IV
		Behavior Assessment System for Children
		AD/HD Rating Scale-IV
		Semi-Structured Background Interview
		Developmental Health and History form
		Child and Family Information Sheet
Parent	Self and family	Parenting Scale
		Parenting Stress Index—Short Form
		Symptom Checklist-90-Revised
		Adult AD/HD Rating Scale-IV
		Dyadic Adjustment Scale-Revised
		Parenting Alliance Inventory
Teacher	Child	AD/HD Rating Scale-IV
		Academic Performance Rating Scale
		Behavior Assessment System for Children
Child	Self	Wechsler Intelligence Scale for Children-III
		Wechsler Individual Achievement Test
		Conners' Continuous Performance Test

Note: AD/HD = Attention-deficit/hyperactivity disorder.

logical testing that routinely includes administration of the Conners' CPT. If intelligence or educational achievement testing has not been done recently, the WISC-III and either the WIAT or the WJ-III can be added. If recently completed IQ and achievement test results are available, a brief screening procedure consisting of the Vocabulary and/or Block Design subtests from the WISC-III will usually suffice.

Generally speaking, we have found that this assessment battery is an exceptionally comprehensive yet cost-effective way to evaluate AD/HD, and it is a useful model for many points we wish to make in this and the following chapters. But first, we must acknowledge that this battery is designed primarily for use in initial evaluations of children 6–11 years old. Children whose clinical needs or life circumstances are different or whose age lies outside this range may need a different combination of procedures. In view of this possibility, we now shift our attention to factors that can alter the final appearance of a multimethod battery.

Factors Affecting the Selection Process

The comprehensive assessment battery described above is a useful starting point for most clinical situations. Modifications can be made depending on a variety of factors, including reason for referral, age of the child, family circumstances, and family health insurance coverage.

One of the most important factors affecting the selection process is the referral question. Depending on the nature of this question, many different directions can be taken when putting the battery together. For initial evaluations, there is little reason to modify the battery we've described. If, however, the referral is for a different reason, the battery may need to be changed to reflect the desired outcome. For example, some children have already undergone comprehensive assessments and received diagnoses as well as treatment recommendations. Such a child might be referred for a second evaluation because the parents disagree with the original diagnosis, the treatment, or both. Hence, what they are requesting is a *second opinion*. To the extent that this follows closely on the heels of the first evaluation, clinicians should avoid duplicating assessment procedures, unless of course those are the procedures in question. In that case clinicians should select alternative or parallel forms. Thus, one might administer the ADDES rather than the AD/HD Rating Scale-IV, or the Stanford Binet Intelligence Scale rather than the WISC-III.

Another common situation is when a child has never undergone an AD/HD assessment but has been evaluated for other reasons, such as concerns about learning disabilities. In these situations the child's records are often available summarizing the previous intelligence and achievement testing results. When such procedures have been recently administered, there is little reason to repeat them. Instead, one can add the results to whatever new findings are obtained to sharpen the diagnostic picture.

Another common referral situation is that of the child who has already been diagnosed with AD/HD or is already receiving treatment for it. Often questions remain as to whether other diagnostic conditions are interfering with the child's functioning. Similarly, there may be questions about the adequacy of the treatments already in place. In such situations it is often possible to reduce the size and scope of the assessment battery by eliminating procedures that duplicate what is already known about the child. Thus, clinicians may not need to administer the AD/HD module of the DISC-IV or ask parents and teachers to complete the AD/HD Rating Scale-IV. Depending on the nature of the referral question, other assessment procedures can be put into place to determine the presence of impairments (e.g., central auditory processing difficulties) not covered by the original assessment.

Another consideration in selecting procedures is the child's age. Clinicians need to select a procedure whose age range covers the child in question, not only at the time of the evaluation but in the immediate future as well, because such data may serve as a baseline for gauging treatment. To illustrate how age might come into play, assume for a moment that a 4-year-old child has been referred for evaluation. Although preschool norms for the AD/HD Rating Scale-IV are being developed, they are not yet available. Until they are, one might instead use McCarney's ECADDES, whose norms cover children 2–6 years of age.

Similar age adjustments need to be made for many of the other procedures. For example, due to the low incidence of conduct disorder in very young children, a clinician may decide not to ask questions from the Conduct Disorder module of the DISC-IV if the child is 4 or 5 years old. Similarly, for an 8 year old it may be unnecessary to administer the Eating Disorders module. Likewise, there is little need for clinicians to include the APRS or the short PSI-SF when evaluating teenagers, because neither has norms for adolescents. One could, however, address parenting stress with the upward extension of the PSI that was developed recently (Sheras & Abidin, 1998). Another common adjustment for adolescents is the completion of self-report ratings, such as the Conners–Wells Adolescent Self-Report form.

Family circumstances also come into play. When a parent is without a partner, there is no need for marital satisfaction or parenting alliance questionnaires. Similar modifications can be made for children living with grandparents or in foster care placements. For foster care placements in particular, gaining insight into the psychological functioning of the caretakers is seldom necessary if it appears that the child will only be in their care temporarily. So measures such as the SCL-90-R or the Adult AD/HD Rating Scale—Self-Report Version need not be administered.

One final factor that can have a tremendous impact is health insurance coverage. For families with no health insurance, out-of-pocket resources may not cover the cost of a comprehensive assessment battery. Even families who have health insurance may find that it does not cover some of the procedures. Some insurance companies also limit the amount of assessment time that they will cover (e.g., only reimbursing two 1-hour sessions). Under such constraints, clinicians must make a difficult choice. Do they pare down the length and breadth of the assessment battery, or do they administer a multimethod battery anyway, knowing that much of their time and effort will not be reimbursed?

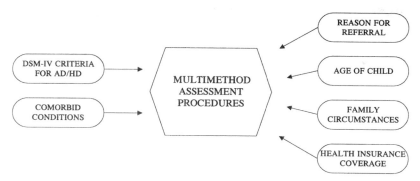

FIGURE 5.1. Factors affecting multimethod assessment procedures.

As summarized in Figure 5.1., many circumstances must be taken into account when deciding on assessment procedures. First and foremost, one must select measures with outstanding psychometric properties that comprehensively address the *DSM-IV* criteria for AD/HD as well as comorbidities. Next, the child's age and family circumstances must be factored into the selection equation. Once this is done, the clinician must determine whether the procedures are affordable.

COLLECTING ASSESSMENT DATA

Once the components of the assessment battery have been selected, the next step is to administer them in a reliable and valid way. For the most part this can be accomplished easily by simply following the standard test administration guidelines set forth by its developers. In this age of managed care, clinicians must also administer them cost-effectively. Therein lies the challenge for clinicians who wish to administer a particular combination of procedures for which they may not be fully reimbursed. Very often they must decide how to pare down the assessment protocols to stay within the insurance boundaries. Thus, efficient data collection is important.

Having frequently worked under such reimbursement constraints, we have developed a method of data collection that reduces clinician time and effort without sacrificing critical portions of the assessment battery. We divide the data collection process into two phases. The first phase begins when referral is initiated. In our university setting, this is when a parent telephones the clinic and requests an AD/HD evaluation. Demographic and insurance information is collected at this time, and parents are informed of the clinic's procedures and policies pertaining to billing and registration matters, confidentiality issues, and the manner in which our evaluations are conducted. Special care is taken to clarify our reasons for sending out questionnaires that request information about the parents' personal functioning and marital satisfaction. In particular, the intake person tells parents that this information allows us to screen for any circumstances that may interfere with their efforts to implement home-based treatments. We also ask who will be completing the questionnaires. At the very least this will involve sending a packet to the child's mother or whoever else identifies themself as the primary caretaker or legal guardian. Whenever possible, packets are sent to both parents, or to any other caretakers in the home.

The home packets include various broad-band and narrow-band rating scales discussed earlier. Assuming our child in question is 8 years old and living in a two-parent home, the mother's packet would typically contain the BASC, the AD/HD Rating Scale-IV, the Parenting Scale, the Parenting Stress Index— Short Form, the Symptom Checklist-90-Revised, the Adult AD/HD Rating Scale—Self-Report Version, the Revised Dyadic Adjustment Scale, and the Parenting Alliance Inventory. Primary caretakers would also be asked to fill out the Child and Family Information Form and the Developmental and Health History questionnaires. Any other caretaker would not need to complete another Child and Family Information Form or Developmental and Health History questionnaire. Attached to these packets is a cover letter (Appendix M) and an instruction sheet (see Appendix N) to assist completion of the forms. Although parents are told during the telephone intake that they will be asked to reveal information about themselves and their family, the instructions are a reminder of why we request it. If for some reason a clinician is concerned about sending the parent self-report ratings, they can be completed at the clinic after the clinician has further clarified their purpose.

During the telephone intake, staff also explain to parents the importance of teacher input and the manner in which it is obtained. With the parent's verbal consent, rating scale packets are then sent to one or more of the child's teachers. For preschool and elementary school children, one teacher packet often suffices. Two or more packets may be sent if two or more teachers have frequent contact with the child, such as when a child receives instruction from both regular and special-education teachers. For teens, we customarily send packets to two teachers, usually the English and the math teachers, or whomever else the parent and intake staff deem appropriate. The main reason for this is that middle and high school teachers spend considerably less time with their students than do elementary teachers; therefore, a teacher may not know the student as well. Although the exact packet can vary, a typical packet for an elementary school student includes the teacher versions of the BASC and the AD/HD Rating Scale-IV, as well as the APRS. The same combination of procedures is used with teens, minus the APRS. Like the parent packets, teacher packets contain a cover letter (Appendix O) and instructions (Appendix P).

Because of the critical role that parent- and teacher-completed ratings play in our multimethod assessments, we inform parents during the telephone intake that we will not schedule the next phase of our assessment until we have received completed packets. This motivates parents and teachers to complete them in a timely fashion. It also eliminates the possibility that the clinician will provide hours of direct contact and then be unable to finish the evaluation because the forms and rating scales have not been returned.

There are further advantages to collecting assessment data this way. Many parents prefer this approach because they can fill out the forms at their convenience. The same is true for teachers, who often cannot meet with the clinician during the school day. From the clinician's point of view, a tremendous amount of assessment data can be collected with little time or effort. Also, the questionnaires can be scored before the child and parents ever come to the clinic. Some clinicians prefer to examine this information beforehand as a guide to issues of clinical concern. Others take a different approach, deliberately not looking at the results until after they have met with the family, which precludes clinician bias that might alter the assessment outcome. Either way is acceptable.

In the second phase of our data collection process, we gather information directly from children and parents. This includes administration of the DISC-IV and the semistructured background interview with parents. Our preference is to administer the semistructured interview first. One reason for doing so is that it provides a nice historical backdrop for the DISC-IV questions about current functioning. Equally important is the fact that the semistructured interview allows parents ample opportunity to say as much as they please, after which they are usually more amenable to the restricted range of responses imposed by the DISC-IV's standard administration. During this phase of the data collection process, clinicians also administer the Conners' CPT and any IQ or educational achievement tests that might be necessary. In addition, they routinely speak with the child about his or her understanding of the reason for the evaluation. They also address the child's self-perception of behavior, emotional functioning, academic performance, peer relations, and family functioning.

When two or more clinicians are involved, one can interview the parents while the other interviews and tests the child. More often than not, only one is available to administer these procedures, greatly increasing the time required to complete the assessment process. In this case, some families prefer to spread the assessment across two separate contacts, an especially attractive option when full IQ and educational achievement tests are given, because they can take up to 3 hours. Even if family preference is not at issue, clinicians often insist on two sessions because many children with AD/HD have difficulty sitting unsupervised in a clinic waiting room for the duration of the parent interviews (which can take up to 2 hours).

When splitting the assessment into two sessions, clinicians must decide the order in which to proceed. One option is to see the parents in the first session, the child in the second. Alternatively, clinicians may work with the child first. This is often more convenient, because the clinician has time to score child results before the parents come back for the second session. After parents finish giving their responses to both the DISC-IV and the semistructured interview, the clinician may be able to give feedback about the entire evaluation before they leave, depending in part on the clinician's comfort with analyzing data and drawing conclusions rapidly. For experienced clinicians, this is a reasonable possibility, and many parents prefer receiving feedback at that time rather than coming back for another visit.

INTERPRETING ASSESSMENT DATA

Once the assessment data have been collected, it is time to determine whether the *DSM-IV* criteria for AD/HD have been met. At face value this seems relatively simple and straightforward, but it is not. One factor complicating this process is the manner in which *DSM-IV* presents the criteria. Other potential problems include the inconsistencies that often arise across informants, as well as missing or incomplete data.

Re-ordering the *DSM-IV* Criteria

With their assessment data before them, the first thing that most clinicians look for is evidence that the child is displaying 6 or more symptoms of either inattention or of hyperactivity-impulsivity (Criterion A). If so, they next examine their assessment data for indications that these symptoms were present prior to 7 years of age (Criterion B). Assuming that such evidence exists, clinicians then conduct similar analyses to determine if Criteria C, D, and E have been met. If they are, an AD/HD diagnosis is made. If they are not, alternative explanations for the child's reported difficulties are then considered.

Although one can certainly address these criteria in the order in which *DSM-IV* presents them, such an approach is rather awkward and cumbersome, and moreover, runs counter to the realities and logic of clinical practice. Why? Consider how most children with AD/HD come to the attention of child health-care professionals and educators. Such referrals occur not so much because of inattention, impulsivity, or hyperactivity *per se*, but because parent and teacher expectations for daily behavior and performance are not being met. The child may be working below his or her academic potential or having difficulties interacting with peers or with family members. Deficits in psychosocial functioning, more than the AD/HD symptoms themselves, are what prompts most parents and teachers to seek professional consultation. Thus we believe that the best starting point for addressing the *DSM-IV* guidelines is the criterion dealing with functional impairment, Criterion D.

If Criterion A is not addressed first, at what point should it be considered? And what about the remaining criteria? Is there any basis for re-ordering them as well? In our opinion, the *DSM-IV* ordering of the remaining criteria is also inconsistent with what makes sense clinically. Therefore, to smooth the decision-making process, we have developed our own order of addressing the criteria. A summary of this revised approach appears in Figure 5.2.

Assuming for a moment that there is clear evidence of functional impairment, we next ask, "Is the child displaying any symptoms of inattention, impulsivity, or hyperactivity that might reasonably be connected to this functional impairment?" If there is no evidence of symptoms, or if they are present but seem unrelated to the impairment in the child's functioning, there is little need to proceed to the remaining criteria, because the impairment is probably not due to AD/HD. If, on the other hand, AD/HD symptoms are present at least to some degree, and if they appear to be either causing or contributing to the functional

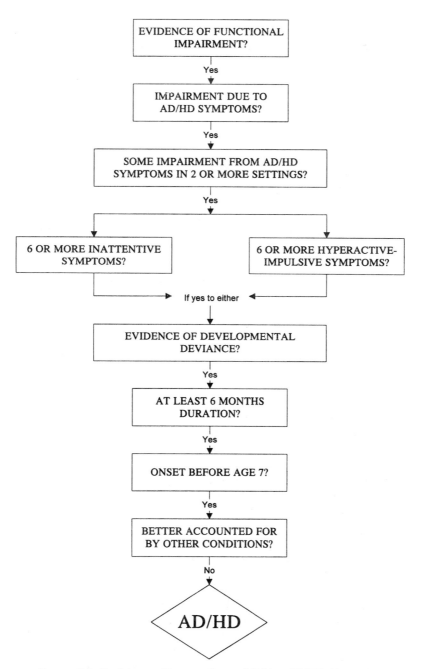

FIGURE 5.2. Decision-making tree for establishing AD/HD diagnosis.

impairment, the possibility of AD/HD remains. In which case we then determine whether these symptoms are of sufficient magnitude to be considered manifestations of AD/HD.

Having established a possible connection between these symptoms and the child's psychosocial difficulties, thereby addressing portions of both Criteria A and Criteria C, we next ask whether the symptoms are causing impairment in two or more settings. If not, the review of the AD/HD criteria may cease, necessitating consideration of other explanations for the child's problems. If, however, there is clear evidence of impairment in multiple settings, then the symptom pervasiveness requirement (Criterion C) has been fully met and we move on to the next criterion.

At this point the symptom frequency requirement, which is part of Criterion A, comes into play. Fundamentally, the question that needs to be asked here is, "Are there enough symptoms to consider the possibility of AD/HD?" If there are fewer than 6 inattention symptoms *and* fewer than 6 hyperactive-impulsive symptoms, AD/HD is ruled out. If, however, there are 6 or more of either, the symptom frequency portion of Criterion A has been met and the criteria review continues.

Related to this issue of frequency is the notion of developmental deviance. As noted earlier, nowhere does *DSM-IV* provide any guidance on how to make this determination. In the next section we attempt to shed light on this matter. In the meantime, the point that we wish to make here is that some determination needs to be made about developmental deviance, because without such evidence, no further criteria need be addressed. However, if the data suggest that the symptoms deviate significantly from expectations for children of same age and gender, the developmental deviance requirement is fulfilled.

Although documenting the frequency and developmental deviance of the symptoms addresses a major portion of Criterion A, we must still decide whether these symptoms meet the first of two temporal requirements imposed by *DSM-IV*—namely, the duration requirement. If symptoms have not been present for 6 months or longer, some other condition, such as an adjustment disorder, might be responsible for the child's difficulties. It is also possible that AD/HD is truly present but not yet fully emerged. In clinical practice, duration is seldom a sticking point, so we will assume that this requirement is met, fulfilling the final portion of Criterion A, thereby allowing us to move on to the next criterion.

The second temporal requirement of the *DSM-IV* is age of onset. If we have little reason to believe that AD/HD symptoms were present before age 7, we could technically stop the review and begin considering other explanations. On the other hand, if such evidence exists, the onset criterion (Criterion B) is met and our analysis shifts to the final *DSM-IV* criterion.

Thus far we have addressed Criteria D, C, A, and B. Together, these are the *DSM-IV* inclusionary criteria for AD/HD. Before deciding that these symptoms *are* due to AD/HD, we must consider that the clinical presentation might better be accounted for by some other diagnostic condition. If no other conditions are present, or if they are but do not seem connected to the child's difficulties, we can conclude that AD/HD best accounts for the child's symptoms and functional impairment.

Before moving on, a word of caution is in order. In the preceding discussion we frequently referred to stopping the review of the *DSM-IV* criteria if any one criterion was not met. Technically speaking, this is the correct way to proceed with respect to the Combined, Predominantly Inattentive, and Predominantly Hyperactive-Impulsive subtype classifications of AD/HD. Hypothetically, it might be possible to encounter a child or adolescent who does not meet a particular criterion in the middle of this decision-making sequence, but nevertheless meets all other criteria both before and after the one that's not met. For this type of situation we might use the Not Otherwise Specified classification, thereby signaling the need for clinical intervention. In view of this possibility, some clinicians may wish to address all of the *DSM-IV* criteria even if one is not met along the way.

Addressing the *DSM-IV* Criteria

We now turn our attention to how data are extracted from the assessment battery to address the *DSM-IV* criteria. We begin by identifying which procedures generate the data necessary for meeting these criteria in the order that we have presented them. Along the way, we provide suggestions for objectively determining whether the criteria have been met.

Criterion D—Functional Impairment

> There must be clear evidence of clinically significant impairment in social, academic, or occupational functioning.

Implicit in this statement is the idea merely having symptoms of inattention and hyperactivity-impulsivity does not warrant an AD/HD diagnosis. When accompanied by impairment, however, they do.

Unfortunately, the *DSM-IV* criteria for functional impairment are somewhat vague and limited in scope. Of particular concern is that *DSM-IV* defines impairment exclusively from the point of view of the individual child. From a systems perspective, one could broaden the definition of impairment to include AD/HD-related disturbances in various areas of family functioning, such as parenting stress, sibling relationship difficulties, and marital discord. Independent of this or any other psychosocial domain, uncertainty exists about what constitutes a "clinically significant" level of impairment. With no clear guidelines to follow, practitioners must rely on their own interpretation of how to address this particular criterion, which makes for even more variability in the way that AD/HD evaluations are conducted.

Assessment procedures are needed that allow for a more objective and uniform approach to determining clinically significant levels of impairment. As depicted in Figure 5.3. many of the measures in our assessment battery can address impairment in several areas, including home, school, and social functioning.

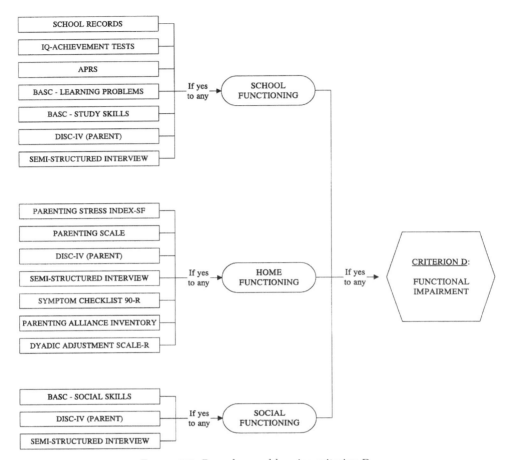

FIGURE 5.3. Procedures addressing criterion D.

With respect to school functioning, records are perhaps the best source of information. Report cards often show that a child's achievement is well below that of peers. School records may also contain information concerning special-education services, retentions, suspensions, and expulsions. Summaries of testing completed by school-based assessment teams are also commonly found in school records. Results of educational achievement testing, for example, can help determine whether a child's academic performance is commensurate with peers. Educational testing results can also be used in conjunction with IQ results to determine if the child is working up to his or her capabilities. Such comparisons are possible because the results of intelligence and achievement testing can be expressed as standard scores. The standard score from the IQ test can be used to predict the standard score for the educational achievement test. When achievement test scores are at least 15 points lower than what the IQ score predicts, it is considered clinically significant, thereby reflecting academic impairment.

Another way to assess school functioning is through teacher responses to the APRS. Of particular interest here is the academic productivity score, which provides an estimate of how much work the child is completing on a daily basis. Although there are no clear guidelines for interpreting data from this measure, academic productivity scores that are more than 1 standard deviation from the mean may reflect a level of productivity significantly lower than that of peers. The teacher-completed BASC can also show school impairment. In particular, one can look at the T scores from the Learning Problems and Study Skills sub-scales to see if impairment was present. Although the deviance cut-point is somewhat arbitrary, most clinicians and researchers agree that T scores of 65 and above reflect impairment.

Less-direct evidence of impairment in school functioning can be derived from parent responses to school-related questions in the DISC-IV and in the semistructured interview, but neither is an objective way of determining academic impairment. Moreover, both are limited to input from parents, who may not know many details of a child's performance in school. Thus clinicians are well advised to use information from these interviews primarily to corroborate impairment findings from other procedures.

Many measures are also available to address impairment in home functioning. The Parenting Stress Index is perhaps the one most sensitive to the effects of raising a child with AD/HD. According to the developers of the short version, Total Stress scores at or above 91 indicate clinically significant levels of stress. The Parenting Scale (PS) is another measure that may be sensitive to the effects of raising a child with AD/HD. As was the case for the APRS, scores on the PS that fall more than 1 standard deviation beyond the mean are considered evidence of functional impairment. Clinicians may also find evidence of impairment in the home from parental responses to the DISC-IV and the semistructured interview, but again, such evidence is subjectively interpreted based on parent responses to the interview questions. Scores on the SCL-90-R, the PAI, and the revised version of the Dyadic Adjustment Scale (DAS-R) can often be elevated for reasons other than the difficulties of raising a child with AD/HD. But because it is possible that these scores can be deviant due to having such a child, they should be reviewed as well. Used cautiously, abnormal scores on these measures may provide additional documentation of functional impairment at home. According to the developer of the SCL-90-R, any global or subscale T score at or above 63 indicates clinically significant psychological distress. Although similar guidelines are unavailable for either the PAI or the DAS-R, clinicians can still employ a statistical approach, looking for scores that are 1 standard deviation or more beyond the means.

Fewer measures are available for determining impairment in social functioning. Among them, the SSRS is an excellent measure to employ whenever there are major concerns about a child's social functioning. Standard scores below 85 on the social skills portion suggest deficits in social functioning. When the SSRS is not given, clinicians can turn to other measures for addressing impairment in peer relations. One such measure is the BASC Social Skills subscale. As is the case for other BASC subscales, T scores of 65 and above suggest clinically significant social difficulties. More subjective evidence can be obtained from parental responses to the DISC-IV and the semistructured interview.

If any of the procedures that address school functioning indicate abnormalities, it is considered evidence of functional impairment in the academic domain. Likewise, all that is required for documenting functional impairment at home or in social situations are abnormal results on any one measure from each of these domains. Evidence of impairment in any domain meets Criterion D. Having established this, clinicians can examine the next *DSM-IV* criterion in our decision-making sequence.

Criterion C—Impairment in Multiple Settings

Symptoms of AD/HD appear across multiple settings. The way that *DSM-IV* addresses cross-situational pervasiveness is through its requirement that:

> some impairment from the symptoms is present in two or more settings (e.g., at school and at home).

The clinical intent of this criterion is often misunderstood. It's not so much that there needs to be evidence of inattention or hyperactivity-impulsivity in two or more settings. More to the point, what is required is evidence of functional impairment in two or more settings—impairment that very likely is caused by, or at the very least exacerbated by, AD/HD symptoms.

Another potentially confusing point pertains to the range of settings. *DSM-IV* provides an example of one particular combination of settings that would fulfill this requirement for cross-situational pervasiveness—namely, *at school and at home*. Although no other child examples are given, it is a mistake to view *at school and at home* as the only combination of settings to consider. Recreational and social situations with peers should certainly be on this list. So too should various public settings, such as stores and restaurants. The practitioner's office is yet another setting. Even within the same general setting there may be specific subsettings that further attest to cross-situational pervasiveness. For example, AD/HD symptoms in the classroom and on the playground could meet the two-setting requirement. This requirement might also be met when AD/HD symptoms arise at both the dinner table and in church.

With this expanded range in mind, it is possible to document cross-situational pervasiveness through combinations of settings that may not include both school and home situations (e.g., at home and in social situations with peers). To allow for this possibility, clinicians must incorporate procedures that sample a child's behavior in settings beyond those two physical boundaries.

As shown in Figure 5.4., meeting the requirements of the next criterion, Criterion C, is a multistep process. First, there must be evidence of functional impairment co-occurring with AD/HD symptoms within the same setting, with the additional stipulation that the symptoms apparently contribute to that impairment. Furthermore, this combination of symptoms and impairment must be pervasive, occurring in two or more distinct settings.

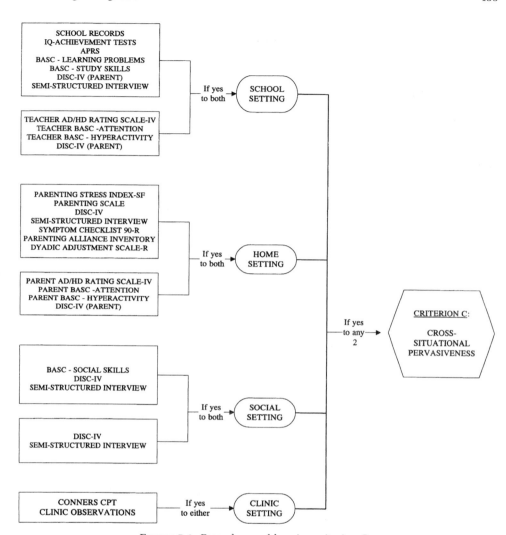

FIGURE 5.4. Procedures addressing criterion C.

Based on the analysis of criterion D (functional impairment), we first identify settings where impairment is evident. If impairment is occurring in two or more settings, the first part of the Criterion C is established. Now the presence of AD/HD symptoms in those same settings must be established, along with their contribution to impairment. Objectively documenting the co-occurrence of functional impairment and AD/HD symptoms is a relatively straightforward process. More challenging, and far more subjective, is establishing a connection between the impairment and the symptoms. To some extent, observations can call attention to this possibility, but even so, it is still necessary to infer the existence of such a connection. Therefore, meeting the requirements of Criterion C primarily involves documenting the *co-occurrence* of impairment and AD/HD symptoms within each of two or more settings.

For example, if impairment is occurring in school, as evidenced by APRS findings, the teacher-completed AD/HD Rating Scale-IV and the BASC Attention Problems and Hyperactivity subscales can document the existence of abnormally high levels of AD/HD symptoms in the same setting. Additional information about the existence of AD/HD symptoms in school settings can come from parent responses to the DISC-IV and the semistructured interview, which can also provide insight into the existence of symptoms that may be contributing to elevated parenting stress or to other impairment in the home. Although this information is helpful, an even more detailed and objective way to document the presence of AD/HD symptoms at home is through the parent-completed AD/HD Rating Scale-IV and BASC. However, when social situations are one of the two settings, fewer options exist. Clinicians must turn to the DISC-IV and the semistructured interview for parent responses suggestive of AD/HD symptoms during peer interactions. Another setting in which the co-occurrence of AD/HD symptoms and functional impairment can be established is the clinic itself. For example, a connection can be made when the child's performance on the Conners' CPT is abnormal *and* the clinician observes symptoms of inattention and hyperactivity-impulsivity both during the testing and at other times during the clinic visit.

Criterion A—Frequency, Developmental Deviance, and Duration of Symptoms

Having established that AD/HD symptoms are present and that they likely contribute to difficulties in the child's daily life, we would then ask:

> Are these observed symptoms of inattention and/or hyperactivity-impulsivity of sufficient clinical intensity to warrant consideration of being labeled AD/HD?

As shown in Figure 5.5., this is determined by frequency, developmental deviance, and duration.

We must first see whether the AD/HD symptoms are frequent enough to be clinically significant. More specifically, we must answer the following questions:

> Are 6 or more symptoms of inattention present in the settings where functional impairment has been detected? Similarly, is there any evidence that 6 or more hyperactive-impulsive symptoms are present in the settings where functional impairment has been detected?

To answer these questions, we need symptom counts, which come primarily from the DISC-IV. Frequency can also be addressed by informally examining the AD/HD Rating Scale-IV. More specifically, clinicians can count the odd-numbered items endorsed as *2* (*often*) or *3* (*very often*) for a simple, cost-effective estimate

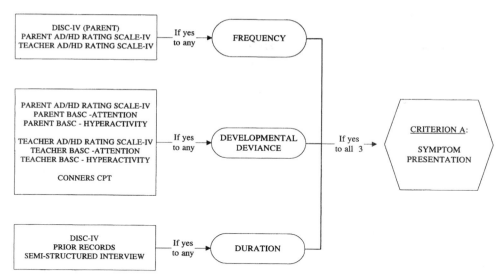

FIGURE 5.5. Procedures addressing criterion A.

of the number of frequently occurring inattention symptoms. Likewise, the hyperactive-impulsive symptoms are counted by tallying even-numbered items endorsed as *2* or *3*. These estimates may be obtained from one or both parents, from one or more teachers and, in some cases, directly from children or adolescents themselves. If 6 or more symptoms are endorsed from either list, the frequency aspect of Criterion A is met.

Along with specifying that a certain number of symptoms must be present to consider an AD/HD diagnosis, *DSM-IV* stipulates that these symptoms must be:

Maladaptive and inconsistent with developmental level.

This is extremely important, not only for establishing an AD/HD diagnosis but also for evaluating other childhood psychiatric disorders.

Despite the fact that *DSM-IV* recognizes this developmental issue, nowhere in its diagnostic criteria are there any guidelines on how to determine whether AD/HD symptoms deviate from developmental expectations. Thus, clinicians must draw on their own clinical experiences, which often results in idiosyncratic handling of this matter.

This situation becomes even more complicated when one considers how developmental considerations come into play. For example, if parents report that their child is very inattentive, impulsive, and hyperactive, is that sufficient to consider an AD/HD diagnosis? If the child is 10 years old, perhaps. But what if the child is 4 years old? In that case, the answer would be far less definitive, because normal preschoolers characteristically display many of these same behaviors. Would it make any difference whether the child was a boy or girl?

Most developmental research suggests that it would. An especially good example of this gender consideration is that boys typically display more physical activity than do girls. What about intellectual ability? Would it make a difference if the child was developmentally disabled? Although there are no clear-cut answers to this, it is presumably relevant, because children with significant intellectual delays often behave more like children of the same mental age, rather than the same chronological age.

How do clinicians take such matters into account when determining whether symptoms are developmentally deviant? Without clear guidelines, most intuitively make comparisons with the developmental norms they carry in their heads, a subjective method of questionable validity that increases the variability with which AD/HD is diagnosed.

For reasons such as these, we need a more objective approach. As a first step toward achieving this, clinicians should use assessment procedures with well-standardized norms, thereby allowing for more-accurate chronological age and gender comparisons.

To determine whether the developmental deviance aspect of Criterion A has been met, clinicians must answer the following questions:

> As a group, do the endorsed inattention symptoms deviate significantly from developmental expectations based upon a consideration of chronological age and gender? Likewise, as a group, do the endorsed hyperactive-impulsive symptoms deviate significantly from developmental expectations based upon a consideration of chronological age and gender?

How much does an AD/HD symptom have to deviate from the norm to be considered significant? This is not well-understood or well-researched. Some researchers suggest that scores above the 90th percentile should be considered significant deviations (DuPaul et al., 1998). Others contend that the 93rd or 95th percentile is a better demarcation line (Barkley, 1998). Still others advocate a more stringent cut-point, the 98th percentile (Achenbach, 1991a). The answer to this question varies partly as a function of differences from one measure to the next. Age, gender, and ethnicity may also exert an influence. For now clinicians should consider adopting a definition of developmental deviance that lies somewhere between the 90th and the 98th percentiles.

Which procedures allow for this determination? The parent- and teacher-versions of the AD/HD Rating Scale-IV serve this purpose well. Clinicians can look at the inattention and hyperactive-impulsive scores to see if they deviate significantly from expectations for children of the same age and gender. According to the scale's manual, a reasonable cut-point is at or above the 90th percentile on either factor. Parent and teacher versions of this questionnaire can be examined separately. The parent- and teacher-completed BASC can also be used to make this determination. In particular, clinicians can examine the Attention Problems and Hyperactive subscales to see if the T scores are 65 or higher (93rd percentile). If so, this would serve as evidence of developmental deviance. Like the AD/HD Rating Scale-IV estimates, the BASC percentiles are derived from age- and gender-appropriate norms and are therefore more precise estimates of developmental deviance than those from the DISC-IV. Developmental deviance can also be established via the Conners' CPT *T* scores and other of its indices that lie within the clinically significant range as determined by the test's developers.

Assume for a moment that a child does exhibit at least 6 symptoms from either list, and that such symptoms are developmentally deviant. This alone does not fully satisfy the requirements of criterion (A), which also stipulates that:

> six (or more) of the ... symptoms have persisted for at least 6 months.

Meeting this requirement is not usually difficult, but there are times when it can be. This might be the case for a preschool child, for whom only a few of the reported 6-plus symptoms have had a duration longer than 6 months. In such a situation, even though the evaluating clinician might strongly suspect the presence of AD/HD, he or she would not be technically entitled to make this diagnosis. Although it may seem overly restrictive, the main reason for this requirement is to differentiate AD/HD symptoms from both normal developmental behavior patterns and behaviors resulting from various short-term psychosocial stressors.

What this means for practitioners is that they should use assessment procedures that allow for clarifying the duration of every item contained in both the inattentive and hyperactive-impulsive lists. The DISC-IV does this. In a less objective way, similar information can be obtained from parent responses to the semistructured interview. Although less definitive than either of these two interview methods, the child's records may contain information that also helps to address this criterion.

Criterion B—Symptom Onset

Throughout its long history, AD/HD has been conceptualized as a disorder whose symptoms arise in early childhood. Although there is currently a debate about exactly when AD/HD symptoms first appear (Barkley & Biederman, 1997), the current criteria require that:

> Some hyperactive-impulsive or inattentive symptoms that cause impairment were present before age 7 years.

At face value, this seems relatively straightforward. Indeed, it usually is, but occasionally it is not. Not everyone agrees on what is meant by "symptoms that cause impairment." Taken literally, it implies that the symptoms were evident before age 7 and that they were associated with some type of impairment in the child's life. Documenting both of those conditions is only possible through interviewing parents or reviewing records, neither of which is an especially reliable way to assess these matters. Especially problematic is finding objective evidence of functional impairment before age 7. Clinical experience suggests that many parents were aware of their child's symptoms before that age, but they

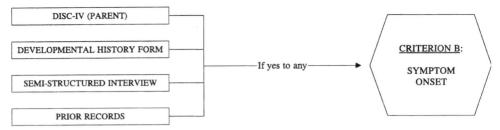

FIGURE 5.6. Procedures addressing criterion B.

may not have labeled them "problems." Does the mere fact that a parent notices AD/HD symptoms constitute a problem? Given these sorts of definitional debates and methodological limitations, it is inadvisable to impose a stringent interpretation of this *DSM-IV* phrasing. In keeping with conclusions drawn by Applegate et al. (1997), it instead seems best to look for evidence of AD/HD symptoms prior to age 7, whether or not they were clearly associated with impairment.

Obviously, this onset requirement does not need to be assessed with a procedure when a child younger than 7 arrives for an AD/HD evaluation, but with children older than 7, it does. The closer a child is to age 7, the easier it is to address this criterion. The further beyond age 7, the more challenging this becomes. As can be seen in Figure 5.6., information about AD/HD symptom onset comes from a limited number of assessment procedures. Generally speaking, onset information may be found in parental responses on the DISC-IV and the semistructured interview. Hints of AD/HD symptoms existing prior to 7 years of age can sometimes be uncovered in reviews of medical and school records. Although much less reliable, parental responses to the Infant Health and Temperament section of the Developmental and Health History Information form (Appendix K) may also shed light on this matter. In particular, *yes* answers to item 10 (*Difficult to keep busy*) and item 11 (*Overactive, in constant motion*) may indicate that AD/HD symptoms were present during the child's first 12 months.

Criterion E—Exclusionary Conditions

Before making an AD/HD diagnosis, clinicians must also rule out other mental, developmental, and medical conditions whose symptoms and psychosocial impact can mimic AD/HD. As stated in *DSM-IV*, the question that needs to be asked is:

> Are these symptoms of inattention and hyperactivity-impulsivity a manifestation of Pervasive Developmental Disorder, Schizophrenia, or other Psychotic Disorder? Or better accounted for by a Mood Disorder, Anxiety Disorder, or other mental disorder?

As depicted in Figure 5.7., only a few procedures can rule out exclusionary conditions. Fortunately, they do a very good job of it. Parental responses to the

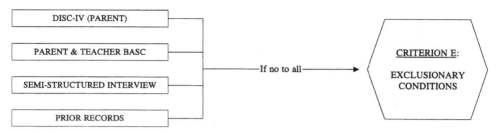

FIGURE 5.7. Procedures addressing criterion E.

DISC-IV are especially valuable in determining the presence or absence of such mental health conditions. To a lesser extent, parental responses to the semistructured interview can do this. Parent and teacher completion of the BASC yields a wealth of clinical information relevant to non-AD/HD psychopathology. Particularly helpful is the fact that the BASC subscales address these different types of psychopathology from a dimensional point of view, thereby providing a mechanism for examining the developmental deviance of these conditions. At times, reviews of records may reveal information about the existence of diagnostic conditions (e.g., learning disorders) that might better account for observed AD/HD symptoms and functional impairment. If information from these procedures produces no evidence of any other condition, Criterion E is automatically met. If other diagnostic conditions are detected, it is necessary to determine whether they realistically provide a better explanation for the child's symptoms and functional impairment. Although not foolproof, an excellent way to determine this is through careful documentation of the historical unfolding of each possible disorder, which often allows clinicians to rule them out because their onset occurred long after the child's AD/HD symptoms and functional impairment appeared.

Addressing Comorbidity Concerns

Assume we have administered our multimethod assessment battery and scored its data. Further assume that we have analyzed these data and have concluded that AD/HD was present. Arriving at this conclusion might end the assessment process for some child health-care professionals, but this would be a serious mistake, because many children and adolescents with AD/HD exhibit secondary diagnostic concerns that require therapeutic attention. As noted in Chapter 3, up to 60% of children and adolescents with AD/HD have additional behavioral complications, including ODD and CD, and a relatively high percentage has mood disorders, anxiety conditions, and learning disabilities.

If a clinician simply wants to screen for AD/HD, the possibility that such comorbid features might be present is not a major assessment concern. To the professional conducting a more comprehensive evaluation, it takes on tremendous clinical importance. Knowing which comorbid features are or are not present clarifies the overall severity of a child's psychosocial impairment, which can have a significant effect on treatment planning.

Thus, clinicians must include assessment procedures that address the question:

> Above and beyond AD/HD, are there any additional behavioral, emotional, social, learning, or psychiatric problems present?

All the procedures that addressed Criterion E (exclusionary conditions) would be suitable for this purpose as well, including the DISC-IV, the semistructured interview, the parent- and teacher-completed BASC, and record reviews (see Figure 5.7.). Clinicians might also need to test for learning disorders. Less often, observations of peer interaction may be conducted to evaluate social skills. Though it is not our intention to describe the exact manner in which every possible comorbid condition is diagnosed, many of the same principles for diagnosing AD/HD apply to the assessment of comorbidities. Particularly critical is the issue of developmental deviance. As with AD/HD, there should be documentation of the developmental deviance of any comorbid symptoms. Consistent with this principle, we would not establish a comorbid diagnosis of Oppositional-Defiant Disorder on the basis of parental responses to the DISC-IV alone. We would, however, make this diagnosis if these DISC-IV results were corroborated by evidence of developmental deviance, as defined by *T* scores at or above 65 on the Aggression subscale of the parent- or teacher-completed BASC.

Addressing Parent and Family Problems

In addition to determining whether any secondary conditions are present, clinicians must also clarify the extent to which parents and other family members have psychosocial difficulties of their own. Although this was covered in part in the earlier discussion of impairment in home functioning (Criterion C), here the emphasis is on the possibility of family complications that exist independent of the child's or adolescent's AD/HD. Left unchecked, they could exacerbate the child's problems or seriously interfere with the family's efforts to implement the child's recommended treatment strategies. Clinicians must therefore incorporate procedures that allow them to answer the question:

> Is there any evidence of parenting stress, parental psychopathology, marital discord, or other disruptions in family functioning, due to factors other than the child's AD/HD?

Many procedures that assess functional impairment at home can be used for this (see Figure 5.4.). Among them are the PSI-SF, the SCL-90-R, the PAI, and the DAS-R. Although not used to address functional impairment, the Adult AD/HD Rating Scale—Self-Report can also screen for parental AD/HD problems. Knowing whether the parents themselves have AD/HD, other psychological problems, or relationship difficulties is essential for treatment planning, because steps can be taken to address these problems either prior to or concurrent with whatever interventions are implemented on behalf of the child. This puts parents in a better position to provide whatever therapeutic assistance their child might need, thereby enhancing the child's prognosis.

Inconsistent, Incomplete, or Missing Data

When data are gathered via a multimethod assessment battery, there is an excellent chance that inconsistencies will arise across informants, across methods, or across both. If some of the data suggest that the *DSM-IV* criteria have been met but some do not, what conclusion should be drawn? Faced with such a dilemma, some clinicians might reason that, as long as some of the data indicate the presence of AD/HD, the diagnosis should be made. Others might instead argue that the diagnosis should not be considered in the face of contradictory evidence. Still others might contend that the best way to resolve this situation lies somewhere in between these two arguments. Unfortunately, there are no empirically validated guidelines for addressing inconsistencies, so clinicians handle it subjectively.

Differences of opinion across informants is the most common inconsistency. This can include discrepancies between mothers and fathers, between parents and teachers, and between teachers. Such discrepancies do not necessarily mean that one informant is being truthful and the other is not. More likely, both informants are accurately reporting what they see, with the discrepancies reflecting the different conditions under which they observe the child. This is consistent with AD/HD's situational variability. As noted earlier, AD/HD symptoms are much more likely in repetitive, familiar, boring situations. They are also more evident in group situations and in situations where children are left unsupervised or given infrequent, delayed feedback about their performance. Finding the differences in situational demands can help to make sense of discrepant data.

For example, a mother might report that her child displays AD/HD symptoms, whereas the child's father does not. Might the different demands that each parent places on the child provide an explanation for their difference of opinion? As described by one couple who recently came to our clinic, the mother was responsible for getting her son up in the morning; for helping him get breakfast, get cleaned up, and get dressed for school; for accompanying him to and from the bus; for giving him a snack and then overseeing completion of his homework; for reminding him to do afternoon chores; for getting him to sit down at the table for dinner; for asking him to shower, brush his teeth, and change into pajamas before bed; and for getting him to bed on schedule. What about the father? His role centered around having breakfast with his son in the morning, eating dinner with him in the evening, and then talking or playing with him after dinner. Although this is an extreme, rather stereotyped example, it highlights the different daily demands that each parent can place on a child. The father primarily did things that the child enjoyed; the mother was responsible for getting the child to do many things that might best be described as repetitive, familiar, and boring. It is easy to see why the mother would report

AD/HD symptoms and the father would not. Many other cross-informant differences can be resolved when situational variability is considered.

When situational variability is not the explanation, however, other factors must be considered. Among these are family and parental influences. For parents in the midst of serious marital tensions, differences in how they describe their child's behavior may relate more to playing out marital battles than to accurately reporting what they see. Perceptions of child behavior can also be affected by parental psychopathology, especially depression. Commonly, depressed parents view their child's behavior as more negative than it actually is. Thus personal and marital difficulties can explain why one parent sees things a certain way and the other does not.

The potential for parental bias has led some to propose that teacher input is more accurate and should be given more weight in the assessment process. Although there may be some merit to this based on the child development training that most teachers receive, it is a mistake to side routinely with teachers, because they too are subject to psychological distress and interpersonal problems. For obvious reasons, one cannot assess the psychological status of the teacher. Thus, clinicians can never really be sure if the information they're receiving from teachers is biased or not. The point is that it can be. Thus, clinicians should not automatically give greater weighting to teachers whenever differences of opinion with parents arise.

Data inconsistencies are not limited to discrepancies across informants. Sometimes they arise within the same informant. If the data from the same informant via two different procedures (e.g., interview and rating scale) are not that discrepant or contradictory, it is usually safe to go with the procedure suggestive of greater pathology. If, on the other hand, the information is vastly discrepant, one must examine the conditions under which the data were collected. Such an examination might, for example, reveal that interviews were conducted several weeks after rating scales were completed, during which time the child's behavior changed. In situations like this, it is often best to give greater weight to the more recent data.

Inconsistencies can also emerge in comparisons between rating scale results and findings from clinic-based testing. Some argue that more weight should be placed on the clinic results because they provide a more objective picture of the child's behavior and performance. Others counter that clinic-based tests have limited ecological validity. Remembering situational variability can again help to resolve this difference of professional opinion. The novel, one-to-one, highly structured nature of clinic-based testing increases the likelihood of relatively normal findings. So it seems reasonable to place less emphasis on clinic-based results when they differ from parent and teacher ratings. Additional reason for weighting parent and teacher input more heavily stems from a consideration of how children come to professional attention in the first place. Referrals are prompted not because children do poorly on tests that purportedly measure AD/HD symptoms, but because the child is not behaving or performing according to parent or teacher expectations. Thus, biased or not, input from parents and teachers is ecologically important and should be treated as such.

Another diagnostic obstacle is when data do not adequately address certain portions of the *DSM-IV* criteria. Although the intent of the multimethod approach is to eliminate this, it is sometimes unavoidable. An example of how this might occur is when a ten-year-old child arrives for an evaluation with a stepparent who has little knowledge of the youngster's early history and is therefore unable to address the onset criteria. One obvious solution is to administer additional assessment procedures to elicit the missing information, perhaps telephoning one or both of the child's biological parents to clarify symptom onset. Sometimes parent and teacher rating scales are returned with missing information. Fortunately, this is not a serious problem. Given the usual lag time between receipt of the rating scales and face-to-face contact with child and family, there is ample opportunity to see what's missing and obtain it. This usually is when the scales are being scored. If the packet is incomplete, the clinician can mail the packet back for completion, complete it over the phone, or simply have the parent finish it during the face-to-face evaluation. Similar attempts can be made to retrieve missing teacher data.

Sometimes obtaining additional assessment data is not an option. Such is often the case for children in foster care. For example, an older child may arrive for an evaluation with a foster parent who has known the youngster for less than 6 months. This might be just the most recent in a long string of foster-care placements, and the child may have been enrolled in multiple schools and had several different case managers. Obviously, trying to address the AD/HD duration and onset criteria—not to mention many other clinically relevant matters—would be an enormous challenge.

Inconsistent, incomplete, or missing data are certainly not a regular feature of every evaluation, but they do occur often enough to complicate the diagnostic process. Regardless of which complication might arise, one very important fact remains—a decision regarding the presence or absence of AD/HD must still be made, albeit with varying degrees of certainty.

PUTTING THE PIECES TOGETHER

Establishing a diagnosis is like putting a puzzle together. If there are enough pieces and if they fit together properly, they will form a clear, unmistakable picture—in this case, either an AD/HD diagnosis, as depicted in Figure 5.8., or some other diagnostic explanation. At times, pieces may be missing or may not fit (due to incomplete or inconsistent data). As long as enough pieces are assembled, it may still be possible to recognize the picture (see Figure 5.9.). If, on the other hand, too many pieces are missing, discerning the picture may be impossible (see Figure 5.10.), in which case no diagnosis can be established.

Implicit in the preceding discussion are several important points. First and foremost is the notion that the more assessment data that are available to a clinician, the more likely it is that he or she will be able to render an accurate diagnostic decision. Related to this issue of diagnostic accuracy is the matter of diagnostic certainty. The more pieces of evidence that converge on a particular diagnostic criterion, the more confidence one can have in the validity of the diagnosis.

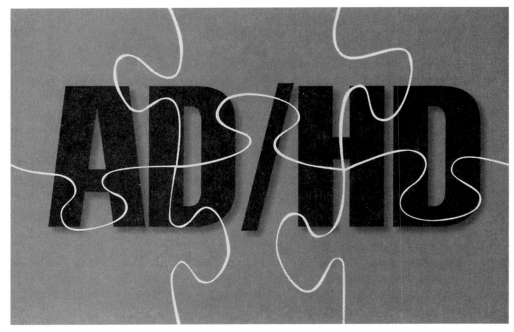

Figure 5.8. Clear diagnosis of AD/HD emerging from the assessment puzzle.

In many ways this is the driving force behind the multimethod assessment battery. The multimethod approach generates an enormous amount of data covering not only the *DSM-IV* criteria for ADHD, but also various comorbid conditions, and problems that may exist in the home. This approach has numerous checks and balances; nowhere is there reliance upon a single procedure. On the contrary, multiple assessment procedures address every one of the *DSM-IV* criteria, and likewise, reveal any comorbidities or family problems.

Little Puzzle Pieces

In keeping with this spirit of "more is better," we would now like to call attention to additional, somewhat obscure sources of information that can be gleaned from our multimethod assessment battery. One would not normally think to include them because they have little direct bearing on the *DSM-IV* criteria, but they can serve as little pieces of our diagnostic puzzle. Combined with the larger pieces, they further sharpen the picture, facilitating the diagnostic process.

The first of these smaller pieces is found in the anecdotal comments that parents and teachers sometimes make, during interviews and other informal contacts; spontaneous remarks of diagnostic significance. Some of these comments have already been mentioned earlier in this text. For example, one parent

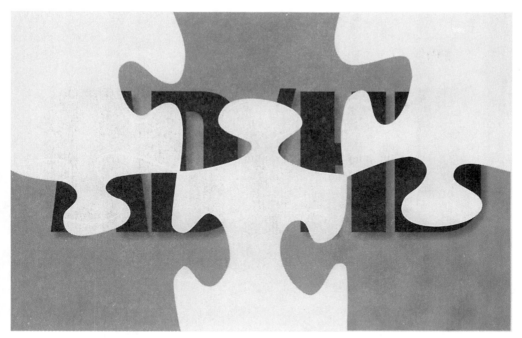

FIGURE 5.9. Probable diagnosis of AD/HD emerging from the assessment puzzle.

once remarked, "Once he learned how to walk, all hell broke loose." Another quipped, "These kids are a lot like helium balloons, you let go of them for one second and they're all over the place." Still another lamented, "She goes to bed talking and wakes up talking ... do you have any idea how hard it is riding in a car with her for three hours?" Such comments do not directly address the *DSM-IV* criteria, but they increase a clinician's confidence in the validity of the data captured through the multimethod procedures.

Comments from teachers can do the same. Sometimes these comments appear in school records. This might be revealed in the comments section of a first grade report card where a teacher has written, "has trouble following directions," "does work carelessly," "not working up potential," or "needs to settle down." Another place where incidental teacher comments may be found is along the rating scale margins. An excellent example of this appeared on the back of an AD/HD Rating Scale-IV returned by a dedicated and insightful third grade teacher, who wrote:

> Michael is a child with great potential. He appears to be very bright, has much general knowledge, a wonderful oral vocabulary, and seems to absorb a lot even if I think he is not listening. *But* he will not produce unless an adult is standing right next to him. When left on his own after work is thoroughly explained, nothing gets done. It is difficult to evaluate where he stands as far his grade level because many times work is incomplete or hurried at the last minute. I have no doubt, however, that Michael could easily produce above grade level in all areas if he applied himself.

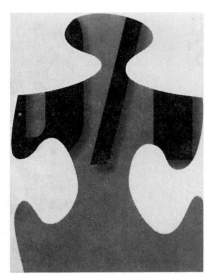

FIGURE 5.10. Uncertain diagnosis of AD/HD emerging from the assessment puzzle.

This teacher comment is unusual in its length and clinical detail, but variations of this type of teacher input are commonplace.

Additional diagnostic information can come from the semistructured interview and the Developmental and Health History form, which both contain data having etiological implications. In the family portion of our Semi-Structured Background Interview, many questions deal with the psychiatric and medical histories of the immediate and extended family. Many times such questioning reveals that family members either have been diagnosed with AD/HD or are strongly suspected of having it. Included in the Developmental and Health History form are questions about maternal smoking and drinking during pregnancy, as well as about lead poisoning and head injuries. Commonly, mothers of children with AD/HD indicate that some of these circumstances have occurred. These data alone are not proof of an AD/HD etiology, nor are they intended to be, but they are certainly consistent with an AD/HD diagnosis.

The main point is this: In addition to producing large puzzle pieces, multimethod assessments very often contain small pieces that are clinically useful. Their inclusion sharpens the picture, building a stronger case for whatever diagnostic conclusion is ultimately made.

CASE EXAMPLES

With this puzzle analogy in mind, we now give examples of how to establish an AD/HD diagnosis—not just when all the pieces are in place and fit well together, but also when pieces are missing, due to inconsistent, incomplete, or missing data. In each case we follow the order of the *DSM-IV* criteria that we outlined earlier, addressing each criterion with the aid of the decision trees presented in Figures 5.2. through 5.7. As part of this discussion, we also address comorbidity issues and family problems.

Ross D.

Ross D. is an 8-year-old Caucasian boy enrolled in a regular third grade classroom. He was referred by his parents because of numerous home and school difficulties including excessive fidgeting, difficulty following through on assigned tasks, and working below his potential. He was evaluated for these same concerns about a year earlier by a local psychologist, who found no evidence of AD/HD or any other psychological problem. Because their concern persisted, Mr. and Mrs. D. decided to have him evaluated again.

Background Information

Ross's developmental history was unremarkable. He has been in good health throughout his lifetime. He does not take any prescription medications for behavior management purposes. He and two younger half-siblings live with their parents in a home where the family has resided for the past year. Ross maintains typical relations with his siblings, neither of whom has any major medical, behavioral, or learning problems. Mr. and Mrs. D. have been together for nearly 7 years and married for the last 3, with no major difficulties in their relationship. No psychosocial stressors have occurred in the past year. There is no extended-family history of AD/HD, but several maternal relatives have displayed conduct problems and antisocial behavior, as well as learning disorders.

Throughout his schooling Ross has performed at grade level to somewhat below grade level academically. His parents and teachers believe that his achievement is well below his potential. Despite such concerns, he has not undergone any school-based testing, nor has he received special-education assistance.

Apart from the assessment done a year ago by the psychologist, Ross has had no psychological testing. Thus, he carries no diagnoses and has received no psychotherapy.

Assessment Results

A summary of the parent- and teacher-completed rating scale results appears in Table 5.2. Ross's testing results are presented in Table 5.3. Based upon these findings and other information from the assessment battery, we will now consider whether Ross meets *DSM-IV* criteria for AD/HD using the order shown in Figure 5.2. Simultaneously, we will also determine whether any comorbid disorders are present.

Criterion D.   A review of Ross's school records revealed consistent comments that he was perhaps not working up to his potential. Although the APRS re-

TABLE 5.2.   Summary of Parent and Teacher Rating Scale Results for Ross D.

Rating scale	Rater			
	Mother	Father	Teacher A	Teacher B
AD/HD Rating Scale-IV				
Inattention	24	21	17	3
Hyperactive-Impulsive	26	23	24	6
Behavior Assessment System for Children				
Hyperactivity	83	74	74	52
Aggression	72	53	67	53
Conduct Problems	57	54	49	46
Anxiety	45	68	51	44
Depression	67	59	68	55
Somatization	47	47	42	42
Atypicality	61	57	64	64
Withdrawal	42	55	64	48
Attention Problems	71	68	57	46
Learning Problems	*	*	51	39
Adaptability	36	36	37	50
Social Skills	34	52	49	54
Leadership	50	55	63	66
Study Skills	*	*	52	59
Academic Performance Rating Scale				
Academic Success	*	*	27	30
Productivity	*	*	26	38
Parenting Stress Index—Short Form				
Total Stress	97	110	*	*
Parenting Scale				
Total	2.4	2.9	*	*
Symptom Checklist-90—Revised				
General Severity	63	*	*	*
Adult AD/HD Rating Scale				
Total Severity	29	*	*	*
Revised Dyadic Adjustment Scale				
Total Score	52	*	*	*
Parenting Alliance Inventory				
Total Score	76	*	*	*

Note: * = not applicable or not available.

vealed no deficit in his Academic Success score, his Academic Productivity score was 1 standard deviation below the mean for his grade and gender. The IQ and achievement tests gave even stronger evidence for academic impairment. There was a substantial discrepancy between his predicted achievement (129 ± 15) and his actual achievement in reading, math, and spelling, which ranged from 91 to 96. Additional evidence came from Mrs. D.'s responses to DISC-IV and semistructured interview questioning. The PSI-SF results from both parents revealed high levels of parenting stress; both were well above the clinical cut-point of 91. Impaired home functioning was evident from Mrs. D.'s responses to the DISC-IV and the semistructured interview. Her elevated SCL-90-R score

TABLE 5.3. Summary of Child Testing Results for Ross D.

Test	Score	Test	Score
Wechsler Intelligence Scale for Children-III		Wechsler Individual Achievement Test	
Verbal IQ	129	Reading Standard score	91
Performance IQ	123	Math Standard score	96
Full Scale IQ	129	Spelling Standard score	93
Verbal Comprehension Index	136	Conners' Continuous Performance	
Perceptual Organization Index	133	Test	
Freedom fron Distractibility Index	98	Omission Errors	57
Processing Speed	86	Commission Errors	60
Picture Completion	17	Hit Reaction Time	58
Information	16	Standard Error for Hit Reaction	55
Coding	5	Time	
Similarities	16	Variability of Reaction Time	52
Picture Arrangement	9	Attentiveness	54
Arithmetic	10	Risk Taking	58
Block Design	19		
Vocabulary	15		
Object Assembly	17		
Comprehension	18		
Symbol Search	9		
Digit Span	9		
Mazes	*		

Note: * = not available.

raised the possibility that she was experiencing psychological distress that might be related to raising a difficult child. Deficits in Ross's social functioning were found in Mrs. D.'s BASC responses, which produced a Social Skills sub-scale score 1.5 standard deviations below the mean. Taken together, these findings provided ample evidence for impairment in Ross's school, home, and social functioning. Thus, Criterion D was met.

Criterion C. Evidence for AD/HD symptoms in school was reported by the first of two teachers providing input on Ross. This came from Teacher A's hyperactive-impulsive score on the AD/HD Rating Scale-IV and hyperactivity score on the BASC. Coupled with the impairment in his academic achievement, this provided evidence consistent with the notion that Ross's functional impairment in school might be related to his AD/HD symptoms. Likewise, the AD/HD Rating Scale-IV results from both parents produced inattention and hyperactive-impulsive scores suggestive of AD/HD problems at home. Their BASC Attention Problems and Hyperactivity subscale scores further corroborated such symptoms. Ross's CPT also yielded evidence of impulsivity problems, shown by his higher-than-expected commission error score. Overall, these findings revealed evidence of AD/HD symptoms in multiple settings where functional impairment was also found. Thus the cross-situational pervasiveness requirement of criterion C was met.

Criterion A.   Mrs. D.'s responses to the DISC-IV indicated that Ross frequently displayed 7 of 9 inattention symptoms and 9 of 9 hyperactive-impulsive symptoms, meeting the frequency requirement of Criterion A. As for the developmental deviance aspect, evidence suggested that it too had been met: Both parents' inattention scores from the AD/HD Rating Scale-IV fell above the 98th percentile, as did their hyperactive-impulsive scores. Mr. and Mrs. D.'s BASC responses produced Attention Problems subscale scores between the 93rd and 98th percentiles and Hyperactivity subscale scores well above the 98th percentile. Additional evidence of the developmental deviance of Ross's inattention and hyperactivity-impulsivity came from Teacher A's BASC Hyperactivity subscale, which fell above the 98th percentile. On the Conners' CPT, Ross's high commission error score was not quite as deviant (84th percentile), but together such findings showed that Ross's inattention and hyperactive-impulsive symptoms were developmentally deviant. Mrs. D.'s responses to the DISC-IV and to the semistructured interview left little doubt that Ross had been displaying symptoms of inattention and hyperactivity-impulsivity for the past 6 months. In sum, frequency, developmental deviance, and duration of Ross's AD/HD symptoms were all clinically significant, fulfilling the requirements of Criterion A.

Criterion B.   Mrs. D.'s responses to the DISC-IV and the semistructured interview showed that she was well aware of Ross's difficulties dating back to approximately 6 years of age. School records indicated that his teachers were concerned about his behavior and academic performance when he was in first grade. Thus, onset of symptoms before age 7 was established.

Criterion E.   Mrs. D.'s responses to the BASC produced a Depression subscale score for Ross that was in the clinically significant range. Mr. D.'s BASC responses suggested the possible presence of clinically significant anxiety. Input obtained from Teacher A was in line with Mrs. D.'s responses, revealing a BASC Depression subscale score in the clinically significant range. Despite the fact that hints of depression and anxiety emerged from the BASC, there was no evidence whatsoever of clinically significant levels of depression or anxiety from the DISC-IV or from the semistructured interview conducted with Ross or Mrs. D. Although there were never any concerns about learning disorders, his WISC-III performance hinted at visual–motor problems, as evidenced by his focally low score on the Coding subtest, but even if this indicated a motor-based learning disorder, it would not by itself account for the spectrum of problems Ross was having. Thus, there was little reason to believe that a learning disorder or any other condition might be accounting for his difficulties. Criterion E was therefore addressed.

Comorbidity

Although no exclusionary condition was detected, there was ample evidence from the current evaluation that Ross might be displaying a secondary condition. More specifically, Mrs. D.'s responses to the DISC-IV indicated that he was displaying a total of 5 out of 8 symptoms of ODD, including noncompliance with requests, argumentativeness, and frequent temper outbursts. Evidence for the developmental deviance of these oppositional-defiant features came from parent and teacher rating scale responses. The BASC Aggression subscale fell above the 95th percentile for Mrs. D. and for Teacher A. Together, these interview and rating scale results raised the possibility of comorbid ODD. As noted above, there was also a possible motor-based learning disability.

Parent and Family Concerns

Mrs. D.'s score on the SCL-90-R was clinically significant, suggesting a high level of psychological distress. Likewise, her adult AD/HD Rating Scale score fell more than 2 standard deviations outside the mean for her age and gender, indicating that she may have been affected by both personal problems and by adult AD/HD symptoms.

Diagnostic Conclusion

The assessment results produced clear evidence that Ross met *DSM-IV* criteria for a diagnosis of Attention-Deficit/Hyperactivity Disorder, Combined Type (314.01). In addition, he met the *DSM-IV* criteria for a secondary diagnosis of Oppositional-Defiant Disorder (313.81). Together, these conditions were likely responsible for his diminished academic productivity, the significant gap between his predicted and actual educational achievement, his peer relationship problems, and the elevated parenting stress reported by both parents. No other major diagnostic concerns emerged from this evaluation, but evidence suggested that depression and anxiety might be emerging. Moreover, the possibility of a visual–motor problem was raised. In addition to these child concerns, there was reason to believe that his mother might be having adult AD/HD difficulties and other psychological distress.

Assessment Issues of Interest

Several important points are evident in this case presentation. First, given the many pieces in Ross's assessment puzzle, the diagnostic picture that emerged was akin to that in Figure 5.8. In other words, the picture was clear and there was little doubt about the AD/HD and ODD diagnoses. This case example shows the importance of a comprehensive, multimethod assessment. The likelihood that Ross was not displaying clinically significant AD/HD or ODD problems when he was evaluated by the local psychologist is slim. According to Mr. and Mrs. D, the psychologist evaluated Ross primarily by interviewing and testing him in his office. The particular assessment methods used very likely account for the faulty diagnostic conclusion that this psychologist made. Another point this case illustrates is that despite Mrs. D.'s elevated level of personal distress, her input was nonetheless very much consistent with what her husband and Teacher A provided. Thus, one should not discount parent input just because the parent has personal difficulties. Of additional interest is that

Teacher B's perspective not only differed from that of Mr. and Mrs. D., but also from that of Teacher A, again highlighting the situational variability of AD/HD symptoms, even within the same setting. One final point is that Ross's WISC-III freedom from distractibility score was significantly lower than his verbal comprehension and perceptual organization scores. Although this type of discrepancy is often not apparent in testing results obtained from most children with AD/HD, in this case it was.

David H.

David H. is a 10-year-old Caucasian male enrolled in a regular fifth grade classroom. His pediatrician referred him because of long-standing concerns about his short attention span, behavioral immaturity, and other home and school problems suggestive of AD/HD.

Background Information

David's early developmental history was unremarkable. Throughout his lifetime he has maintained excellent physical health. He has a three-year-old sister with whom he gets along quite well. No behavioral or medical problems were reported for this sibling. Both of David's parents were high school educated and working full time. Mr. and Mrs. H. had been married for 11 years and their relationship was relatively stable. Neither had a history of significant psychiatric difficulties. There was no report of AD/HD or other psychiatric problems among the extended relatives. Over the past 12 months there were no major psychosocial stressors affecting the immediate family.

Due to concerns about David's lack of progress in reading and his behavioral immaturity, he underwent school-based testing in the second grade, which showed him to be of normal intelligence in the absence of specific learning disabilities. He has received no special-education assistance. Despite his normal intelligence, David's academic achievement has consistently been somewhat below grade level.

Except for the school-based testing, David had not undergone any psychological assessment. Likewise, he had received no individual therapy. Apart from occasional assistance from school personnel, Mr. and Mrs. H. received no on-going advice about managing David's behavior problems at home.

Assessment Results

Summaries of the rating scale results and of David's psychological testing results appear in Tables 5.4. and 5.5., respectively. These data will be used in combination with other findings from the multimethod evaluation to determine whether David meets the re-ordered criteria for AD/HD. Comorbidity and various parent and family concerns will be addressed as well.

Criterion D.   Evidence for impairment in school functioning came primarily from a review of school records, which showed David to be working at least a

TABLE 5.4.   Summary of Parent and Teacher
Rating Scale Results for David H.

Rating scale	Rater		
	Mother	Father	Teacher A
AD/HD Rating Scale-IV			
Inattention	25	19	12
Hyperactive-Impulsive	4	9	10
Behavior Assessment System for Children			
Hyperactivity	48	50	61
Aggression	45	41	53
Conduct Problems	60	50	52
Anxiety	45	45	42
Depression	66	67	61
Somatization	36	36	51
Atypicality	55	46	53
Withdrawal	59	49	41
Attention Problems	71	73	67
Learning Problems	*	*	53
Adaptability	53	59	46
Social Skills	35	40	46
Leadership	37	39	47
Study Skills	*	*	45
Academic Performance Rating Scale			
Academic Success	*	*	21
Productivity	*	*	34
Parenting Stress Index—Short Form			
Total Stress	99	82	*
Parenting Scale			
Total	4.2	2.8	*
Symptom Checklist-90—Revised			
General Severity	65	49	*
Adult AD/HD Rating Scale			
Total Severity	14	1	*
Revised Dyadic Adjustment Scale			
Total Score	38	51	*
Parenting Alliance Inventory			
Total Score	82	89	*

Note: * = not applicable or not available.

half-grade level below his peers. The evaluation produced no other evidence of impairment in his school functioning. David's APRS scores were within normal limits, and there were no significant discrepancies between his actual academic achievement and that predicted by his intelligence test results. In contrast, there was ample evidence of impairment in home functioning. Mrs. H.'s PSI-SF score of 99 was above the clinical cutoff of 91, indicating elevated parenting stress. Her SCL-90-R score was also elevated significantly, raising the possibility that she was experiencing other types of personal distress, including depression and anxiety, that might be related to the stress of raising David. Mrs. H.'s PS score

TABLE 5.5. Summary of Child Testing Results for David H.

Test	Score	Test	Score
Wechsler Intelligence Scale for Children-III		Wechsler Individual Achievement Test	
Verbal IQ	101	Reading Standard score	101
Performance IQ	87	Math Standard score	97
Full Scale IQ	94	Spelling Standard score	105
Verbal Comprehension Index	103	Conners' Continuous Performance	
Perceptual Organization Index	89	Test	
Freedom fron Distractibility Index	90	Omission Errors	65
Processing Speed	*	Commission Errors	53
Picture Completion	10	Hit Reaction Time	50
Information	11	Standard Error for Hit Reaction	66
Coding	8	Time	
Similarities	10	Variability of Reaction Time	61
Picture Arrangement	10	Attentiveness	58
Arithmetic	9	Risk Taking	54
Block Design	6		
Vocabulary	10		
Object Assembly	6		
Comprehension	11		
Symbol Search	*		
Digit Span	7		
Mazes	*		

Note: * = not available.

was more than 2 standard deviations beyond the mean suggesting difficulties in managing his home behavior. Additional evidence of home-based difficulties came from Mrs. H.'s responses to the DISC-IV and the semistructured interview. Input received from Mrs. H., and to a lesser extent from Mr. H., suggested that David's peer relations were below average, based on Mrs. H.'s BASC Social Skills subscale score, which fell 1.5 standard deviations below the mean. Though less extreme, Mr. H.'s BASC score on this subscale was in the same direction. Thus, there was sufficient evidence for impairment in multiple domains, meeting the requirements for Criterion D.

Criterion C. David's history showed some indication of impairment in school functioning, so the next question was whether David was displaying AD/HD symptoms in school. His teacher's BASC Attention Problems subscale provided this evidence. The existence of AD/HD symptoms in the home was shown in the DISC-IV, in the inattention scores from the AD/HD Rating Scale-IV completed by both parents, and in the BASC Attention Problems subscales of both parents. Informal observations of David during the clinic-based testing did not reveal any AD/HD symptomatology, but indications of inattention emerged from the Conners' CPT results. Overall, the evidence revealed AD/HD symptoms in the settings where functional impairment had been detected, thus Criterion C was met.

Criterion A.   Mrs. H.'s responses to the DISC-IV indicated that David had frequently been displaying 8 of 9 inattention symptoms, but only 2 of 9 hyperactive-impulsive symptoms. Thus, the frequency aspect of Criterion A was met. Developmental deviance for these symptoms was apparent from multiple sources. The AD/HD Rating Scale-IV inattention score obtained from David's mother fell above the 98th percentile; the same score from his father was above the 93rd percentile. The BASC Attention Problems subscale scores from both parents were more than 2 standard deviations above the mean, falling above the 98th percentile. The BASC Attention Problems subscale from David's teacher was at the 93rd percentile. The omission error score and several other inattention indices from the Conners' CPT also fell beyond the 93rd percentile. Together these data documented the developmental deviance of David's inattention symptoms but not of his hyperactivity-impulsivity symptoms, which were minimal. The 6-months' duration requirement was met through Mrs. H.'s DISC-IV responses, her responses to semistructured interview questioning, and from a review of David's school records. In sum, these findings showed that the frequency, developmental deviance, and duration of David's AD/HD symptoms were clinically significant. All aspects of Criterion A were therefore addressed.

Criterion B.   Mrs. H.'s responses to the DISC-IV and to the semistructured interview questioning indicated that she was aware of David's inattention during kindergarten. Moreover, she recognized that he was having learning difficulties stemming from his inattention beginning in first grade; in fact, these difficulties were the reason he was referred for school-based testing at the start of second grade. Taken together, this information established an onset of AD/HD symptoms prior to 7 years of age, thereby meeting Criterion B.

Criterion E.   Nothing in David's school or medical records suggested significant learning or medical problems, nor did the current evaluation produce evidence of clear-cut learning difficulties. However, Mrs. H.'s responses to the DISC-IV revealed that David often seemed sad and irritable, and that this had been occurring fairly regularly for the past 2 years. Moreover, during this time his self-esteem was low, he had trouble concentrating and making decisions, and he expressed feelings of hopelessness, raising the possibility of Dysthymic Disorder. Concentration problems are part of this condition, so we had to consider the possibility that Dysthymic Disorder might provide a better explanation for David's problems. Because most of these depression symptoms surfaced approximately 2 years after his inattention symptoms were first noticed, his inattention probably existed independent of depression. Thus, Dysthymic Disorder did not rule out AD/HD. No other major diagnostic concerns emerged from the evaluation, so there was no viable alternative explanation for the concerns that prompted it. In the absence of any exclusionary condition, Criterion E was met.

Comorbidity

As noted above, the DISC-IV results indicated Dysthymic Disorder might be present. Further evidence for this was found in the BASC Depression subscale results from both parents and to a lesser extent, from David's teacher. The scores from his parents on this BASC index fell above the 93rd percentile and the score from his teacher was above the 84th percentile. Together with the DISC-IV results, these BASC findings indicated that Dysthymic Disorder was present. No other comorbid diagnoses emerged.

Parent and Family Concerns

No major family relationship problems were evident, but there was a substantial amount of parenting stress reported by David's mother, and her Parenting Scale responses showed less-than-effective parenting strategies. Moreover, Mrs. H.'s SCL-90-R suggested personal problems characterized by depression and anxiety, though how much these symptoms stemmed from her difficulties raising David was not clear.

Diagnostic Conclusion

The above findings warranted a diagnosis of AD/HD, Predominantly Inattentive Type (314.01), along with Dysthymic Disorder (300.40), the cause of which was not entirely clear. No obvious psychosocial stressors seemed to be at work, though possibly it was a consequence of his AD/HD impairment. Whatever the reason, these conditions together were viewed as factors contributing to David's difficulties in school, at home, and to a lesser extent, in peer relationships. No other major learning, behavioral, or emotional difficulties emerged from the evaluation, at least with respect to David, but concerns did surface regarding his mother's elevated levels of personal distress and parenting stress.

Assessment Issues of Interest

This case nicely illustrates a commonly encountered subtyping variation of AD/HD, coupled with comorbid internalizing problems. There was fairly good agreement across all 3 informants with respect to AD/HD and dysthymic symptoms. The inattention indices of the Conners' CPT corroborated the parent- and teacher-completed rating scales. Somewhat surprisingly, the teacher-completed AD/HD Rating Scale-IV was not in line with the teacher's BASC results or with the input obtained from either parent. Another discrepancy was that neither the APRS nor the psychological testing results showed any impairment in school functioning, contrary to what was consistently reported in school records. In view of such inconsistencies, the diagnostic picture emerging from this evaluation is analogous to that depicted in Figure 5.9. As in the preceding case presentation (Ross), Mrs. H.'s elevated personal distress did not cloud her perception. Her evaluation responses were in line with those of her husband and her son's teacher, again highlighting the importance of not automatically discounting input from a parent experiencing personal problems. Of additional interest is that David's WISC-III freedom from distractibility score was not significantly lower than either his verbal comprehension or perceptual organizational factor index scores. In contrast with our previous case, Ross, this case highlights why sole reliance on this index often leads to incorrect diagnostic conclusions.

Mark L.

Mark L. is a 16-year-old African American male in 10th grade, with a history of behavioral and academic problems. He was referred primarily to determine whether these difficulties were due to Attention-Deficit/Hyperactivity Disorder. A secondary purpose was to assess his intellectual functioning.

Background Information

Mark was the product of a normal pregnancy, but his delivery was complicated by skull trauma that resulted in brain hemorrhaging. The remainder of his neonatal course was unremarkable. Mark reached most developmental milestones at age-appropriate times. Apart from his delivery complications, Mark has been in good health throughout his lifetime. Mark and his 12-year-old stepsister live with their biological mother and stepfather. Mark's biological father died unexpectedly more than 10 years ago. Mrs. L. and Mark's stepfather have been married for the past 9 years, during which time their relationship has been stable. Both parents are college-educated and employed full time. Neither has a history of significant medical or psychiatric difficulties. No major lifestyle changes or psychosocial stressors have occurred over the past 12 months. Among the extended biological relatives there is a maternal family history of AD/HD, antisocial behavior, and dyslexia.

Mark attended regular preschool before enrolling in a public school kindergarten at age 5. From 2nd through 10th grades he attended three different parochial schools; two of these school changes occurred over the past 2 years. Upon returning to public school this year, Mark was deficient in many academic areas, so it was recommended that he repeat 10th grade for most classes. Throughout his schooling his academic grades have been mostly Cs, with occasional Ds and Fs. Despite this, Mark has never undergone formal psychological testing, nor has he received any special-education assistance.

Assessment Results

The parent- and teacher-completed rating scale results appear in Table 5.6. Mark's psychological testing results are presented in Table 5.7. As seen in Table 5.6., two teachers were asked to provide input. Apart from the AD/HD Rating Scale-IV and a few subscales of the BASC, most of the forms that these teachers returned were incomplete, and efforts to contact them to retrieve this missing data were unsuccessful. Thus, we had to evaluate him based primarily on input from Mark and his parents and from a review of his records. Bearing this limitation in mind, we will now review the results with respect to the *DSM-IV* criteria for AD/HD. We will also address comorbid problems and parent and family difficulties.

Criterion D. Two sources of information revealed impairment in Mark's school functioning, one being school records, which showed a long-standing pattern of academic failures and frustration and achievement well below grade level. Hints of academic difficulties were also evident from Mrs. L.'s responses to the

TABLE 5.6.   Summary of Parent and Teacher Rating Scale Results for Mark L.

	Rater			
Rating scale	Mother	Father	Teacher A	Teacher B
AD/HD Rating Scale-IV				
Inattention	23	19	12	14
Hyperactive-Impulsive	15	16	8	12
Behavior Assessment System for Children				
Hyperactivity	56	67	*	57
Aggression	78	78	*	*
Conduct Problems	75	86	*	*
Anxiety	37	49	*	*
Depression	39	57	*	*
Somatization	44	47	*	*
Atypicality	50	55	*	*
Withdrawal	37	44	*	*
Attention Problems	76	68	52	57
Learning Problems	*	*	*	*
Adaptability	41	28	*	*
Social Skills	38	25	*	*
Leadership	45	34	*	*
Study Skills	*	*	*	*
Symptom Checklist-90—Revised				
General Severity	50	*	*	*
Adult AD/HD Rating Scale				
Total Severity	6	5	*	*

Note: * = not applicable or not available.

DISC-IV and the semistructured interview, which were the primary sources for documenting the existence of deficits in Mark's home functioning. These procedures revealed that Mark frequently engaged in disagreements with both parents over a variety of daily activities, above and beyond what they felt was typical of boys his age. Of particular concern to them was his reluctance to do homework, which necessitated constant parental reminders. Mark's responses to interview questioning corroborated the existence of conflict with his parents, which he too deemed excessive. In their semistructured interview responses both Mark and his parents said that he had long-standing difficulties getting along with peers. Social problems were also evident in the BASC Social Skills subscales results from both parents, which placed Mark's social skills more than 2 standard deviations below the mean, corresponding to less than 2% of the general population of boys his age. Viewed together, these findings provided clear evidence of academic and social impairment. Although marginal, impairment in home functioning seemed present as well. On the basis of these findings, Criterion D was met.

Criterion C.   Readily apparent in Mark's school records and in Mrs. L.'s responses to both the DISC-IV and the semistructured interview were numerous

TABLE 5.7. Summary of Child Testing Results for Mark L.

Test	Score	Test	Score
Wechsler Intelligence Scale for Children-III		Wechsler Individual Achievement Test	
Verbal IQ	101	Reading Standard score	109
Performance IQ	75	Math Standard score	99
Full Scale IQ	87	Spelling Standard score	93
Verbal Comprehension Index	100	Conners' Continuous Performance	
Perceptual Organization Index	77	Test	
Freedom fron Distractibility Index	115	Omission Errors	69
Processing Speed	*	Commission Errors	57
Picture Completion	9	Hit Reaction Time	38
Information	12	Standard Error for Hit Reaction	64
Coding	6	Time	
Similarities	9	Variability of Reaction Time	55
Picture Arrangement	9	Attentiveness	58
Arithmetic	11	Risk Taking	55
Block Design	1		
Vocabulary	10		
Object Assembly	5		
Comprehension	9		
Symbol Search	*		
Digit Span	14		
Mazes	*		

Note: * = not available.

references to inattention and hyperactivity-impulsivity concerns. Mark himself acknowledged significant inattention problems in school that made it difficult to complete his work. Moreover, he said that he would often impulsively blurt out comments that caused trouble with his teachers. Although there was no direct evidence of AD/HD symptoms from either teacher, input obtained from Mark, his mother, and his records was enough to document their existence in the school setting. Mrs L.'s responses to the DISC-IV and the semistructured interview corroborated the existence of AD/HD symptoms in the home. Further evidence came from Mr. and Mrs. L.'s AD/HD Rating Scale-IV Inattention and Hyperactive-Impulsive subscales, as well as from their BASC Attention Problems and Hyperactivity subscales. Clear-cut evidence of AD/HD symptoms in social situations was not readily available, but Mark's CPT performance fell into the abnormal range on numerous indices of inattention, thereby providing evidence of impairment in another setting. Together, these results documented the presence of AD/HD symptoms in at least two settings where functional impairment had been detected. Thus, the cross-situational pervasiveness requirement of Criterion C was fulfilled.

Criterion A.   Input from Mark's teachers was of limited value. In contrast, Mrs. L.'s responses to the DISC-IV showed that Mark was frequently displaying seven of nine inattention symptoms and five out of nine hyperactive-impulsive symptoms, confirming that symptom frequency was clinically significant. The developmental deviance of these inattention symptoms was established in part through the parent rating scales. Mr. and Mrs. L.'s Inattention scores from the AD/HD Rating Scale-IV fell above the 93rd percentile, as did their ratings on the Hyperactive-Impulsive subscale from this same measure. Additional evidence of developmental deviance was found in their BASC responses, which produced Attention Problems subscale scores approximately 2 standard deviations beyond the mean for his age and gender, roughly corresponding to the 98th percentile. Similarly, the Conners' CPT results were developmentally deviant scores for the Omission Errors score and the Standard Error for Hit Reaction Time score; they fell above the 95th and 90th percentiles, respectively. As for the duration requirement, Mark's and his mother's responses to semistructured interview questioning indicated that his symptoms had been present for well over 6 months. This was further corroborated by Mrs. L.'s DISC-IV responses.

With respect to Mark's inattention symptoms, the findings suggested that they were of a sufficient frequency, developmental deviance, and duration to be considered clinically significant. Although both the duration and the developmental deviance of Mark's hyperactive-impulsive symptoms were clinically significant, there was no evidence that they met the *DSM-IV* frequency criteria. Mrs. L.'s endorsement of 5 hyperactive-impulsive symptoms fell just short of the required 6. Thus, although there were certainly elements of both inattention and hyperactivity-impulsivity, only the inattention symptoms met all of the requirements for Criterion A.

Criterion B.   Mrs. L.'s responses to the DISC-IV and to semistructured interview questioning indicated she was aware of Mark's AD/HD difficulties when he was approximately 4 years old. Careful reviews of Mark's school records showed that as early as first grade, teachers noticed his difficulties following through on instructions, finishing assigned work, and sitting still. The Developmental and Health History form revealed that Mrs. L. had endorsed item 11 in the temperament section, indicating that Mark was overactive and in constant motion during his first 12 months. Based on all the findings, it was clear that the onset of Mark's AD/HD symptoms occurred prior to 7 years of age, thereby meeting Criterion B.

Criterion E.   Mrs. L.'s responses to the DISC-IV indicated that Mark was frequently displaying 4 out of 8 symptoms suggestive of ODD, including being argumentative, noncompliant with rules, frequently angry, and prone to blame others for his own mistakes. Such problems were first evident when he was 10 years old, long after he had begun to display AD/HD symptoms, so this condition did not better account for Mark's lifelong pattern of problems. No other major behavioral, emotional, or psychiatric concerns emerged from either the DISC-IV or the semistructured interview, but results of the psychological testing raised the possibility of a learning disorder. In part this was based on the large and significant discrepancy between Mark's verbal comprehension abilities, which were average, and his perceptual organizational abilities, which were approximately 1.5 standard deviations below the mean. A more detailed analysis of the WISC-III subtest results highlighted his significant organizational difficulties, as shown by his focally low scores on the Block Design and Object Assembly subtests, a pattern consistent with nonverbal learning disabilities. This could account for some of Mark's inattention and long-standing academic problems, but certainly not all. Moreover, a nonverbal learning disability would not account for Mark's subclinical levels of hyperactivity-impulsivity. In view of such circumstances, it did not appear that a learning disorder or any other condition could better account for Mark's symptoms of inattention, hyperactivity-impulsivity, or history of functional impairment. Thus, the exclusionary requirement of Criterion E was considered met.

Comorbidity

Although there was insufficient evidence to conclude that exclusionary conditions existed, many signs pointed toward the presence of comorbid conditions. As noted above, Mrs. L.'s DISC-IV responses revealed concerns about Oppositional-Defiant Disorder. Corroboration was found in Mr. and Mrs. L.'s BASC Aggression subscale results, which fell between 2.5 and 3.5 standard deviations beyond the mean, above the 98th and 99th percentiles, respectively. Also elevated were their BASC Conduct Problems subscale scores, which fell above the 98th percentile. In addition to these secondary behavioral concerns, the psychological testing results strongly suggested that Mark had a nonverbal learning disability, characterized by substantial organizational difficulties.

Parent and Family Concerns

What limited information was available did not indicate the presence of any clinically significant parent or family problems.

Diagnostic Conclusion

Though teacher input was sparse, we could still make a diagnosis based on input from Mark's parents, from Mark, and from a review of school records. This information provided clear documentation of all *DSM-IV* criteria. In regard to Criterion A, the frequency, development deviance, and duration of his inattention symptoms were clinically significant. His hyperactive-impulsive symptoms, though developmentally deviant and of long duration, fell short of the clinical frequency threshold (i.e., 5 symptoms instead of the required 6). Being so close to the threshold makes it tempting to give Mark a "combined" subtype classification, but that would be stretching *DSM-IV*'s rules a bit. Of additional concern is that a Combined classification might saddle him with a label that reflects where he's been rather than where he's going, given that many teenagers display fewer hyperactive-impulsive symptoms as they get older. For reasons such as these, we gave Mark a diagnosis of Attention-Deficit/Hyperactivity Disorder, Predominantly Inattentive Type (314.00). In the report summarizing this diagnosis, we noted that although Mark received this classification, he was still displaying subclinical levels of hyperactivity-impulsivity that might also require therapeutic attention.

Along with Mark's AD/HD diagnosis, there was sufficient evidence to establish a secondary diagnosis of Oppositional-Defiant Disorder (313.81). The parent-completed BASC also raised the possibility that symptoms of Conduct Disorder might be emerging. Because this concern did not surface in the DISC-IV, no such diagnosis was made. Nonetheless, these antisocial features were taken seriously, potentially signaling a Conduct Disorder in emergence.

The results of IQ and educational achievement testing raised the strong possibility of a nonverbal learning disorder. Because our multimethod assessment battery is not designed to diagnose learning disabilities, we did not diagnose it. Concerns about this possibility were nevertheless raised.

Mark's predominantly inattentive AD/HD, his ODD, and his presumed nonverbal learning difficulties very likely account for many of the academic difficulties that he has had throughout his lifetime. His AD/HD and ODD symptoms may also be largely responsible for his difficult interactions with his parents and, to lesser extent, his peers.

Assessment Issues of Interest

Mark's case illustrates a rare situation in which a substantial amount of requested teacher input is missing. Had such input been available, it may have added greater clarity to the final outcome, perhaps making the subtyping differentiation clearer. But it wasn't available, so we proceeded without it. Fortunately, both parents contributed to the assessment process in a highly consistent way. Mark's self-report during the interview and his psychological testing results also played a major role in the evaluation, contrary to what is often the case with younger children. Also emerging from the evaluation was the fact that Mark had relatives with AD/HD and learning disorders, as well as a birth history with a risk factor for AD/HD and learning disorders (i.e., the brain injury). These small pieces of information added detail to our assessment puzzle that helped sharpen the ultimate diagnostic focus. Overall, the picture resembles that of David, our last example, but with fewer pieces in place (Figure 5.9.). One final point: Mark's freedom from distractibility score was anything but abnormal, once again highlighting the unreliability of this index as a sole criterion for establishing an AD/HD diagnosis.

CONCLUSION

Emerging from the preceding discussion are several important points. First, and foremost, the assessment of AD/HD is neither easy nor straightforward. Pitfalls may arise at any point, thereby complicating the evaluation process and making it difficult to rule in or rule out an AD/HD diagnosis. This in turn hinders treatment planning and implementation.

Much of this complexity is due to the fact that AD/HD is not defined by any single feature. On the contrary, it is a disorder for which a particular *pattern* of symptoms and behaviors must be present to arrive at a diagnosis. What this means for the assessment process is that no one procedure—whether it be psychological, medical, or otherwise—can address all of these complexities. Multiple procedures are indeed necessary to accomplish the formidable task of diagnosing AD/HD.

6

Planning Treatment

"He just needs to spend a little bit more time with his Dad, that's all."

Clarifying the diagnostic picture is important in and of itself, but an accurate diagnosis should lead to effective treatment for the disorder as well. Given this, how do clinicians implement treatment strategies on behalf of children and adolescents with AD/HD? Although there is no "correct" way of doing this, a good starting point is the comprehensive, multimethod assessment (Barkley, 1998).

To the extent that clinicians are able to gather detailed information about a child's performance in school, at home, and with friends, they are in an excellent position to make an accurate determination not only of the presence of AD/HD, but also of its severity and cross-situational pervasiveness. Information obtained from multimethod assessments can also shed light on the presence and severity of the various comorbid features that have a high probability of accompanying AD/HD. Furthermore, multimethod assessments generate important information about the child's family, and thus about a parent's capacity to implement treatment. Taken together, such assessment data make it possible to get a more complete picture not only of the child's problems, but also of the settings in which they occur and of the factors that exacerbate or maintain them, which is invaluable in putting together a treatment plan.

Because it is highly unlikely that any single treatment approach can meet all the clinical management needs of children with AD/HD, clinicians must often employ multiple treatment strategies, each of which addresses a different aspect of the child's difficulties. Thus, the assessment information becomes the foundation for treatment planning.

EMPIRICALLY SUPPORTED TREATMENTS

Where does one start when determining treatment options? The first place is the research literature. That is, what has empirical support for its use with the particular symptoms? Especially with AD/HD, there are many possible options. Due to its high rate of occurrence relative to other childhood disorders, AD/HD attracts a large share of intervention attention. Unfortunately, many of the interventions lack adequate empirical support and burst onto the therapeutic scene with unsubstantiated promises of a cure. Families and even therapists, eager to help the child, may choose one of these treatments, hoping for positive results. Unfortunately, lack of therapeutic progress, and sometimes even a deterioration in functioning, can result when research is not used in the decision-making process.

Considerable attention has been given to documenting the empirically supported interventions for childhood disorders. Several pharmacological, school-based, and home-based treatments have resulted in clinically significant improvements in child and family functioning. Among those with adequate, or at least preliminary, empirical support are pharmacotherapy, parent training and counseling, teacher applications of contingency management techniques, and cognitive-behavioral training (Pelham, Wheeler, & Chronis, 1998). Even so, these treatments should not be viewed as curative of AD/HD. Their value lies in their temporary reduction of AD/HD symptoms and related behavioral or emotional difficulties. When the treatments are removed, AD/HD symptoms very often return to pretreatment levels. Thus, their effectiveness presumably rests on maintaining them for a long time.

Pharmacotherapy

For many years, clinicians and researchers have used medication in their management of children with AD/HD on the assumption that neurochemical imbalances are involved in its etiology. Although the exact neurochemical mechanisms of its therapeutic action are unknown, research has shown that at least two classes of medication—namely, stimulants and antidepressants—can reduce AD/HD symptomatology.

Numerous studies demonstrate that stimulant medications are highly effective in managing AD/HD symptoms for many children and adolescents who take them (Greenhill, Halperin, & Abikoff, 1999). By some estimates, as many as 80–90% respond favorably, and most will display relatively normal behavior (Rapport, Denney, DuPaul, & Gardner, 1994). Somewhat lower response rates are reported for preschoolers (Byrne, Bawden, DeWolfe, & Beattie, 1998). In addition to bringing about improvements in primary AD/HD symptoms, these medications very often help the child become more compliant and less aggressive (Hinshaw, Henker, & Whalen, 1984). Side effects tend to be mild (e.g., decreased appetite), and most children tolerate them without great difficulty, even over extended periods (Zeiner, 1995). Thus, many child health-care professionals incorporate stimulant regimens into their clinical practice.

Historically, Ritalin, Dexedrine, and Cylert have been the most commonly prescribed stimulants. Of these, Ritalin is often the medication of choice. In its standard form, Ritalin acts rapidly, producing effects on behavior just 30–45 minutes after oral ingestion. Therapeutic effects peak within 2–4 hours, and it typically dissipates within 3–7 hours, even though minuscule amounts remain in the blood for up to 24 hours (Cantwell & Carlson, 1978). It is usually pre-scribed in twice-daily doses, but recent research shows that a third dose is tolerated fairly well by most children (Kent et al., 1995). Although children often take this medication exclusively on school days, it can also be used on week-ends and during school vacations, especially if the symptoms seriously interfere with home functioning.

A major disadvantage of using Ritalin in its standard form is that it must be administered two to three times a day. Although a sustained release version has been available for years, it has not been widely used, primarily because it does not deliver therapeutic benefits for a full 6–8-hour duration, as intended. A new stimulant medication, Adderall, was recently put on the market. Preliminary research suggests that Adderall delivers therapeutic benefits evenly over 6–8 hours (Swanson et al., 1998b). An additional advantage to using Adderall is that it comes in a variety of doses, thereby allowing physicians to tailor medication regimens more precisely to the needs of individual children and adolescents.

Despite their overall utility, stimulants may not be appropriate for some children with AD/HD who require a medication component in their overall clinical management. To meet the needs of such children, child health-care professionals have turned to tricyclic antidepressants, such as imipramine and Wellbutrin. Most often, these medications are employed in situations where certain side effects known to be exacerbated by stimulants (e.g., motor tics), are of concern or where significant mood disturbances accompany AD/HD symp-tomatology (Plizska, 1987). As a rule, antidepressants are given twice daily, usually in the morning and evening. Because they are longer acting than stimu-lants, it takes more time to evaluate the therapeutic effectiveness of a given dose (Rapoport & Mikkelsen, 1978). Despite this limitation, recent research shows that low doses can increase vigilance and decrease impulsivity, as well as reduce disruptive and aggressive behavior. Mood elevation may also occur, especially in children with significant pretreatment levels of depression or anxiety (Pliszka, 1987). Such treatment effects can diminish over time. Thus, antidepressants are usually not the medication of choice for long-term AD/HD management.

Parent Training

As discussed earlier, AD/HD is now viewed as a condition characterized by deficiencies in behavioral inhibition (Quay, 1997; Barkley, 1997). Stated some-what differently, children with AD/HD have difficulty regulating their behavior in response to situational demands. Such demands include not only the stim-ulus properties of the settings, but also the consequences of their behavior. To the extent that these situational parameters can be modified, one might reason-ably anticipate corresponding behavioral changes. Assuming this is valid, it provides justification for using behavior therapy techniques in the clinical management of children with AD/HD.

Despite the plethora of research on parent training, few studies have exam-ined its efficacy specifically with children who have AD/HD. What few studies exist can be interpreted with cautious optimism as supporting its use with such children (Anastopoulos et al., 1993; Pelham et al., 1988; Pisterman, McGrath, Firestone, & Goodman, 1989). Most of these interventions involved training parents in general contingency management tactics, such as positive reinforcement, response cost, and time-out strategies. Some have combined this training with didactic counseling aimed at increasing parental knowledge and understanding of AD/HD (Anastopoulos et al., 1993). In addition to producing changes in child behavior, parent training interventions have also led to improvements in various aspects of parental and family functioning, including decreased parenting stress and increased parenting self-esteem (Anastopoulos et al., 1993; Pisterman et al., 1989).

Classroom Modifications

Another clinically appropriate method for treating AD/HD is through classroom modifications. Somewhat more research has addressed the use of behavior management methods in the classroom, and it suggests that contingent use of positive reinforcement alone can produce immediate, short-term improvements in the student's behavior, productivity, and accuracy (DuPaul & Stoner, 1994). For most children with AD/HD, tangible reinforcers are more effective at improving their behavior and academic performance than are teacher attention or other social reinforcers (Pfiffner, Rosen, & O'Leary, 1985). Combining positive reinforcement with various punishment strategies, such as response cost, typically leads to greater behavioral improvements than either alone (Barkley et al., 1996; Barkley et al., in press; Pfiffner & O'Leary, 1987).

Despite the promising nature of such findings, many of these treatment gains subside when the treatment is withdrawn (Barkley, Copeland, & Sivage, 1980; Barkley et al., in press). Of additional concern is that these improvements in behavior and performance seldom generalize to other settings where treatment is not in effect. As a result, researchers have recently directed their attention to the development of interventions with generalization potential. For example, Barkley (1990) noted that children with AD/HD usually respond well to daily report card systems, which involve having teachers rate two or three target behaviors throughout the day; parents then convert these ratings into tangible reinforcers. Zentall (1985) has also found benefits to altering the properties of the educational stimuli (e.g., highlighting instructions in color). Recognizing that it is not always possible to modify the classroom for a single child, DuPaul and associates (DuPaul, Ervin, Hook, & McGoey, 1998) recently demonstrated that class-wide peer tutoring is an effective, nondisruptive way to bring about academic and behavioral improvements in children with AD/HD.

Cognitive-Behavioral Therapy

Over the past 20 years clinicians and researchers have employed a large number and variety of cognitive-behavioral interventions with children manifesting AD/HD symptoms. Included among these are various self-monitoring, self-reinforcement, and self-instructional techniques. Much of their clinical appeal stems from their apparent focus on some of the primary deficits of AD/HD, such as impulsivity, poor organizational skills, and difficulty with rules and instructions. Also contributing to their popularity is a presumed potential for enhancing treatment generalization.

Research on self-monitoring shows that it can improve on-task behavior and academic productivity in some children with AD/HD (Shapiro & Cole, 1994). A combination of self-monitoring and self-reinforcement can also lead to these improvements, and to improvements in peer relationships as well (Hinshaw, Henker, & Whalen, 1984). For self-instructional training, the picture is less clear; many recent studies (Abikoff & Gittelman, 1985) have failed to replicate earlier reported successes (Bornstein & Quevillon, 1976; Meichenbaum & Goodman, 1971).

Readily apparent in these recent studies are several potential limitations. For example, to achieve desired treatment effects in the classroom, children with AD/HD must be reinforced for using self-instructional strategies. Hence, this form of treatment does not free children from control by the social environment, but merely shifts the control to a slightly less direct form. Another limitation is that treatment effects seldom generalize to settings where the self-instructional training is not in effect, or to academic tasks not specifically part of the training process (Barkley et al., 1980). In this regard, self-instructional training does not, as had been hoped, circumvent the problem of situation specificity of treatment effects, which has plagued the use of contingency management methods for many years.

Combined Interventions

Single-treatment approaches, whether pharmacological, behavioral, or cognitive-behavioral, do not, by themselves, meet all of the clinical management needs of children with AD/HD. For this reason many researchers and child health-care professionals have recently begun to employ multiple treatments in combination.

Despite the intuitive appeal of this clinical practice, there is currently little empirical support for such treatment combinations. Many early studies that addressed this concluded that, regardless of the combination used, the therapeutic effect of a combined treatment package (e.g., stimulants with classroom contingency management) is typically no greater than the effect of either treatment alone (Gadow, 1985). Similar findings have emerged from studies examining the use of stimulant regimens in combination with cognitive-behavioral interventions (Hinshaw et al., 1984). Prior to drawing any definitive conclusions about combination treatments, it would be wise to await the findings from the recently completed multisite multimodal treatment of AD/HD (MTA) outcome study that has been in progress under the sponsorship of the Child and Adolescent Branch of the National Institute of Mental Health. Preliminary data from that project have suggested that for some children and their families, a combination of medication and intensive psychosocial treatment is superior to either alone.

From a somewhat different perspective, there have been attempts to evaluate, retrospectively, the long-term effects of individualized multimodality intervention on AD/HD outcome (Satterfield, Satterfield, & Cantwell, 1980). Such
multimodal interventions have included medication, parent training, individual counseling, special education, family therapy, and other treatments as
needed. The results indicated that an individualized program of combined
treatments, when continued over several years, increased social adjustment of
children with AD/HD, decreased their antisocial behavior, and improved their
academic achievement.

Adjunctive Procedures

In the preceding sections, we discussed numerous treatment strategies that
directly target the needs of children with AD/HD. Not covered was how comorbid features are typically addressed. When certain comorbid features, such as
aggression, are present, they will often diminish in frequency and severity along
with the targeted symptoms. This does not always occur, however. Moreover,
there are numerous occasions when secondary emotional or behavioral features
arise independent of the primary AD/HD diagnosis, and therefore are unrespon-
sive to AD/HD interventions. In such situations it is necessary to consider the
use of adjunctive intervention strategies. For example, individual therapy may
aid a child or adolescent in adjusting to parental divorce.

Due to the increased incidence of various psychosocial difficulties among
the parents of such children, clinicians must sometimes suggest that they too
receive therapy services, such as individual or marital counseling. In addition
to benefiting the parents themselves, these adjunctive procedures can also indirectly benefit their children. For example, when parental distress is reduced,
parents very often become better able to implement recommended treatment
strategies, such as parent training, on behalf of their child. Although intuitively
appealing and clinically sound, such adjunctive procedures have yet to be
addressed empirically, making this a fertile area for further research.

FROM RESEARCH TO PRACTICE

Progress has been made in developing treatments for AD/HD, but what may
not be so readily apparent is the degree to which clinicians have incorporated
these treatments into their practices. There are no published reports on how
these practitioners assemble and implement treatment plans for children and
adolescents with AD/HD. Thus, much of what is known about typical clinical
practice is best described as speculation.

Clinical experience suggests that a surprisingly large number of practitioners are simply not aware of recent scientific advances in the field, which
might explain why some children with AD/HD are placed on dietary regimens
(e.g., food-additive restrictions), for which there is little empirical validation. It
might also explain why some children and their parents expend a great deal of
time, energy, and money pursuing neurobiofeedback training, for which there

is, at best, weak empirical justification. Even when using treatments for which there is some empirical justification (e.g., medication), some clinicians surprisingly opt for variations (e.g., Prozac) that work well for other conditions but not for AD/HD.

For clinicians who employ empirically validated approaches, uncertainties remain, because of a large gap between research and practice. Contributing to this gap is that treatment outcome studies generally assign subjects to a certain type of treatment, whereas in real life, parents and children have some choice over the type of treatment they receive. Also, most AD/HD treatment research has examined single-treatment approaches rather than combinations of treatment, but in real life, treatments are typically used in combination. Even among those treatment outcome studies that have employed combined interventions, little regard was paid to the timing and sequential ordering of treatments (e.g., should medication be started before or after psychosocial treatment?). Moreover, almost no research has addressed the question of which treatments work best for which children, under which conditions, for which target behaviors, and so on. Thus, the moderating influence of age, gender, socioeconomic status, and cultural diversity, among many other factors, remains unclear.

An excellent example of how to employ an empirical approach is found in pharmacotherapy studies, which typically assess the efficacy of different doses of medications using highly controlled, double-blind, drug–placebo trials, in which objective measures assess not only therapeutic benefits but also potential side effects. Unfortunately, most clinicians who recommend medication as a treatment for AD/HD do not follow this research lead. Instead, they recommend medication with little systematic assessment of the drug's initial or sustained effectiveness. It is certainly understandable why a clinician may not be able to conduct such a trial in its entirety, due to limited access to placebo preparations and other obstacles, but some attempt should be made to assess a medication's effectiveness. A clinician who cannot access placebos can still conduct a reasonably objective assessment by systematically introducing different doses over equal time intervals. To approximate blind conditions in the assessment of school performance, parents can inform teachers that a trial is underway but not inform them of which dose is in effect at a given time. At the end of each dosage interval, relevant clinical data may then be obtained in the form of parent/teacher ratings of the child's behavior and of any side effects. Although not up to the standard of a formal double-blind, drug–placebo trial, data collected in this way can nevertheless provide a relatively objective assessment of a medication's efficacy at the outset. Once treatment is underway, trials of this sort can be done periodically (e.g., annually) to determine whether a child should be taken off medication or perhaps switched to a therapeutically more effective dose.

TAILORING TREATMENT OPTIONS

Armed with the knowledge of what might be a reasonable treatment, the next step is to begin tailoring the options to the particular child and family. Child, family, and system issues come into play, as do treatment philosophies.

Child Factors

In choosing interventions, one must consider the characteristics of the child. Again, comprehensive assessment data are essential. How old is the child? What specific AD/HD symptoms does the child have? What is the severity and pervasiveness of the symptoms and in which areas are they causing impairment? Are there any comorbid conditions? What are the child's strengths? Unfortunately, research on child treatment outcome in general, and with respect to AD/HD specifically, may not address all of these factors. However, by mapping the child's characteristics onto the available research, one can at least be aware of which options have clear empirical support, which ones have promising support, and which ones are too new to endorse.

Family Factors

Of equal importance are family factors. This was highlighted in the rationale for the assessment battery and is no less important in planning treatment. What is the family structure? Who is likely to participate in treatment? What is known of the parenting strengths, needs, psychopathology, and marital stability?

If family problems exist, they will probably have been detected while reviewing the child's functional impairment, and they should be considered not only in choosing which interventions to include, but also for how they will affect the intervention itself. For example, significant marital difficulties may hinder a parent training intervention. Likewise, parents with significant depression or other psychological concerns may not be able to adequately oversee their child's medication regimen.

What are the family's financial resources? For families with no insurance and little money, getting to a clinic to have a child or adolescent treated for AD/HD just may not be feasible. Even if they can get there, they may not be able to pay the cost of long-term clinical management. This may necessitate streamlining some of the highly specialized treatments. Delivering services in community settings can increase their accessibility, particularly for economically disadvantaged families (e.g., Community Parent Education program; COPE; Cunningham, Bremner, & Boyle, 1995; Cunningham, Bremner, & Secord-Gilbert, 1997).

Even for families who can get such services, obstacles may arise. Parents with limited education may have trouble adhering to a child's medication regimen or reading and understanding the handouts or between session homework assignments in parent training programs. Similar comprehension difficulties may occur among parents for whom English is not the primary language. When such situations arise, clinicians must try to find interventions with support materials in other languages or on audiotape or videotape (e.g, Webster-Stratton, 1998). Other options include identifying family friends or relatives who are willing to provide assistance as translators or interpreters. This, of course, introduces the possibility that something may "get lost in the translation," thereby complicating the treatment process. It is unacceptable for a clinician to recommend an intervention without considering these constraints. If such obstacles are ignored, the family is not likely to access the treatment. In many instances, they are then regarded as noncompliant or uninterested in helping their child, when the real problem is a lack of consideration for pertinent family factors.

Just as child strengths are important in treatment planning, so too are family strengths. Families who have adequate financial resources, strong social support, good educational background, and so on, usually have more treatment options available. One would want to ensure that the intervention does not undermine these strengths but rather supports them.

School Factors

For many children with AD/HD, school-based interventions will be a part of the treatment package. As with home-based treatments, one should consider the characteristics of the teacher, the classroom, and even the school in deciding which empirically supported treatments are likely to be feasible. Size of the class, availability of supportive services, and the willingness of the teacher to implement an intervention—all will help to target possible treatments.

System Factors

Although not usually part of the assessment, system factors do affect treatment planning and the ultimate success of the treatment. Factors such as school redistricting, mental health agency changes, even changes in the current research literature, can affect treatment planning. Perhaps most notable is the issue of managed care. Although treatment should be not dictated by reimbursement considerations, it is unrealistic to ignore them.

Some managed care plans specifically list AD/HD as a condition that they do not cover. When it is accompanied by comorbid conditions for which coverage is allowed, clinicians often make the comorbid conditions the focus of the treatment to reduce the financial burden on families and to receive reimbursement for their services. But what if there are no comorbid conditions? Some clinicians may then be tempted to list a comorbid diagnosis for symptoms that are present but subclinical in nature. Others may reduce their fees. Still others may not have the luxury of making such a fee adjustment and do not feel comfortable listing a subclinical condition as an intervention focus, so they are forced to refer the family to another practitioner.

Even when coverage is available, managed care often restricts the number of visits that can occur in a single year or over the course of a lifetime. Commonly, the number of contacts allowed falls far short of what most children with AD/HD require. Once again, this places clinicians in the uncomfortable position of having to decide between drastically reducing their fees to continue working with the child and the family versus referring them elsewhere for services that are more affordable.

Relying on treatments with empirical support can, in some cases, improve the reimbursement picture. Demonstrating in the original request for approval, or even during an appeal, that a certain treatment for AD/HD is not only effective but will reduce the need for more-costly services in the future, is often a compelling argument. Thus, using empirically validated treatments is not only more likely to be successful in human terms, but in dollar terms as well.

Philosophy Guiding Treatment

In addition to various child, family, school, and system issues, the manner in which an intervention is conducted is very much influenced by one's philosophy regarding treatment. Our own experience and what we have learned from recent research findings confirm that treatment plans that are strength-based, that consider antecedents and consequences, and that address the goodness-of-fit issue are likely to be the most successful.

Strength-Based Approaches

In developing any treatment plan for a child with AD/HD, certain behaviors are targeted. Clearly the plan will target behaviors that are maladaptive and inappropriate, with the goal of reducing or eliminating them. Choosing a proven intervention is likely to result in some improvement in child functioning, family functioning, or both, but ameliorating maladaptive behaviors is only half the picture. It is important to target positive behaviors and competencies as well. Although decreasing a maladaptive behavior (e.g., task-irrelevant activity) might increase a more appropriate alternative (e.g., attention to task), it might not. Targeting behaviors that should be increased as well as those that should be decreased is more likely to result in success. This more balanced approach to treatment planning should proceed nicely from the information on strengths, as well as on difficulties, emanating from the multimethod assessment battery.

Strength-based treatment planning involves considering child, family, and system strengths. Strengths can be used to develop interventions. For example, in planning a school-based intervention, if a child is very interested in and skilled at computers, computer access could be incorporated into a token economy system designed to reduce disruptive classroom behavior. Strategies should also be considered to insure that interventions are not counterproductive. Using a school-based example again, recess or playing on an athletic team is often used in token economy programs: The child loses access if a behavioral goal is not reached. This approach is chosen because these activities are highly valued by the child and likely to be motivating. But, what if the child's strength, and primary (or only) area of accomplishment and success, is on the playing field? It may be the one place where peer relations are successful. It would be unwise to jeopardize this rewarding aspect of the child's life when other motivators could be used.

Strength-based approaches are often appealing to the child and family, which increases the likelihood that treatment will be effective. Evidence is accumulating that strength-based approaches are not only more effective than traditional pathology-driven interventions (Burns, Goldman, Faw, & Burchard, 1999; Dunst, Trivette, & Deal, 1994), but are more acceptable to children, parents, and teachers (e.g., Jones, Eyberg, Adams, & Boggs, 1998; Miller & Kelley, 1992; Power, Hess, & Bennett, 1995; Tarnowski, Simonian, Park, & Bekeny, 1992).

Addressing Behavioral Antecedents and Consequences

Typical interventions work primarily by altering the consequences of the child's behavior. Although this is certainly effective, this approach has inherent limitations. For example, as children get older it is increasingly difficult to identify positive classroom consequences that can be administered promptly. One option is to move the consequences to a home-based incentive system. Yet success can also be achieved by addressing the conditions that trigger the behavior in the first place. Understanding what precedes, or triggers, a behavior— whether positive or negative—as well as what follows and maintains it, is the foundation of functional behavioral analysis. By addressing both sides of the behavioral equation, one can develop a more comprehensive treatment plan that will likely work.

Goodness-of-Fit

A philosophy related to treatment planning is *goodness-of-fit*. Originally applied to temperament, this concept has relevance to treatment planning as well. Optimal development is thought to occur when there is a match, or goodness-of-fit, between a person's skills and the environment's demands. In many ways, a lack of fit characterizes the whole issue of functional impairment in a child with AD/HD. The child's AD/HD symptoms negatively impact his or her ability to develop or use competence to meet the demands of the environment. Difficulty complying with parental requests, difficulty negotiating peer relations, and difficulty persisting with a challenging academic task are all examples of this. The whole purpose of a treatment plan is to increase the fit between the child and the environment. This can be done in two ways.

First, one can include interventions that decrease the AD/HD symptoms (e.g., medication), increase the child's skills (e.g., social skills training), or both. Second, one can alter the environment such that the child is more likely to be successful. Parent training, where parents learn more-effective ways of presenting a command or request, is one example. So too are alterations in the classroom environment, such as preferential seating, lowering task demands, or reducing the amount of individual desk work. Just as addressing both antecedents and consequences results in "more bang for the buck," so too does addressing not only skill-building, but environmental change.

PLANNING COLLABORATIVELY WITH PARENTS

By now one should have a list of potential treatments that have empirical support, that are tailored to the specific child and family, that are strength-based, that consider both antecedents and consequences, and that are aimed at improving the goodness-of-fit between the child's abilities and the child's environment. With this list in hand, the final and most important step in developing the treatment plan is *collaboration with the family.*

There is a growing recognition that successful mental health services for children require successful partnerships between families and their service providers. Defined as working together or joining in the pursuit of a common goal (DeChillo, 1993), these partnerships are relatively new in service delivery. In the fields of developmental disabilities, early intervention, pediatrics, and mental health there has been a gradual shift from viewing the child's family as the source of the problem, to making the family the focus of therapy but not a part of decision-making, to seeing the family as a fully participating partner in design, delivery, and evaluation of care (e.g., DeChillo, Koren, & Schultze, 1994; Dunst, Johanson, Trivette, & Hamby, 1991; Shelton & Stepanek, 1994).

This shift has positive outcomes for children, families, and professionals. When adequate information is gathered from parents about preferences and adequate information is provided about the empirical support and reasoning behind an intervention, that intervention is more efficacious. Families who are respected members of their child's treatment team report increased satisfaction with services, and collaborative treatment planning is related to both improved service coordination and to successfully addressing children's needs (e.g., Koren et al., 1997; Rosenblatt, 1996).

Collaborative goal setting is the key to providing culturally competent treatment and to maintaining and refining efficacious interventions for children (e.g., Dunst, Trivette, Davis, & Cornwell, 1988; Hernandez, Isaacs, Nesman, & Burns, 1998; Hodges, Nesman, & Hernandez, 1999). It is the primary vehicle for developing interventions that truly reflect the family's priorities, values, and hopes for their child. It has intrinsic merit as well, in that it "satisfies an ethical obligation to parents and families in our society" (Heflinger, 1995, p. 6).

Satisfaction with the Treatment Plan

Even when empirically supported treatments are available, one must still consider whether they will be implemented. Satisfaction with and acceptance of interventions play a considerable role in the degree to which a particular intervention will even be initiated. They may also determine whether treatment will be implemented with enough fidelity to evaluate its success. In some cases, these beliefs are crucial in determining whether any intervention, even an effective one, will be continued long enough to result in significant clinical change.

For example, parental satisfaction with treatment has been shown to be related to changes in child compliance and to improved parent behavior ratings (Brestan, Jacobs, Rayfield, & Eyberg, 1999). Adolescent satisfaction has also been associated with change in parent-reported behavior problems, parental satisfaction, parental ratings of treatment progress, therapist ratings of progress, and *DSM* Global Assessment of Functioning scores (Shapiro, Welker, & Jacobson, 1997).

Acceptability is equally important in designing an intervention package. There are remarkably consistent findings across studies that parents, teachers, and children prefer positive interventions. Reinforcement, positive attention, and other positive treatments are more favorably received than such interventions as time-out and response cost, and sometimes, medication (e.g., Fairbanks & Stinnett, 1997; Jones, Eyberg, Adams, & Boggs, 1998; Miller & Kelley, 1992; Power, Hess, & Bennett, 1995; Tarnowski et al., 1992). Information about what the intervention can do and why it is being recommended can also increase its acceptability, a point nicely made in a recent study by Bennett, Power, Rostain, and Carr (1996), who found that knowledge of AD/HD was positively related to parent acceptance of medication as a treatment.

As with any research, results that apply to groups may not apply to individuals. Nonetheless, trends do show that a strength-based approach is likely to be an acceptable option. In addition, when recommending what may be perceived as negative interventions, it is important to provide justification for them, along with information for parents to use in making an informed decision.

DEVELOPING A PLAN

Given the complexity of AD/HD in its clinical presentation, multiple treatments should be used in combination to bring about optimal therapeutic benefits. Unfortunately, little research has been conducted that addresses which treatment combinations should be used for which children. Until such research is done, practitioners must rely on their own clinical judgement to guide them in putting together multimodal treatment plans to meet the needs of individual children and their families. When doing so, they should also make every effort to use treatments for which there is at least a modicum of empirical validation. Among the many treatments available, stimulant medication therapy is perhaps the one used most often and most effectively. Although not yet empirically validated, combining stimulant medication with other treatments, such as parent training or classroom modifications, is regarded as acceptable and desirable clinical practice.

Before starting any intervention, one must first present a preliminary treatment plan to the child and the family. After soliciting their reaction, one can then invite the family to suggest additions or subtractions. By proceeding in this collaborative fashion, clinicians increase the likelihood that the treatment will be successful. What might this preliminary plan be? How does one engage the family in a treatment planning dialogue? The latter question is addressed in the next chapter. The remainder of this chapter illustrates how preliminary treatment plans are constructed.

Identifying Target Problems

AD/HD may be mild, moderate, or severe. It may occur in some settings but not in others. Its presentation may be mild in one setting but moderate in another. Children with AD/HD may also have one or more comorbid conditions. Many have an Oppositional-Defiant or Conduct Disorder. Some have depression, anxiety, or other internalizing problems. Others have learning disabilities. Still others have combinations of these. Some come from stable homes with ample financial supports and resources. Others live in homes where there is parental psychopathology, domestic violence, and child maltreatment.

The point is, that children with AD/HD come in many shapes and sizes, which is why a one-size-fits-all approach is inappropriate. For the same reason, no single treatment approach is likely to address the multiple needs that many of these children and adolescents bring with them. Thus, multiple treatments must be used to maximize therapeutic outcome.

Which treatments should be used in combination? The exact treatment plan for a given child depends in part on the overall severity of the clinical presentation. Overall severity is determined by considering several factors, including the severity and pervasiveness of their AD/HD symptoms, the presence or absence of comorbid conditions, and the nature and existence of family problems. Such problem areas are in turn mitigated by the strengths of the child and the family. Once the severity of the clinical presentation is known, a useful way to conceptualize the process of developing a treatment plan is to invoke a variation of the puzzle analogy that was applied to diagnostic assessment. Specifically, putting together a treatment plan can be thought of as another puzzle to assemble. Like most puzzles, this one will have at least two pieces, but it usually has more. For children with mild symptoms and few (if any) comorbid problems, fewer treatment pieces need to be in place, as shown Figure 6.1. For those whose AD/HD is more problematic and whose difficulties go beyond AD/HD, additional treatment pieces will need to be included, as illustrated in Figure 6.2. Because some children with AD/HD present with multiple problems, one must often expand the treatment plan to include an even larger number and variety of intervention strategies, as shown Figure 6.3.

Case Example

To illustrate how a preliminary treatment plan might be developed, we refer back to the case of Ross in Chapter 5. In brief review, Ross was an 8-year-old, third-grade boy who received a dual diagnosis of AD/HD, Combined type, and ODD. Additional concerns emerged with respect to subclinical levels of depression and anxiety symptoms and a possible motor-based learning disorder. In addition, evidence suggested that Ross's mother was experiencing high levels of parenting stress, personal distress, and possibly features of adult AD/HD as well.

Ross's AD/HD and ODD seemed to be jointly contributing to the highly significant discrepancy between his actual academic achievement and that predicted by his IQ. The same two conditions were presumably responsible for some of the difficulties he was having with peers, and with respect to the high level of parenting stress reported by both parents.

Given the multiple problems inherent in Ross's clinical presentation, it was

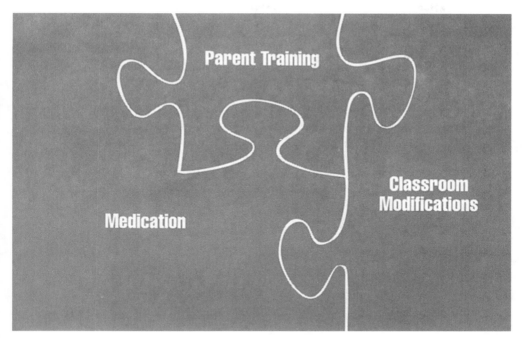

FIGURE 6.1. Sample treatment plan for mild clinical presentation.

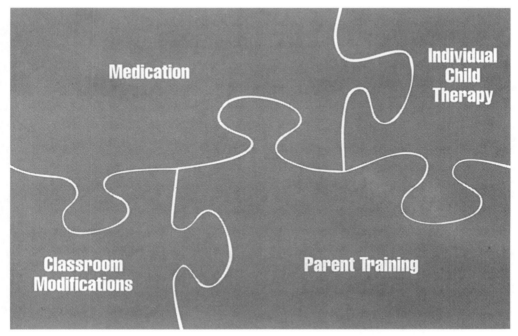

FIGURE 6.2. Sample treatment plan for moderate clinical presentation.

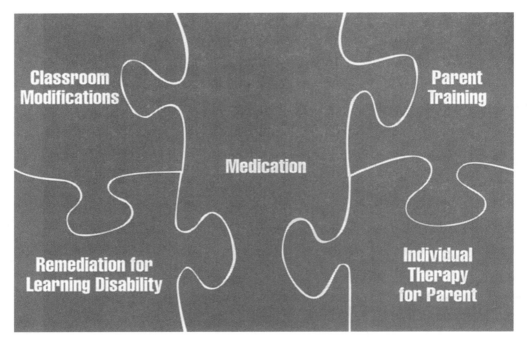

Figure 6.3. Sample treatment plan for severe clinical presentation.

clear that no one treatment could address everything. Thus, a multimodal intervention strategy was adopted, analogous to the one shown in Figure 6.3.

To deal with Ross's AD/HD symptoms in school, a trial of stimulant medication was recommended. In addition, changes in his classroom were recommended to create conditions that would reduce the impact of his AD/HD, thereby maximizing his behavior and performance. This included compensatory strategies such as providing Ross with opportunities to receive academic instruction on a computer, reducing his workload, attaching an index card with classroom rules to his desk, and using high-interest curriculum. Because compensatory strategies alone are not always sufficient, additional motivational strategies were recommended. This included giving Ross more immediate and more frequent feedback throughout the day. Along the same lines, suggestions were made for incorporating meaningful incentives into his daily programming; a daily report card system was identified as one means of accomplishing this.

To deal with Ross's AD/HD and ODD problems at home, which were identified by his parents as a treatment priority, training in specialized behavior management strategies was recommended. Books on this topic and the availability of a 9-week, clinic-based parent training program were made known to Ross's parents. Because Ross also visited with his biological mother fairly regularly, his father and stepmother were encouraged to include her in the process.

To facilitate implementation of all of the above recommendations, Ross's parents and teachers were encouraged to learn more about AD/HD through reading and through videotaped presentations.

Given that Ross may have been displaying a motor-based learning problem, further assessment of this matter was recommended.

Also noted during the evaluation was that Ross was experiencing mild depression and anxiety symptoms, as well as peer relationship problems. Although the exact etiology of the mild depression and anxiety symptoms was unclear, there was reason to believe that they might be secondary manifestations of Ross's primary AD/HD and ODD symptoms. Thus, interventions for them were deferred to see whether the above treatments lessened his primary symptoms. If the primary symptoms improved but the other symptoms did not, we would then consider targeting these social and emotional areas more directly, using school-based social skills training and individual therapy, respectively.

One last finding from the multimethod assessment bears mentioning. Because there was evidence that Ross's mother might be experiencing personal difficulties, as well as adult AD/HD problems, this too needed to be addressed. Thus, we recommended that she consider an evaluation to determine whether treatment should be initiated. To the extent that she successfully addressed these personal difficulties, she would be able to more effectively provide treatments to Ross.

CONCLUSION

Multimodal interventions must be used to bring about optimal therapeutic benefits. These will vary from child to child as a function of many factors, including the severity and pervasiveness of the AD/HD and the presence of comorbid conditions. Also critical to the success of any intervention is the inclusion of families in designing the treatment plan.

Regardless of the starting point, it is important to keep in mind that initial treatment plans are just an approximation of what will probably be in effect later. Thus, like researchers, clinicians must systematically collect clinical data to test their "hypotheses," which in this case is the effectiveness of their treatments. Such data then become the basis for deciding whether to adjust an ongoing treatment, add a new treatment, or remove a treatment whose effectiveness is questionable.

7

Providing Feedback

"How can he possibly have AD/HD? He can play Nintendo for hours!"

Thus far we have outlined a comprehensive process of choosing assessment methods, applying the *DSM-IV* criteria, and deciding on a diagnosis and course of treatment. What links all this with meaningful outcomes for the child and family is feedback. Done well, feedback enhances family and teacher understanding of the child's strengths and needs. Feedback also helps them to understand how AD/HD affects the child's functioning, and it facilitates accessing and using appropriate interventions.

The success of any therapeutic encounter directly relates to the thoroughness of the initial planning. This is no less true of evaluation feedback. If feedback occurs immediately after evaluation, there is little time to plan for it, in which case feedback planning is done right at the start, as part of the process of planning the assessment itself. This means anticipating frequently asked questions, common referral issues, and so forth. If the feedback session is to be held later, more-extensive planning can take place, enabling the session to be tailored to the specific results that need to be communicated. Regardless of timing, several things must be considered before giving feedback. Planning increases the likelihood that the encounter will be successful.

As the Boy Scout motto states, "Be Prepared." Although it is impossible to be prepared for every question or referral need that may arise during a feedback session, many things can be anticipated. For example, many parents do not know much about AD/HD, so they often ask for more information. Many also ask about treatment in general and medication in particular. At one end of the medication preference continuum are those who do not want to leave without a prescription; at the other end are those who are worried that an AD/HD diagnosis automatically means medication and who adamantly oppose it. When questions like these arise parents need scientifically based information. If the child has been having trouble at school, there are often questions about what kinds of changes teachers can make, or about the types of special services for which the child may be eligible. Whatever the questions, feedback is of paramount importance to the family and to other referral sources, thus there is no excuse for "winging" a feedback session. A lack of preparation can negate even the most insightful evaluation.

What follows is a more detailed discussion of the many factors that contribute to providing successful feedback. Examples of the type of feedback that can be given, as well as the various ways it can be presented, are described below.

PROVIDING FEEDBACK TO PARENTS AND CHILDREN

Once a decision has been made about the child's diagnosis and treatment options, the next step is to schedule a feedback session. Face-to-face feedback is best. It permits a discussion of testing, conclusions, and recommendations. It affords an opportunity for questions and answers regarding what's next. It is the end of the assessment process and the beginning of collaborative treatment planning. To make the session successful, one can take as a guide the research examining parental satisfaction with feedback. Although most of this research was done on parents of children with developmental disabilities or chronic illness, some of its findings apply to psychiatric diagnoses as well. AD/HD can, in many respects, be considered a type of developmental disability, because the child does not outgrow it and must learn to adapt in order to be successful.

When one reviews the literature, it is surprising to see how often parents are dissatisfied with the feedback they receive about their child's diagnosis. Given how frequently clinicians give feedback, one would think they would be better at it, but it continues to be problematical. To address this, Cunningham, Morgan, and McGucken (1984) examined the efficacy of a model program for providing feedback to parents about the diagnosis of Down syndrome. They found that their approach was much more satisfying to parents (e.g., 100% satisfaction) than the usual approach, which resulted in only 20% satisfaction. The key components of their program included scheduling adequate time; ensuring that parents' questions were answered; including as many family members as possible, or at least both parents in a two-parent family; providing information as soon as possible after the assessment; and providing follow-up support and services. These findings have been echoed in other studies as well. This literature and our own experience lead us to conclude that several things will optimize a feedback session.

First, although managed care places constraints on time, it is important to schedule enough time so to create an atmosphere that encourages questions. A thorough explanation, given in a way that lays the groundwork for establishing a collaborative relationship with the child's family, is the most efficient choice in the long run.

Second, one needs to determine who will participate in the feedback session. As part of the multimethod assessment process, important individuals in the child's life will have already been identified. If at all possible, families should be given the option of scheduling the feedback session for a time when these individuals can attend. Having multiple family members present has several advantages. More people in the child's life hear the information firsthand, reducing the need for parents to be the only ones communicating feedback to the family. Another advantage is social support. To the extent that the family *is* supportive, having them present can be very helpful, particularly if the findings upset the parents. Finally, including grandparents and other extended family may be very important in what unfolds following the feedback, because very often they are key players in the treatment plan.

Scheduling feedback requires flexibility on the part of the clinician. Nevertheless, this step ensures that the information reaches those who will be supporting the child. When it is not possible to include these individuals, other steps can be taken, such as giving feedback via telephone or setting up a later session. Once it is determined who should be part of the session, the clinician can see whether other accommodations are needed. For example, is an interpreter needed for a non-English-speaking or hearing-impaired family member? One might assume that, in the case of the parents anyway, such information would already be known, but sometimes parents for whom English is not the primary language can complete rating scales and even structured interviews, but may still lack sufficient understanding of the language to fully comprehend the feedback.

Third, it is important to remember that the child needs information too. Sometimes it's best to give feedback to a child while the parents are present, particularly with a younger child. One benefit of this approach is that it models for the parents how to anticipate and answer a child's questions. Another benefit is that it shows the child that questions are not only permissible but welcome. Also advantageous is that the family hears the same information, so each knows what was told to the others. This is especially important if the child gave information as part of an interview, because he or she may be wondering what has been shared with the parents. A good rule of thumb is to address confidentiality issues with both the child and the parents during the interview. Although issues arising in AD/HD evaluations are not usually a problem in this regard, it is always possible the child may share information that is sensitive (e.g., drug use) or that requires the suspension of confidentiality (e.g., child maltreatment, threat of harm to self or others). These issues of shared feedback are especially challenging with adolescents.

Although joint sessions have advantages, so do separate ones. When there is particularly negative or unsettling information to convey, separate sessions may be best. It can be difficult and inappropriate for a child to hear certain appraisals arising from an assessment. Let's say, for example, that the information provided by a child's teacher was especially negative. Even if the teacher's perception is valid and the child is already aware that things are not going well, it may still be hard to discuss this information in front of the child. This does not imply that one wouldn't share a summary with the child, but doing so in an individual session allows one to tailor the presentation. Similarly, if information is likely to be especially upsetting for the parents, they may feel more comfortable having a session alone with the clinician, where they can react honestly and ask questions such as those about prognosis. Also, older children and adolescents may feel more comfortable raising certain issues in private. Individual sessions also set the stage for an adolescent to take a more active role in managing the AD/HD. If individual sessions are scheduled, scheduling the adolescent's session after the parents' tends to facilitate trust a bit more than if this session had been scheduled first. In any event, the goal of all feedback is an open discussion about the assessment findings and the treatment options, which empowers the child and family to move forward.

Sometimes it is impossible to cover everything in one session, such as when one must give feedback immediately following the evaluation or when one wants to schedule individual sessions with the parents, the child, and possibly with other family members as well. It is imperative that one knows how much time is available; one can then decide what to share in the initial session.

Feedback Content

How does one prioritize what information to share in the face of time constraints? The guiding principle is to address the family's priorities first (e.g., what is their most immediate need for information?). Addressing the family's priorities has at least two advantages. First, it respects the family's unique and essential role in the child's life. Second, it lessens the chance of increasing their anxiety and frustration because it ensures that issues of paramount importance are addressed.

The clinician must also attend to feedback issues that he or she deems essential to communicate as soon as possible. In many cases, these will be the same issues prioritized by the family, but sometimes there are other pressing issues that must be discussed. For example, if decisions are to be made in the next week about the child's classroom placement for the next year, this should be addressed. Keeping these caveats in mind, there are several things that should be discussed in any initial feedback session.

Results of the Assessment

First and foremost, the results of the assessment must be discussed. Let's say that an AD/HD diagnosis is confirmed. One would want not only to communicate this diagnosis but also to explain the process by which this was determined. Parents should already have some understanding of the multimethod assessment process by virtue of having just gone through it. Nevertheless, it is important to explain what information was obtained, any inconsistencies in the data, and how they were resolved. In short, one would describe the process outlined in Chapter 5. This is critical, because parents need to understand how and why an AD/HD diagnosis was established.

Several concepts critical to the diagnostic process are unfamiliar to parents. One relates to developmental deviance. Even the term "deviance" can be misleading, particularly if parents equate it with "delinquency." Parents need to know that "deviance," as used in an AD/HD diagnosis, is a statistical term meaning "more frequent and severe than would be expected for children of the same age and gender." *T* scores, translated into percentiles, are often the benchmark for this determination, but percentile rankings may not be familiar either. To explain percentiles, it is often helpful to use an example. Let's say that the child's AD/HD symptoms, averaged across ratings, fell above the 95th percentile. One way to depict this is to have the parents imagine that their child is in a group of 100 children of the same age and gender. Next, they are asked to imagine that the children were evaluated to see how inattentive, impulsive, and hyperactive each one was. Based on the results of this evaluation, the children were then rank ordered. Child number 1 in this line-up showed these behaviors the least often. Child number 100 showed them the most often. Child number 50 displayed an average amount. The clinician would then note that if the child in question was number 65 in the lineup, he or she would show more AD/HD features than an average child, but would still be close to the middle of the pack. Therefore, we would consider this to be within normal limits and would not initiate any intervention. Referring back to our multimethod data, we might point out that their child was at the 95th percentile, meaning that 95 children in the group displayed fewer of the problem behaviors. Less than 5 out of 100 would have similar difficulties. Because this lies far away from the middle of the pack, it is unlikely to be normal variation. As such, it is considered developmentally deviant, which gives us reason to believe that it is a manifestation of a clinically significant problem, in this case AD/HD. A visual aid, such as that depicted in Figure 7.1., can be very helpful in illustrating this.

Once the process of arriving at an AD/HD diagnosis has been described, a similar discussion can take place with regard to any comorbid conditions that are present. The concept of developmental deviance and its application to diagnostic criteria apply here as well, but there are additional considerations for giving feedback about comorbid conditions. For many families whose children undergo an evaluation, someone, either themselves or a teacher, has thought about the possibility of an AD/HD diagnosis. In fact, it is hard to find a parent who has not heard of this diagnosis.

What can come as a surprise, however, is the presence of additional difficulties. Sometimes parents are comfortable with the idea of an AD/HD diagnosis but become quite dismayed when they hear about conduct or anxiety disorders, for example. If one is not careful, the feedback session starts to sound like a litany of the child's problems. Parents may leave with the impression that everything is wrong with their child. This can be devastating, greatly limiting the parents' capacity to move beyond assessment to treatment, and perhaps more importantly, this deficit-only approach would be an unrealistic picture of the child. But how can one communicate all the results accurately yet in a way that respects the parents' feelings?

First, one must take a balanced approach. All children have strengths. Some

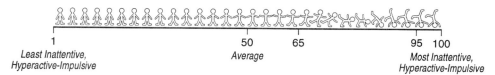

| 1 | 50 | 65 | 95 | 100 |
| *Least Inattentive, Hyperactive-Impulsive* | *Average* | | *Most Inattentive, Hyperactive-Impulsive* | |

FIGURE 7.1. Visual aid illustrating developmental deviance.

of these strengths relate to their personal characteristics, such as a good sense of humor, an upbeat demeanor, or high intelligence. Some strengths relate to their family, such as a strong marriage, concerned parents, and adequate social support. Still others relate to environmental strengths, such as concerned teachers and an excellent school system. These must be discussed in the feedback session as well. In fact, it is often a good idea to start the feedback session with them, because it lays a good foundation for discussing problems. As detailed earlier, the BASC was chosen for the core diagnostic battery partly because it identifies behavioral strengths. Identifying strengths as well as weaknesses is more accurate and thus results in more-effective treatment planning and better parent–clinician collaboration (e.g., Dunst et al., 1994; Hodges et al., 1999).

Another strategy is to explain why the comorbid disorders are present, if this is known. For example, it is easy for most parents to understand why many children with AD/HD also have ODD. Alerting parents to the fact that children with AD/HD often avoid, delay, or actually refuse to do repetitive or boring things not only helps them to understand the source of the ODD diagnosis, but lays the groundwork for intervention. As with the concept of developmental deviance, explaining psychological terms and avoiding superfluous jargon is important. The term "comorbid" is usually unfamiliar and may convey an image of morbidity and death. One would not want the family to infer that the child's comorbid condition was terminal. Although helping professionals are quite fond of acronyms, which provide a useful shorthand between professionals, they can be confusing to parents at best, misleading at worst. For example, verbal or written feedback that with no explanation uses "ODD" for oppositional-defiant disorder may be upsetting to a parent who mistakes the term for a comment on the child's personality. One must put comorbid conditions into a cohesive framework that ties directly back to symptoms and problems already known to the parents.

Finally, one must always remember that the feedback session is a time for shared information. It is not only a time for the clinician to talk, it is also a time for the clinician to listen and to understand what the diagnosis means to this particular child and family. To some, the diagnosis is a relief of sorts: There is a name for the problem and a sense that something can be done about it. For others, the diagnosis is devastating, implying a lifelong parenting challenge or perhaps reminding the parents of horror stories they have heard about other children with AD/HD. One must never make assumptions about how a child or a family will take the news. Rather, one must create an opportunity during the feedback session for their views to be expressed and for the clinician to be supportive.

Information about AD/HD and Other Disorders

Once the assessment process and the diagnostic picture have been discussed, the next thing is to provide the family and the child with factual information about AD/HD and any other pertinent concerns. Information is empowering. For the parents and the child to become active partners in the design and implementation of interventions, they need to become knowledge-able about the disorder. This can be done partly through the written report, which will be discussed later, but certain information can and should be provided during the feedback session as well. This is because the information should be timely, and also because some information is too cumbersome to repeat in each report (e.g., a full description of AD/HD and its etiology).

To this end, one can simply provide parents with standard handouts describing what AD/HD is, what we know about it, and how it is treated—particularly important given the enormous amount of popular-media AD/HD *mis*information. If one frequently assesses children for AD/HD, it may be helpful to develop one's own information sheet. One may also want to direct parents to organizations such as CHADD (Children and Adults with Attention-Deficit Disorder; see Appendix Q) or the Association for the Advancement of Behavioral Therapy, both of which have their own AD/HD information sheets. One should also assist the family in understanding and reviewing various AD/HD information. Particularly in this age of the Internet, information with no empirical support is readily available. A good feedback session, then, also assists families in becoming good consumers of information that they might encounter in the future.

Information sheets are very useful as parents attempt to communicate test results to other family members. Although it is preferable to have concerned others at the feedback session, it is not always possible. Cost can preclude scheduling additional sessions, so parents must then become the "resident experts" about their child's assessment and diagnosis. Putting the information literally in their hands increases the likelihood that other family members can support the parents and child effectively.

When considering the written information that is shared with the family, it is imperative that one considers the reading level and primary language of the parents and family. Ideally, information should be written at a sixth grade reading level and if necessary, translated. When literacy is a problem, a brief description of the disorder and an overview of diagnostic conclusions and treatment recommendations may be audiotaped. Another option is to use an already existing videotape about AD/HD (see A.D.D. WareHouse, Appendix Q). What should guide the clinician in this regard is ensuring that the most comprehensive information is provided in the most useable format. When this is accomplished, the feedback session is likely to result in a successful outcome.

Children should also be educated about AD/HD. As mentioned earlier, one can model for parents how to describe it to a child, but sometimes this is not possible. Even when it is, the initial feedback information may not be comprehensive enough as the child gains more insight into AD/HD. One way to address this is through books, often called *bibliotherapy*. There are any number of good books written about AD/HD for children of all ages. Rather than recommend specific ones, we simply advise clinicians to become familiar with several that cover a wide age range and can be used for children and adolescents. The public library and organizations such as CHADD and the A.D.D. WareHouse are just some of the places where children's books and videotapes can be obtained.

Information about Treatment Options

Once information about the assessment and diagnosis has been provided, one needs to discuss treatment options. As mentioned in Chapter 6, there are many treatments for AD/HD, along with resources that help the child and family understand AD/HD and any comorbid disorders. Parents need to know what treatment options exist and to what extent they are empirically supported. This applies to treatments for AD/HD as well as for any comorbid conditions that the child may have.

One of the primary treatments for AD/HD is stimulant medication. Regardless of whether the clinician thinks this will ultimately be a part of the child's treatment package, it is a good idea to discuss it. As mentioned, it is rare to find a parent who hasn't heard something about Ritalin. Its frequent mention in print and on television has made Ritalin almost a household word; consequently many parents come to the feedback session with an opinion on it.

In anticipation of this, information should be included about how one determines when medication is appropriate. We have found that a brief overview of the stimulant trial procedure is reassuring to most parents. The stimulant trial highlights an objective way to make the best decision about medication with their child's physician. Next, one should discuss stimulants in general, how quickly they act and how quickly they leave the system. The empirical support, particularly the results from the MTA study, help to dispel misconceptions and answer questions that parents might have. Often, parents are afraid that taking medication will increase the child's chance of drug abuse or addiction in adolescence and adulthood. Information should be given to counter this fear and to explain that any future drug abuse is more likely to be due to other factors (e.g., antisocial personality features) than to taking medication for AD/HD.

Parents also need to know what to expect from the medication. Although stimulant medication can result in tremendous improvements for some children, it cannot address all possible difficulties. For example, stimulants can help children to be more attentive to parental requests and less impulsive in their actions, in turn reducing noncompliance, but it cannot address the major behavioral difficulties of children with conduct disorder. Sometimes the desired effects of medication are delayed. For example, it is unreasonable to expect that stimulant medication would result in immediate improvement of a child's grades. This is particularly true if the child has not mastered certain academic material. It is reasonable, however, to expect that stimulant medication will increase productivity and accuracy. To the extent that a child is free of learning disabilities and has the basic building blocks for the task, increased attention to detail could, in the long run, result in better grades. Outlining what medication can and can't do increases the parents' satisfaction with it and lays the groundwork for discussing why multiple treatments are often the best approach with AD/HD.

This also has bearing on how parents make attributions for the child's behavior. When parents see improvement in their child, and this improvement seems reliably related to medication, they might, understandably, attribute all gains to the medication and all difficulties to being off it. We have frequently heard parents, teachers, and even clinicians, say to children, "You're really having a tough day today. Did you remember to take your medication?" By understanding more fully what medication can and cannot do, parents can take a more balanced approach to recognizing the benefits and limitations of medication. In so doing, they do not rob the child of whatever credit for improvements they deserve or absolve the child of all responsibility for their difficulties.

If the child is to undergo a medication trial, parents should be provided with examples of how to discuss it with their child. As with the diagnosis, children need accurate information and honest answers to their questions about medication. Descriptions should be guided by the child's cognitive level and attention span. It isn't wise to overwhelm a child with technical aspects of the medication that may be beyond his or her understanding, and it is never a good idea to pass medication off as a "vitamin" or something other than what it is. Young children may not question this initially, but eventually they will realize that other children do not take vitamins this way. We have seen many instances where the child finds out from someone other than the parents that it is really medication. Sometimes it's an older child with AD/HD who is also taking medication at school, sometimes a professional who thinks the child already knows. Then the child feels confused at best, deceived at worst. Furthermore, false information does not facilitate trust between parent and child.

So how does one explain the effects of medication to a child? We have found that analogies related to the child's experience are useful in this regard, especially the analogy of running a race. One can ask the child, "Are you a fast runner?" Nearly every child says yes. The clinician then asks, "What are the names of some kids that don't run as fast as you?" After getting a name or two, the clinician then says, "Let's suppose that you and this friend are about to run a race, but in this race, you have heavy weights attached to your ankle. Who would win the race?" Invariably the child says that the friend would, at which point the clinician says, "Having those weights on is a lot like having AD/HD. It keeps you from doing what you can and know how to do. What would happen if we took off those weights?" After the child responds that he or she would run faster, the clinician offers the reason for the medication trial by saying, "Well that's why we sometimes give medication to children. It helps remove some of the 'weight' on you, and that makes it possible for you to be all that you can be." This analogy helps the child to see the benefits of medication without making it sound like magic. Similarly, highlighting that the medication enables the child to "be all that you can be," emphasizes that the child's own skills play an important part in any gains that are made. One also wants to avoid having the child attribute problems to not taking medication. For the child's self-esteem and self-efficacy, the goal here is to help the child understand the medication basics and appraise the benefits in a realistic way.

Information about other treatment options, such as parent training, school-based interventions, social skills training, and individual therapy is equally important. Recommending parent training can be a sensitive issue. If it is not handled well, parents may leave thinking that they have caused their child's AD/HD, thereby creating feelings of despondency, guilt, or perhaps anger at the clinician for suggesting such a preposterous notion. One should remind them of what we know about AD/HD, which is that it is not caused by poor parenting. However, the clinician must also explain that faulty parenting can exacerbate pre-existing AD/HD, and highlight that parenting such a child requires skills above and beyond those that work with most children. If the parent has reported high levels of parenting stress, one can refer back to this as an indication that the parent is putting forth a good effort but without much success. Another way to make this point is to call their attention to the successful manner in which other children in the home have responded to this same parenting approach. With this foundation, parent training can be introduced as a means of developing specialized approaches to parenting that are proven to work for the parents of children with AD/HD.

Parents also need to know which treatments do not have empirical support and which ones may actually be harmful. Just as with information about the AD/HD itself, misinformation on treatment is readily available in the popular press and on the Internet. Families often do not realize that a treatment can appear in print with no basis of support (e.g., chiropractic manipulations, dietary changes). A brief discussion of treatment-outcome research (e.g., double-blind trials, control groups) can aid parents in evaluating present and future treatment options. Parents are often the ones advocating for certain interventions, and they are usually the ones who must explain to other family members why certain options, and not others, are chosen. The goal, therefore, is to provide the parents with not only basic information for making treatment decisions, but with the knowledge of why this particular treatment plan is the best option at this time. Studies have found that an important influence on parents' satisfaction with feedback is the adequacy of the provider's rationale for treatment (Cadman, Shurvell, Davies, & Bradfield, 1984). By using the process outlined in Chapter 6 that links assessment to treatment, one is in a good position to provide this rationale and to develop, with the family, the best treatment plan for their child.

Understanding treatment options, parents and children are in a better position to actively participate in their design. They can work with the therapist to effect a comprehensive plan—one that addresses the symptoms of concern, builds on child and family strengths, and is acceptable to the family and thus culturally responsive. Without such understanding, the family cannot give truly informed consent.

Information about Referrals

Another feedback issue is whether additional referrals will be made. This conversation often follows the treatment discussion and forms the beginning of a treatment plan. What will the child and family need to act on the recommendations? What services are the child and family eligible for or entitled to? If referrals are to be made, it is helpful to have names and phone numbers ready.

Making the referral call while the family is there, or having a contact person (e.g., the therapist leading a parent training group) meet the family during the session, facilitates use of these resources.

COMMUNICATING WITH OTHERS

If it hasn't been addressed already during feedback, the issue of referrals raises the question as to who else needs the assessment information. In addition to providing a written report, one must sometimes communicate results quickly, even before the formal report is ready. Many of the important players in the child's life will already have been identified as part of the assessment process. Some, such as teachers, will have participated in the assessment. Others, such as the child's physician, may need to be contacted because a medication trial is recommended. Thus, some discussion with the parents should take place during the feedback session about who else should be contacted. Releases can be signed on the spot to avoid a delay in getting the information to those who will be assisting the family.

In the case of school personnel, several scenarios can arise. Because *DSM-IV* criteria require that the difficulties be evident in two or more settings, the child's teacher has probably already observed them. It is therefore helpful for the teacher to have timely information about the diagnostic conclusions and recommendations.

Another scenario is when a learning disability is suspected. In these instances, it may be important to schedule an LD assessment as soon as possible. This would necessitate contacting school personnel, such as the school psychologist, to initiate the referral process and to avoid delays. There have been several instances where, as a result of a phone call from us, the school asked that we complete the IQ and academic achievement testing that was started during the AD/HD assessment. Sometimes the clinician can do this more quickly than can the school. Furthermore, parents are spared having to repeat the same information to the school-based assessment team.

Similarly, if an IEP (individualized education plan) meeting is likely to happen before the written report is ready, the clinician should share pertinent results with the school before the meeting so that the recommendations can be considered. Given reimbursement practices under managed care, this will likely be done via phone, but there are times when the clinician should communicate the results in person, particularly if an important part of the treatment package will be school-based interventions, which are more likely to be implemented when the clinician can personally gather information that would be critical to the treatment. Like the parent session, school contact is an opportunity to exchange information. The clinician shares results and recommendations, but also listens to school personnel about their questions, their intervention priorities (which are not always clear from the assessment information), and what is likely to work in that particular classroom.

Sometimes the child's physician also needs immediate feedback, particularly if medication will be a part of the treatment package. Before instituting a medication trial, the child should have a physical or at least a brief check. Contacting the physician promptly is also important when referrals are to be made, because many managed care companies require that referrals be from the primary care physician. Precious time is wasted if the referral is not obtained before scheduling another service. Finally, physicians sometimes do not feel comfortable prescribing the medication, in which case another referral will then be necessary.

WRITTEN REPORTS

All formal assessments must be accompanied by some type of written documentation, which serves as the permanent record of what transpired, and sometimes also as legal documentation. Like oral communication, written reports are a powerful means of communicating assessment results and recommendations. They are the bridge between the family and others who will be assisting the child. Therefore, it would be a shame to conduct a thorough assessment, engage in thoughtful decision-making, give sensitive, comprehensive feedback, and then write a poor report. One should keep in mind that a report is often the clinician's only link to those who will play an important role in the child's treatment.

Timeliness is also essential. One can write an excellent report, but if it's not ready for several months, its utility is limited. Not only are the data old, but valuable treatment time has been lost. Although oral feedback can help bridge the gap between the assessment and the report, there are times when oral feedback will not suffice, such as when a legal document is necessary to proceed with intervention. What follows is a discussion of the key components of a successful report. The sample report at the end of the chapter illustrates one way to combine these components into a cohesive and effective document.

Report Components

The written report is a tool to communicate information—information about the assessment process and procedures, about the diagnosis, and about treatment recommendations. Each section plays an important part in linking the referral problem with its possible solutions.

Identifying Data

Every report must include basic information about the child such as the legal name, date of birth, age, and grade. Other information such as the child's record number, the date of evaluation, and date of the report, can also be included.

Reason for Referral

The reason for referral is essential in a written report, because it frames all else that follows. Among other things, assessment procedures depend on the referral question. Although clinicians need not go into extensive detail, they must give the reader a clear idea of why the child was evaluated. A specific referral question, stated with precision, also shapes how the diagnostic conclusions and treatment recommendations are discussed later in the report.

Services Provided

One purpose of a report is to highlight the multi-method approach. This can be done easily and efficiently by listing the procedures employed, either alone or with accompanying text description.

Test Results and Interpretation

This section of the report should take the reader through a presentation and brief discussion of the test results, highlighting the information gained through multiple methods and multiple sources. This can be done in an order paralleling the assessment procedures listed in the Services Provided section. A convenient way to present results is by informant, starting with the parent. Within this section, the parent interviews are described first. Narrow-band rating scales that address AD/HD criteria and begin to address developmental deviance are listed next, followed by the broad-band rating scales addressing both strengths and needs as well as possible comorbid conditions. For both types of scales, information about T scores and percentiles is included to show where the child's symptoms fall relative to other children.

Next come the data provided by the parents with respect to their own functioning, including areas likely to affect the child's symptoms or to be affected by them. These are most often rating scales that can be grouped according to general categories: such as those covering parenting issues (e.g., Parenting Stress Index, Parenting Alliance Inventory, Parenting Scale); individual psychological symptoms (e.g., adult AD/HD Rating Scale, SCL-90-R, Beck Depression Inventory, Beck Anxiety Inventory); and marital relationship, if appropriate (e.g., revised Dyadic Adjustment Scale).

Teacher information appears next. Results may be described in a similar fashion, that is, narrow-band results appear first, followed by broad-band ratings and any other measures given, such as the APRS.

The remainder of the report describes any individual testing or interviewing that was done with the child, beginning with a brief description of observed behaviors that may have had bearing on the validity of the interview or testing. This is followed by a summary of the intellectual and academic achievement testing results as well as the various clinic-based procedures (e.g., the CPT).

The results of other procedures can be integrated at any point along the way. Often this includes reference to information contained in the child's records.

Summary and Impressions

As outlined in Chapter 5, the decision-making process with respect to diagnostic conclusions is a hypothesis-testing approach. The report should reflect this approach so that the reader understands the rationale for its conclusions. A key element here consists of tying together the assessment results and the reason for the child's difficulties. If it is not AD/HD, the summary must say what it is instead. In short, the diagnostic conclusions must refer back to the referral question. Although this seems obvious, sometimes the decision-making process takes the assessment in a different direction. Even so, one must frame the results as they relate to the referral question.

Strengths must be summarized along with difficulties. Parent and teacher reports and the clinician's own appraisal yield the information for this. As mentioned earlier, strengths are not just the absence of problems (e.g., "no oppositional behavior") nor do they belong only to the child. The report should include child, family, and system strengths (e.g., coping skills, intellectual abilities, caring parents) that will be incorporated into the treatment plan.

Recommendations

A quality report leads the reader from the summary to the treatment plan. A good treatment recommendation section is essential, because a thorough assessment can be overshadowed by a poorly conceived or inadequately described set of recommendations. Even when a clinician has carefully used the multimethod approach to arrive at a thoughtful *DSM-IV* diagnosis, the report loses its impact without realistic and practical recommendations.

In what order should recommendations be listed? The most important ones should be listed first. How is this decided? There are several options, but whatever the choice, there should be some rationale to the decision. Often, the most important recommendations relate back to the referral question, but if issues that arose in the course of the assessment are more pressing, in which case recommendations can tie directly back to the pertinent assessment data, one lists them in order of what *should* be accomplished first. If, for example, a child has not only AD/HD but also Conduct Disorder, one may list treatments for the conduct problems first, because these behaviors are likely to cause both the child and his or her family the greatest distress. Or say a parent is having serious psychological or marital difficulties. The clinician would list individual or marital therapy first, indicating that it should occur prior to, or at least concurrent with, parent training, because parent training requires the parents to work together in addressing their child's difficulties.

Sometimes it is best to start with recommendations that can be accomplished quickly. Quick success can facilitate implementation of other treatments and provide all concerned with a much-needed boost. In any event, the family's priorities should help to guide the listing order.

Once the order is decided, one should write the recommendations in enough detail for the child to receive the services. Merely saying "A school-based intervention should take place" or "The child should receive individual therapy" is not likely to generate any meaningful treatment. Such a brief description provides neither a rationale for the intervention nor how it can be accomplished.

Although recommendations should always be individualized, there are general classes of recommendations that are likely to be appropriate for a child diagnosed with AD/HD. Medication is often an option and thus a medication trial is a frequent recommendation. Because many children with AD/HD also have oppositional behaviors, parent training is often suggested to address them at home. School-based interventions are also often appropriate. They might range from a token economy system, to a home–school communication system, to adaptations of classroom material, to environmental changes such as preferential seating, and more.

To ensure that detailed recommendations are provided, clinicians can develop a recommendations menu that covers medication, parent training, school-based interventions, social skills training, and other common therapies. These can then serve as the basis for a comprehensive list of recommendations that is incorporated into the report, yet tailored to the needs of the child and family.

Sample Report

To illustrate how the results of a multimethod assessment might be communicated in writing, we now give a sample report for Ross, who in Chapter 5 was identified with a dual diagnosis of AD/HD, and ODD, along with features of possible mild depression, anxiety, and visual/motor problems.

PSYCHOLOGICAL ASSESSMENT

THIS REPORT IS CONFIDENTIAL AND IS NOT TO BE RELEASED
WITHOUT THE EXPRESSED WRITTEN CONSENT
OF THE PARENT OR GUARDIAN OF THIS CHILD.

Identifying Information

Client's Name: Ross D.
Record Number: 123456
Date of Birth: 1/28/92
Age: 8 years, 5 months
Education: Third grade
Date of Evaluation: 6/15/2000
Date of Report: 7/20/2000

Reason for Referral

Ross D. is an 8-year-old Caucasian male enrolled in a regular third grade classroom. He was referred by his parents because of numerous home and school difficulties, including excessive fidgeting, difficulty following through on assigned tasks, and working below his potential academically. He was evaluated for these same concerns approximately 1 year ago by a local psychologist, who found no evidence of AD/HD or any other type of psychological problem. Because his difficulties persisted, Mr. and Mrs. D. decided to have Ross undergo another evaluation.

Services Provided

Developmental and Health History form
Computerized Diagnostic Interview Schedule for Children-IV (DISC-IV)—
    Parent version
Semi-Structured Background Interview
AD/HD Rating Scale-IV—Parent and teacher versions
Behavior Assessment System for Children (BASC)—Parent and teacher versions
Academic Performance Rating Scale (APRS)
Parenting Stress Index—Short Form (PSI-SF)
Parenting Scale (PS)
Symptom Checklist-90-Revised (SCL-90-R)
Adult AD/HD Rating Scale—Self-Report Version
Revised Dyadic Adjustment Scale (DAS-R)
Parenting Alliance Inventory (PAI)
Conners' Continuous Performance Test (CPT)
Wechsler Intelligence Scale for Children—Third Edition (WISC-III)
Wechsler Individual Achievement Test (WIAT)
Behavioral observations
School record review

Background Information

Developmental History: Ross was the product of an essentially normal full-term pregnancy and delivery. His neonatal course was complicated by jaundice that required no treatment. As a baby he posed no major health or temperamental problems. He reached all his major developmental milestones at age-appropriate times.

Health History: Throughout his lifetime Ross has maintained excellent physical health. He has no known allergies or chronic illnesses. At no time has he sustained any serious physical injury. His speech, hearing, vision, and motor coordination are age-appropriate. His current patterns of eating, sleeping, and elimination are within normal limits. He is not taking any prescription medication regularly.

Family History: Ross and two younger half-siblings live with their biological father and his stepmother in a home where the family has resided for the past year. Ross reportedly maintains typical relations with his siblings, neither of whom has major medical or developmental problems. Ross's father, Mr. D., and his biological mother were together for 3 years but never married. Ross remained in his mother's care through 6 months of age, at which time he began residing with a paternal aunt. Mr. D. assumed full-time custodial care when Ross was approximately 1 year old, and he received full legal custody when Ross was 5. Ross visits with his biological mother on an alternate-weekend basis. Mr. D. has a high school education and works full time in an auto body shop. Ross's stepmother, Mrs. D., also has a high school education and works full time in a bank. Mr. and Mrs. D. are in good physical health and neither has a history of significant adult psychiatric difficulties. Neither Mr. D. nor Ross's biological mother had documented learning, behavioral, or emotional problems as children. Mr. and Mrs. D. began living together 7 years ago and have been married for the past 3 years. Approximately 4 months ago, Ross's youngest sibling was born. Apart from this and a family move to a new residence earlier this year, there have been no other major lifestyle changes or psychosocial stressors affecting the immediate family over the past 12 months. Among the extended biological relatives there is no known history of AD/HD. There is, however, a reported maternal family history of conduct problems, antisocial behavior, and learning disabilities.

School History: Ross did not attend preschool. At age 5 he began kindergarten in a public school. Thereafter he was placed in a transitional kindergarten/first grade classroom. Since first grade he has been enrolled at the J. School, where he now is in a regular third grade classroom. He has never undergone any school-based assessment. Thus, information about his intellectual level and learning disability status was unavailable. According to Mrs. D., Ross currently is undergoing such an assessment through the school system. To date he has not received any special-education assistance. His academic achievement has been grade level to somewhat below grade level, which his parents and teachers believe is below his potential.

Test Results and Interpretation

DISC-IV/Parent Interview: Mrs. D.'s responses to the structured DISC-IV questioning indicated that Ross displays 7 of 9 inattention symptoms and 9 of 9 hyperactive-impulsive symptoms. These include his difficulties listening to and following through on instructions, distractibility, frequent interruption of others, and constant fidgeting. Many of these have been occurring in a chronic and pervasive fashion since approximately six years of age. In addition, the DISC-IV indicated that Ross displays 5 out of 8 symptoms suggestive of Oppositional Defiant Disorder (ODD), including noncompliance with adult requests, argumentativeness with adults, and frequent temper outbursts. These also have been readily apparent since approximately six years of age. Although the DISC-IV suggested the possibility of a simple phobia, this was in regards to his fearfulness of thunderstorms, which was not judged to be deviant from develop-

mental expectations. No other major behavioral, emotional, or psychiatric diagnostic concerns emerged from the DISC-IV with respect to Ross's psychosocial
functioning over the past 6 months.

Mrs. D.'s responses to semistructured interview questioning indicated that
Ross is happy most of the time. He has never displayed prolonged episodes of
clinically significant depression, anxiety, fearfulness, obsessions, compulsions,
tics, self-injurious behavior, or thought disturbance. He has never experimented
with alcohol, drugs, or cigarettes. There is no reported or suspected history of
physical or sexual abuse. As for his peer relations, Ross generally has been able
to make friends without difficulty. Keeping them, however, has been difficult,
because of his bossy interaction style. Nonetheless, he does have friends and
engages in many age-appropriate recreational activities.

With the exception of the psychological evaluation conducted last year,
Ross has not undergone other assessments of his psychosocial status. He has
never taken medications for behavior management purposes. His teachers reportedly do not employ special strategies to meet his individual behavioral
needs. At home, Mr. and Mrs. D. have been relatively consistent in their use of
various strategies to address his behavior. This has included taking privileges
away, such as toys and TV time, for misbehavior, as well as giving him special
privileges and using a charting system to promote appropriate behavior. Despite
having moderately good control over his home behavior, Mrs. D. indicated that
there was ample room for improvement. Thus, she was receptive to the idea of
receiving additional home management advice.

Parent-Completed Child Behavior Ratings: Mr. and Mrs. D. completed
these forms approximately 1 month before this evaluation. Their AD/HD Rating
Scale-IV results produced inattention and hyperactive-impulsive scores above
the 98th percentile. In line with these findings were their BASC Attention
Problems and Hyperactivity subscales, which generally fell above the 98th
percentile. Further examination of Mrs. D.'s BASC revealed a significantly elevated Aggression score, placing Ross above the 98th percentile on this dimension. Mrs. D.'s BASC Depression subscale and Mr. D.'s BASC Anxiety subscale
raised the possibility of depression and anxiety problems, given that both were
above the 95th percentile. Of additional interest is Mrs. D.'s BASC Social Skills
subscale score, which placed Ross's social skills more than 1.5 standard deviations below the mean. No other rating scale results fell into a clinically significant range.

Parent Self-Report Ratings: Mr. and Mrs. D. completed all of these forms
as well. Their PS results were within normal limits, indicating that they were
using child management strategies that would be appropriate for most children.
In contrast, their PSI-SF results fell into an elevated range, suggesting clinically
significant levels of parenting stress. Somewhat discrepant from her interview
responses, Mrs. D.'s SCL-90-R results fell into an elevated range. Thus, she
would seem to be experiencing levels of personal stress that are higher than that
expected for same-aged adults. Moreover, her Adult AD/HD Rating Scale results

raised the possibility that she herself may be affected by AD/HD. Generally speaking, the DAS-R and the PAI results were within normal limits, suggesting that Mrs. D. is generally satisfied with her marriage and that she perceives a strong alliance with her husband on parenting issues.

Teacher-Completed Child Behavior Ratings: Ross's primary classroom teacher and one of his secondary teachers completed these forms approximately 1 month prior to this evaluation. The ratings were based on observations of Ross in regular classrooms with 1 teacher and approximately 25 students. Generally speaking, none of the results obtained from the secondary teacher fell into a clinically significant range. In contrast, the results from his primary teacher revealed a hyperactive-impulsive score on the AD/HD Rating Scale-IV that fell above the 90th percentile. This finding was generally in line with her BASC Hyperactivity subscale results, which fell above the 98th percentile. Consistent with Mrs. D.'s BASC responses, this same teacher also reported Aggression and Depression scores above the 95th percentile. The APRS results from the primary teacher revealed evidence of diminished productivity, given that the academic productivity score fell more than 1 standard deviation below the mean for Ross's age and gender. No other clinically significant concerns emerged from the teacher ratings.

Behavioral Observations: Ross separated easily for the testing and went to the testing room willingly with the examiner. No problems were evident with respect to his ability to understand or follow directions. His eye contact, affect, and thought processing were within normal limits. He remained cooperative and well-motivated throughout the testing session. At no time did he display any obvious AD/HD symptomatology. Such behavior is somewhat discrepant from parent and teacher reports. Thus, the obtained findings very likely represent an optimal, rather than typical, level of functioning.

CPT Results: Generally speaking, Ross's CPT performance fell within normal limits on most indices of this task. One exception was the commission error score, which fell at approximately the 84th percentile. Although not considered clinically significant, this nonetheless suggests a relatively high degree of impulse control difficulty.

IQ Results: Ross's WISC-III performance yielded a Verbal IQ of 129, a Performance IQ of 123, and a Full-Scale IQ of 129. Further analyses of the WISC-III produced factor index scores of 136 on verbal-comprehension, 133 on perceptual organization, 98 on freedom from distractibility, and 86 on processing speed. Generally speaking, these results suggest that Ross's overall intelligence lies within the high-average to superior range. However, both his freedom from distractibility and his processing speed scores were significantly lower than either the verbal comprehension or the perceptual organizational scores. Thus, these areas represent relative and absolute weaknesses for Ross. A summary of the subtest scaled score distribution appears below:

Verbal Subtests		Performance Subtests	
Information	16	Picture Completion	17
Similarities	16	Coding	5
Arithmetic	10	Picture Arrangement	9
Vocabulary	15	Block Design	19
Comprehension	18	Object Assembly	17
Digit Span	9	Symbol Search	9

With the exception of his coding score, all other scores were of at least average quality, with most falling into a high-average to superior range. Observations of Ross during the testing seemed to suggest that this focally low coding score was due to slowness in his motor functioning rather than to visual memory problems. His relatively high scores on the Block Design and Object Assembly subtests indicate a relative and absolute strength with respect to his nonverbal reasoning and organizational abilities.

Ross's WIAT performance yielded standard scores of 91 in reading, 96 in math, and 93 in spelling. Generally speaking, all of these results are well below expectations for his measured intelligence.

Summary and Impressions

Ross is an 8-year-old boy of high-average to superior intelligence with no prior documented history of learning disabilities. Dating back to six years of age, he has been displaying a chronic and pervasive pattern of inattention, impulsivity, and physical restlessness. Evidence for such behaviors was absent from informal observations of his test behavior. His stepmother's responses to structured interview questioning, her rating scale responses, the rating scale responses from his father, and the rating scale responses from his primary teacher were consistent in identifying the above behavioral concerns as being developmentally deviant. More specifically, the frequency and severity of Ross's inattention, impulsivity, and physical restlessness would not be found in more than 2–5% of the general population of boys his age. Although such problems can stem from underlying Pervasive Developmental Disorders or other psychiatric conditions, such conditions do not affect Ross at present. In their absence, the current evaluation results therefore indicate that he meets *DSM-IV* criteria for a diagnosis of Attention-Deficit/Hyperactivity Disorder, Combined Type (314.01). Relative to other children carrying this diagnosis, Ross seems to possess an AD/HD condition that is moderate to severe in its presentation and manifested across both the home and school settings.

In at least 40% of the AD/HD population, additional behavioral complications are present in the form of Oppositional-Defiant Disorder (ODD). Input from Ross's mother and from his primary teacher were consistent in identifying his noncompliance, argumentativeness, temper outbursts, and other ODD features as being developmentally deviant, that is, above the 95th percentile relative to same-aged boys. Thus, Ross meets *DSM-IV* criteria for a secondary diagnosis of Oppositional-Defiant Disorder (313.81). Relative to others carrying this diagnosis, Ross's ODD appears to be mild. No further diagnostic concerns arose from the current evaluation with respect to other areas of his behavioral, emotional, or psychiatric functioning. However, the parent and teacher completed BASC results did raise the possibility of mild depressive and anxiety features. The exact cause of these is unclear, but they could be related to the frustration that Ross experiences from the daily impact of his AD/HD. Issues related to his biological mother may be at work as well. Ross's focally low coding score on the WISC-III suggests the possibility of visual motor or fine motor difficulties. Although this would not explain all of his school-based problems, having a motor difficulty would certainly serve to complicate matters further.

Ross's AD/HD and ODD very likely have contributed a great deal to the diminished academic productivity and academic underachievement that he displays in school. Moreover, these same conditions probably contribute a great deal to the elevated personal distress and increased parenting stress reported by his parents. The same is true for the emerging peer relationship difficulties that Ross is encountering both at home and at school.

Working in Ross's favor is the fact that he is highly intelligent and has no major learning disabilities. His home life is now quite stable. His parents are motivated to help him in whatever way they can. Although he has not worked up to his own potential, he has achieved academically at a level commensurate with same-aged peers. Of additional significance is that Ross is also in a school system that has traditionally been receptive to modifying the classroom environment of students with AD/HD. For these reasons, there is much basis for predicting that Ross can improve his functioning both at home and at school. To increase the probability that this does indeed occur, consideration should be given to incorporating the recommendations listed below.

Recommendations

1. Given the multiple difficulties that Ross has, multiple treatments will need to be used in combination to address his many needs across the home and school settings.
2. Because proper knowledge and understanding of AD/HD is essential to its effective management, Ross's parents and teachers are advised to increase their awareness of this disorder and its associated features. This may be accomplished in part through selected readings, such as *Taking Charge of AD/HD* by Dr. Russell Barkley. Further educational resources include videotapes by Dr. Barkley and other experts in the field, which may be obtained from the A.D.D. WareHouse. Information about AD/HD can also be acquired through the CHADD Web site (*http://www.chadd.org*).
3. Stimulant medication is often given to children with AD/HD to decrease their inattention, impulsivity, and physical restlessness. Such medication is advisable at the present time due to the severity of Ross's AD/HD and its significant impact on many areas of his functioning, particularly in school. Initially such medication should be administered on a trial basis, preferably in the context of a double-blind, drug–placebo format

in which objective parent and teacher ratings of Ross's behavior, as well as direct performance measures, are used as measures of potential benefits, and side effects. Such a trial should be conducted under the supervision of a child psychiatrist or pediatrician with expertise in this area.

4. Because traditional parenting techniques generally do not work well for children with AD/HD or ODD, their parents often experience a great deal of stress in their parenting roles. This would certainly seem to be the case for the D. family. To reduce such parenting stress and to gain greater control over Ross's AD/HD and ODD problems at home, Mr. and Mrs. D. should consider receiving detailed instruction in the use of *specialized* behavior management strategies. To the extent that Ross's biological mother is interested and available, she too would likely benefit from such instruction. A detailed description of these intervention strategies can be found in Dr. Barkley's recent publication *Taking Charge of AD/HD*. Additional assistance in using such techniques can be obtained through the AD/HD Clinic's 9-week Parent Training Program.

5. According to Mrs. D., a school-based assessment is now in progress. If for some reason this is not occurring, it should be scheduled, because classroom and curriculum modifications will be necessary to maximize Ross's academic progress. Although there is no strong reason to suspect the possibility of learning disabilities, psychoeducational screening measures should nonetheless be given to clarify whether these might indeed be present. In particular, attention should be given to possible visual–motor or fine motor problems. This can be accomplished through an occupational therapy consultation, as well as through a consultation with his family physician.

6. Compensatory strategies can address many AD/HD problems *before* they occur. Use of such strategies initially requires a careful analysis of the situational demands or conditions that precede AD/HD problems. In general, AD/HD symptoms are more likely to occur in situations that are unstructured, ambiguous, boring, repetitive, familiar, or of extremely long duration. Group settings can also exacerbate AD/HD symptomatology. To the extent that such conditions can be changed within the classroom, children with AD/HD can often function more successfully. For this reason, consideration should be given to incorporating the compensatory strategies listed below:

   • To enhance Ross's capacity for completing assigned work, efforts should be made to use curriculum material of high interest. The more that Ross enjoys the work, the less likely it is that AD/HD difficulties will interfere with his performance.

   • In situations where Ross does not benefit from traditional teaching techniques, consideration should be given to providing him with an opportunity to receive similar academic instruction in the context of computerized programming, which may be a more effective way of motivating him to complete assignments.

- In view of Ross's difficulties in completing assigned work, his work-load should be modified to stay within his attentional capabilities. One way this may be accomplished is by reducing lengthy tasks into smaller, more manageable units. For example, a 20-item task might be presented as two separate 10 item tasks. Another option is to have Ross complete just a subset of assigned items. For instance, instead of doing all 20 items, Ross might be asked to complete the first 10 items only. As long as the assigned number of items is sufficient for learning the academic process under consideration, Ross's learning should be enhanced. Similar adjustments may be made with respect to assigned homework.
- In addition to motivational difficulties, children with AD/HD often have trouble adhering to rules. To increase Ross's compliance within the classroom, his teachers should review the rules with him regularly. Index cards with general instructions (e.g., "stay in seat") can also be taped to Ross's desk.

7. Classroom compensatory strategies are not always practical. Where conditions cannot be altered to meet the needs of a particular child, AD/HD symptoms are more likely to interfere with that child's behavior and academic performance. One way to reduce this possibility is by providing the child with clearly stated expectations and consequences for behavior. Of particular significance are the consequences, which provide children with AD/HD with the external motivation that they seem to require to overcome their difficulties. In general, AD/HD symptoms are much less problematic when consequences are dispensed in a clear, meaningful, immediate, frequent, and consistent manner. To the extent that this can be done within the classroom, children with AD/HD very often perform more successfully. For this reason, consideration should be given to incorporating the following motivational strategies:

- Because children with AD/HD are bored easily and lack the motivation to complete uninteresting tasks, it is often necessary to provide them with lots of ongoing feedback about their performance. Thus, Ross's teachers should consider providing him with relatively more feedback, both positive and negative, than would be the case for other children in the classroom.
- As much as possible, incentives should be incorporated into Ross's school programming. Such incentives or rewards should be meaningful to him and should be delivered in a frequent, immediate, and consistent manner. To reduce the possibility that Ross will become bored with this type of programming, target behaviors and consequences should be modified periodically.
- Although classroom applications of behavior management programs are highly desirable, they are often difficult to incorporate for only one child in a regular classroom setting. Thus, it is usually necessary to consider alternative approaches for mainstreamed children with AD/

HD. One such alternative is to incorporate a daily report card system. In this system, teachers monitor various classroom behaviors (e.g., finishes assigned seat work) by providing ratings on an index card that is sent home daily. Parents then convert these ratings into either positive or negative consequences (e.g., loss of television privileges), which, for many children, are more meaningful and effective than those available in school.

8. At the present time, Ross seems to be displaying emerging problems with peer relationships, as well as possible depression and anxiety symptoms. The overall severity of these are not sufficient to warrant immediate intervention. They are, however, of such concern that they ought to be monitored closely over the upcoming months. Should problems in these areas continue after the above interventions are in place, consideration should then be given to having him participate in a school-based group social skills training program, as well as individual therapy to explore the nature of his mild depressive and anxious symptoms.

9. Also emerging from the evaluation were concerns about Mrs. D. having elevated levels of personal distress as well as adult AD/HD symptomatology. Currently she is not receiving treatment for these conditions. To the extent that they may be interfering with her personal life or her efforts to parent Ross, she should consider seeking an evaluation and possibly treatment from a professional with expertise in the area of adult AD/HD. Dr. M. in this clinic is one such individual whom she could contact to explore this possibility.

Disposition

Portions of the above findings and recommendations were discussed with Mrs. D. at the end of the evaluation. Additional feedback will be provided in a follow-up session with her husband present, and possibly with Ross's biological mother present as well. In all likelihood, Mrs. D. and her husband will begin receiving parent counseling and training through this clinic. Thereafter they will likely have Ross undergo a double-blind drug–placebo stimulant medication trial. Any additional consultation or services will be provided upon request.

Arthur D. Anastopoulos, Ph.D.

cc: Medical Records
      Mr. and Mrs. D. (3 copies)

Providing the Report to Others

Reports are commonly shared with parents and other interested individuals. Ideally, a discussion with the parents will take place during the feedback session concerning who should receive the report. Release of information forms can be signed by the child's parent or guardian at that time. It has been our policy to have the parents review the report first and have an opportunity to discuss the results and recommendations before it is sent to others. In most cases, the information contained in the report will not differ from the issues discussed during the feedback session. However, sometimes seeing it in print changes the family's comfort level. Occasionally there are mistakes in the report, such as factual errors in the background history section. It is always better to have these concerns addressed before the report is distributed than to have to make retractions later.

Because of the need for timeliness, it is best if the same report can be distributed to all interested parties. One cost-effective way of doing this is to provide the family with multiple copies. They can then decide when and with whom to share the information and what information to share. Because they have the reports in hand, and thus do not have to sign a release, the report can be shared more readily.

There are times, however, when separate reports may be written. For example, there may be sensitive information that the parents do not want sent to the school (e.g., family history of psychiatric illness). The family's preferences should be respected and a separate report written that omits these sections. In most cases omissions do not hinder the child's treatment. Sometimes, however, such information is important for the teacher to have. In those instances, the clinician should discuss with parents the rationale for including the information and see if a compromise can be reached whereby the core information is shared in a way that is comfortable for the family.

CONCLUSION

Feedback, in whatever form, should provide the child, the parents, and interested others with an understanding of the procedures that were implemented, the process by which the diagnostic conclusions were reached, the rationale for the recommendations, and the interventions suggested. Feedback is a means to an important end: lessening the child's difficulties.

> When handled poorly, the initial diagnostic phase will remain as a bitter memory whose details linger in the minds of the parent for many years thereafter. When handled with sensitivity and technical skill, this experience can contribute to a strong foundation for productive family adaptation and for constructive parent–professional collaboration.
>
> —Thomasgard and Shonkoff, 1998, p. 195

8

Assessing Treatment Outcome

"I've tried this before. It doesn't work."

Ideally, diagnostic assessments are the bridge for developing treatment goals and recommendations. Input from parents, caregivers, and teachers is vital to any AD/HD diagnostic process, as is the perspective of the child or adolescent in some cases. These varying perspectives, gathered through interviews, behavior rating scales, psychological tests, and direct observations offer invaluable information about symptoms, frequency, severity, developmental deviance, and pervasiveness of AD/HD and its impact on functioning. This information, in turn, leads to intervention. But the role of assessment doesn't end there. Assessment procedures can also evaluate the efficacy of treatment, determining when and how to refine it and when to replace it with something else.

In many instances, the data obtained for diagnosis can also serve a double purpose as a baseline for treatment evaluation, but there are times when specific interventions were not clearly articulated at the time of diagnosis. Also, some interventions necessitate specific assessment strategies beyond those carried out during the diagnostic process. In these instances, thought must be directed toward the outcome evaluation. This chapter outlines an 8-step process for designing and conducting a systematic outcome evaluation (see Figure 8.1.). Examples of outcome measures and indicators are provided for the three major AD/HD interventions: pharmacological, school-based, and home-based.

ASSESSING TREATMENT EFFICACY

In order to gather as much data as possible about the benefits of a particular treatment, several things must be considered. Our eight-step process is a systematic way to address these considerations. The first three steps involve the preparation and decision-making that comes before any baseline data are collected. Outcome indicators and benchmarks of success must be defined before evaluation methods are chosen. Baseline data are then collected in Step 4. Step 5

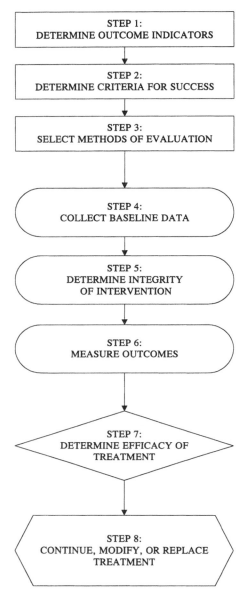

FIGURE 8.1. Outcome evaluation process.

outlines an often overlooked part of the process: the extent to which an intervention is implemented as designed. Without this information, conclusions about treatment are meaningless. Step 6 gives an overview of how to measure outcomes. The last 2 steps address the final decision-making process regarding the treatment's efficacy.

Step 1. Determine Outcome Indicators

Many empirically supported interventions have been described for use with groups of children who have AD/HD. The critical question is to what degree will any of these treatments, alone or in combination, be effective for a *particular* child. To answer this question, one must choose the outcome indicators carefully. In fact, the very design of an intervention evaluation can improve the effectiveness of that intervention. Step 1 forms the foundation of the subsequent steps. Without clearly articulated outcome indicators, it is impossible to carry out an informative efficacy evaluation.

There are several things to consider when choosing the indicators. First, *the outcome indicator must be tied to the intervention*. Initially this statement seems obvious, but there are times when something is implemented for one aspect of AD/HD but the assessment targets another aspect. Take, for example, an intervention designed to increase a child's attention to task. To determine its efficacy, one must identify outcome indicators that are likely to be affected by the intervention (e.g., number of problems completed, accuracy of individual desk work). Although increased attention might also result in decreased disruptiveness in the classroom, this is not the target of the intervention. As a result, one would not look for outcome indicators that measure disruptiveness (e.g., out of seat, talking out of turn). In contrast, for a response cost program whereby the child loses tokens or privileges for disruptive behavior (e.g., out of seat, excessive talking) decreased disruptiveness would be an appropriate outcome indicator.

Second, *the outcome indicator must be specific enough that an accurate evaluation can be made*. For example, parent training might be recommended because a parent reports having constant arguments with a child about chores, homework, friends, or curfew. The goal is to decrease noncompliance and arguing. Although the parent training may well be effective, it is difficult to measure "decreased arguing" because it is such a broad construct. It would be better to tally how many times the child complies with a request the first time it is given in a specific situation. DuPaul and Stoner (1994) suggest that academic output and performance are likely to be more informative than behaviors such as staying in one's seat. The first two examples are more quantifiable and do not violate the "dead-man" test for behavior as described by Lindsley (1991). According to Lindsley, if a dead man could do the behavior in question (i.e., not getting up), it is an inappropriate target for behavior analysis. The absence of a behavior is harder to measure than its occurrence (e.g., raising hand before speaking). In any event, most treatments are designed to affect some aspect of the basic AD/HD symptoms—inattention, impulsivity, hyperactivity—as well as areas of functional impairment (e.g., school failure, parent–child interaction difficulties) that provided the impetus for treatment in the first place.

Third, *the outcome indicator must be likely to change in the time frame outlined for the evaluation*. Take, for example, the use of stimulant medication. A child with AD/HD who responds well to it is likely to be more successful in school. However, it may take a good deal of time to observe actual changes in academic achievement. One would not want to wait through an entire grading period to determine the medication's effectiveness when another index could be observed sooner (e.g., increased work productivity).

Some changes occur only with time. Unless one is conducting a formal research study, a treatment evaluation will generally be done over a fairly short period. For example, it may take several months after the completion of the parent training for the parent to notice changes in the child's behavior. However, if the intervention is successful, one will probably see a significant short-term decrease in parenting stress. This applies to school-based interventions as well. For example, the efficacy of treatment to increase on-task behavior is more likely to be seen first in the number and accuracy of problems completed on a math sheet, and only later will you see improvement in the child's math grades or in scores on a standardized end-of-year testing.

This does not mean that long-term outcomes are not important. Ideally, both short-term and long-term outcome indicators are chosen. However, it is the short-term indicators that are essential, because they ensure that the feedback can be incorporated into the child's treatment protocol in an ongoing manner.

Finally, *the outcome indicators should be of importance to the child, the family, and the teacher.* Indicators should relate not only to AD/HD, but also to the referral concerns. Examples of some outcome indicators that address both symptoms and impairment are presented in Table 8.1.

TABLE 8.1. Sample Outcome Indicators

Intervention target	Sample outcome indicators
Increase attention	Work accuracy
	Task productivity
	Percentage of on-task time
	Sustained attention to task
Decreased impulsivity	Interruptions in conversation
	Turn-taking
	Careless errors
Decrease hyperactivity	Inappropriate vocalizations
	Inappropriate movements
	Subjective feelings of restlessness
	Out-of-seat behavior
Increase social competence	Aggression in peer interaction
	Social skills in peer interaction
Increase behavioral awareness	Matching child–teacher views of behavior
	Accuracy in identifying consequences of behavior
Decrease oppositional behavior	Number of problematic home situations
	Compliance with parental requests
	Number of problematic school situations
	Compliance with teacher requests
Generalize skills	Number of situations skills observed

Step 2. Determine Criteria for Success

After the outcome indicators are identified, the next step is to select the criteria for determining the success of the intervention. One must answer the question, to what benchmark does one compare these ratings? In many cases, intervention evaluations use the child, the family, or the teacher as their own comparison or control. Using an ABAB reversal design, improvements over time or fluctuations in behavior contingent on the initiation or cessation of an intervention will reveal whether the treatment is having the desired effect. Another method is to compare behavior in a setting where the intervention is operating (e.g., classes with Teacher A) with one where it is not (e.g., classes with Teacher B).

Although this type of analysis answers part of the question, the degree to which the behavior represents a meaningful change is still unmeasured. This is critical when deciding whether to continue an intervention. To measure meaningful change, one must identify a norm for the target behavior. That is, has the behavior increased or decreased to the point where the child's functioning is similar to that of peers? This question can be answered in several ways. Let's take a school-based intervention to illustrate. First, the amount of time the child with AD/HD is engaged in on-task behavior can be compared with that of another child in the classroom whose behavior is the norm for that setting. For this, one must choose an observational system such as the BASC Student Observational System (SOS: Kamphaus & Reynolds, 1994). Second, instead of comparing the target child's behavior with baseline, one could compare it with normative data. For this method, one must establish guidelines for success. For example, a successful response to medication might be evidenced by impulsive responding on the Conners' Continuous Performance Test (CPT; Conners, 1994) that is no more than 1 standard deviation above the mean for other children of the same age and gender.

Still another option is to see if clinically significant change occurred. Statistical methods have been developed to assist clinicians and researchers in answering this question. The Reliable Change Index (RCI) is a good procedure for assessing clinical significance (developed by Jacobson and Truax, 1991). In this approach, the RCI is equal to the difference between a child's pretreatment score and posttreatment score, divided by the standard error of difference between the two. When the RCI exceeds 1.96, it is unlikely that the change from pretreatment to posttreatment is due to chance ($p < .05$). Thus, the RCI measures the degree to which an improvement in functioning is likely due to treatment rather than to imprecise measurement. Whatever approach is taken (e.g., subclinical *T* scores, reliable change), all necessitate choosing measurements that have normative data and excellent psychometric characteristics.

Another indicator of a successful intervention is when the child's behavior is no longer severe enough to meet diagnostic criteria. In a comprehensive treatment plan where medication, home-based, and school-based interventions are combined to address the difficulties of a child with AD/HD Combined subtype, one would look for decreased frequency, severity, and pervasiveness of the AD/HD symptoms. In this case, a measure such as the AD/HD Rating Scale-IV, which can be used by parents and teachers, can examine whether parent and teacher ratings of the child's behavior frequently show fewer than 6 inattention or 6 hyperactive-impulsive symptoms following treatment.

Finally, the criterion for success is not always a change in scores or ratings. Sometimes the maintenance of behavior represents success, such as when an improvement is maintained during the fading of a particular program. Whatever the criteria, they must be chosen before proceeding to Step 3, which is deciding on the actual methods to evaluate them.

Step 3. Select Methods of Evaluation

Once outcome indicators are chosen and success criteria defined, the specific methods by which the indicators are evaluated must be determined. The decisions made in the previous steps, and other considerations, will guide these choices.

First, *the method must specifically tap the outcome indicators* identified in Step 1. For example, if one is evaluating an intervention designed to increase positive and decrease negative social interactions, one would choose a rating scale or method that targets that outcome specifically (e.g., number of aggressive exchanges the child initiates during recess), as well as a more global measure of behavioral competence, such as the empirically validated Social Skills Rating System (Gresham & Elliott, 1990).

Second, *the method must be compatible with the process chosen to determine the success of the intervention* (see Step 2). If, for example, the benchmark for success is the target child's performance as compared with a peer's, the methods chosen must be ones that can be used for that peer in the classroom. To compare the target child's performance with a larger sample using normative data, one must use a rating scale or observational system that has norms for children of the same age, gender, and ethnicity as the target child.

Obviously, the most psychometrically sound measures and methods should be chosen, but when several options exist, success criteria should guide the choice. For example, because these measures will be administered repeatedly (at baseline, during treatment, following treatment, and perhaps at follow-up), test-retest reliability is essential. The practice effect of a particular instrument must also be considered. The availability of normative data and a standardization sample comparable to the target child must be considered if norms are to serve as the criterion or to be incorporated into calculations of clinically significant change.

Third, *the methods must accommodate several time factors*. One factor is how often one expects to collect data. Some tools are designed to capture perceptions of a child over several months (e.g., the Child Behavior Checklist). This is not appropriate if the time between baseline and treatment evaluation is short. Other tools, such as the Home and School Situations Questionnaire, are sensitive to short-term changes.

Another time consideration relates to cost, in both dollar and human terms.

This must always be balanced with the usefulness of the information derived. How much training is needed for raters or observers? How disruptive will the evaluation be? What are the ethical concerns when observing a peer? These are just some of the questions to consider when deciding on outcome evaluation methods.

Ideally, *the methods cover the age range of the child across all assessments.* That is, can you use the same measure for baseline, end-of-treatment, and follow-up evaluations? If at all possible, one should choose methods that can be used throughout the evaluation process (e.g., from preschool through early elementary). Many scales, such as the BASC, the Achenbach, and the Conners', are available across a wide age range.

Similarly, *the methods should be available for multiple informants if the intervention is to be evaluated across settings.* Just as information from multiple informants provides a more complete diagnostic picture, it is equally valuable when examining the efficacy of certain interventions. Obviously, there are times when one would not look for changes in multiple settings, such as with a specific school-based intervention or with parent training. However, other interventions, such as stimulant medication, should be evaluated across settings (e.g., home and school).

Finally, as with the diagnostic evaluation, *the methods must be designed to obtain as valid and comprehensive picture as possible.* As such, a multimethod approach, utilizing psychometrically sound methods such as rating scales and direct observation, is likely to yield the most complete picture. Each method has its advantages and disadvantages. The advantages of rating scales include being easy to use, requiring less training to complete, covering a variety of behaviors, and providing normative data. However, sometimes it takes longer for changes in perceptions to show up on rating scales than to show up in direct observation. In addition, the more global items may not adequately tap initial changes in discrete behaviors. Direct observation is less dependent on long-term perceptions, and it may yield more ecologically valid information about initial changes in the discrete outcome indicators chosen to evaluate the intervention, but this method is expensive, requires more training, and may be too intrusive. Deciding how to measure clinically significant change must be done in light of all these issues.

Step 4. Collect Baseline Data

Comprehensive baseline data are essential for a sound evaluation process. The decisions made in the previous steps affect this step as well. For example, if the success criteria involve comparing the target child's performance with that of a classmate, one must obtain baseline data on the classmate. This allows comparisons at two points in time as well as an estimation of typical developmental changes occurring for all same-aged children in the classroom.

One must also decide what will serve as baseline data. Are there data in the diagnostic assessment that can be used? For example, if rating scales were used in the diagnostic process, these could easily serve an outcome evaluation purpose as well. However, time and cost savings from using existing data should not override having timely, appropriate data on the specific outcome indicators. If there was a delay in starting the treatment, data obtained during the initial assessment may no longer be accurate. One must also consider whether the measures and methods chosen are more sensitive to practice effects. If so, multiple baseline assessments may be necessary.

Finally, there is the timing of the baseline data relative to the intervention. For example, one might obtain baseline data on a child during the first 2 weeks of school. The school-based intervention is scheduled to begin the first of October and an initial outcome evaluation is scheduled before Thanksgiving break. However, the behavior of many children during the first 2 weeks of school is not typical. Children often experience a honeymoon period during which their behavior is much better than usual. If so, and baseline data are collected during that time, it may appear that the child's behavior has actually worsened after starting the treatment, and a promising intervention could be inappropriately terminated. For other children, the start of school, particularly if it is a new school, exacerbates behavior problems. If this period is the baseline, the intervention will appear more successful than it actually is. Sometimes baseline data are collected but the intervention does not start at the expected time. One must then collect additional baseline data closer to the start of the treatment. The goal of all this is to determine with as much certainty as possible whether an intervention has resulted in meaningful behavioral changes, so baseline data collection must be scheduled with this goal in mind.

Step 5. Determine Integrity of Intervention

An essential step in evaluating the efficacy of any intervention is to discover if it is actually being carried out as designed. All too often decisions about the effect of an intervention are made without first determining its integrity. Was the intervention implemented as intended? If there are inconsistencies in the delivery of the intervention, an outcome evaluation can serve as a guideline for making adjustments in the program before evaluating its efficacy.

One way to see if an intervention is being implemented as intended is outlined by Gresham (1989). First, all the components of a particular intervention, along with the times during which it should take place, are listed. Next an outside observer or, as a last resort, the person who is to implement the intervention, can check off when the intervention has occurred. How often the treatment component is being implemented can then be calculated for a particular period (e.g., a week). The overall integrity of the intervention package is then computed by averaging the integrity percentages of each of the components. A sample of this analysis is outlined in Table 8.2. using examples from a school-based intervention program for kindergartners (e.g., Barkley et al., 1999).

Even when 100% integrity is not achieved, efficacy evaluations can still be useful, because the information can aid in refining the treatment. The only caveat is that any decisions about continuing the intervention or conclusions about its effectiveness must be examined within the context of its integrity. For

TABLE 8.2. Sample Observation Form for Recording Treatment Integrity

Treatment components	M	T	W	TH	F	% Compliance
1. Describe program daily	○	○	×	○	○	80
2. Unveil color-coded chart	○	○	○	○	○	100
3. Review child's morning progress every 30 minutes	○	○	○	×	○	80
4. Change color based on rule violation	○	○	○	○	×	80
5. Ask child to reflect on rule-following in morning activities	○	○	×	×	○	60
6. Award bonus points for accuracy in behavior matching	○	○	○	○	○	100
7. Award reinforcer at lunch based on color achieved	○	○	○	○	○	100
Total % daily/weekly integrity	100	100	71	71	86	86

Note: ○ = Occurrence; × = Nonoccurrence.

example, if the child's target behaviors worsen on Wednesday, and are generally improved in the morning but not in the afternoon, the integrity data suggest that a less consistent implementation of the program in the afternoons and on Wednesdays may be a factor. Conversely, a more-complete implementation of the program on the other days and in the mornings may be responsible for the child's improved behavior.

If several weeks of integrity data were recorded and this pattern continued, one would examine why it was easier to implement the program in the morning than in the afternoon and why it was harder to implement it on Wednesday. Adaptations to the program could then be made. For example, a discussion with the teacher may reveal that the children have many "specials" (e.g., computer time, music, media center, art) on Wednesday. This may be difficult for the child and result in an increase of problematic behaviors. Also, these transitions, coupled with the fact that the child is spending less time in homeroom, may make it hard for the teacher to employ the program consistently. This information could then lead to a system adjustment. Perhaps fewer behaviors could be targeted so that those recorded are recorded accurately. Another option is to develop an adjunct system that can be used by the various "specials" teachers.

Of course, it is impossible to determine the degree to which periodic integrity evaluations accurately reflect the day-to-day implementation of a program. It is well documented that the mere observation or self-recording of a behavior tends to increase it. Thus, periodic integrity evaluations should be used systematically as part of an ongoing program to maintain the manner, consistency, and frequency of the intervention. At the very least, the numbers can serve as an upper estimate of the program's integrity. Integrity evaluation also provides a type of functional analysis of the child's behavior. Given the helpfulness of this approach for treatment planning, and its necessity with regard to specialized behavioral and educational interventions under the new regulations of IDEA (Individuals with Disabilities Education Act), examining the fidelity of an intervention is as important as examining whether it works.

The level of detail previously described is probably more applicable for school-based interventions or large-scale research investigations, but consideration of treatment integrity is equally valuable for home-based and pharmacological interventions. For example, one might examine the degree to which parent training is effective. These programs often cover information about AD/HD, its effect on parent–child interactions, and how specialized behavior management techniques can improve parenting. To examine its effectiveness, one must have some estimation of how much knowledge the parents have actually acquired about AD/HD and about the key behavioral principles on which the program is based. Rating scales such as the Test of AD/HD Knowledge (TOAK; Anastopoulos, unpublished manuscript) and the Parenting Scale can be helpful for this. How often parents are able to use parts of the program (e.g., special time, time-out) can also be monitored via a short checklist, which can be completed at the end of a therapy session or parent group meeting based on what was reviewed there. Treatment validity applies to pharmacological interventions as well. An estimation of medication compliance is needed to determine the degree to which medication resulted in meaningful change. If medication is to be taken at school, the school nurse can record whether it was given.

Step 6. Measure Outcomes

The next step is to conduct the evaluation (i.e., gather and analyze the data). If the other steps have been completed, the clinician is well positioned to gather data that will help determine whether a certain intervention should be refined, continued, faded, or discontinued. The rationale for the evaluation process should be explained to the individuals who will be providing the outcome data. Because providing data is often time-consuming, respondents need to understand its importance for the child. Ensuring that the outcome indicators are meaningful to parents and teachers also helps to make collecting data a collaborative process.

Although one can never be absolutely sure that changes in behavior are directly linked to an intervention, one should try to rule out as many other explanations as possible. To do so, several factors must be considered before conducting the evaluation.

First, clinicians must decide how long the evaluation will last and then try to schedule data collection for a time when the child's schedule and behavior will be as representative as possible. Taking school-based interventions as example, the following questions should be asked: Are school holidays scheduled? Are there special school activities (e.g., field trips, Halloween parties) that will disrupt the child's routine? Is the child scheduled for any testing or therapy that requires more "pull-out" time than usual? Is the regular teacher scheduled for an extended absence (e.g., maternity leave)? If any of these are likely to occur, postponing the evaluation is preferred. If the evaluation cannot be delayed, at the very least one should be aware of these changes and incorporate that awareness into the decision-making process.

Another timing consideration is whether the child is on medication. If the purpose is to evaluate a psychosocial intervention, the psychosocial interventions should be initiated and evaluated before beginning the medication, or after a regular medication regimen is established. Similarly, if multiple components of an intervention are being examined, the evaluation should coincide with the initiation of these components. For example, if a token economy program is initiated using rewards for the first month and introducing response cost thereafter, one could examine the benefits of the reward aspects after the first month (before the response cost is initiated) and then again after the response cost component is consistently in effect. Similarly, it will be easier to examine the efficacy of parent training if medication is started after parent training is finished, or its effectiveness is established before the training starts.

Finally, the outcome evaluation should be timed such that its data will be maximally helpful to the child. For example, with a little planning, one can often time an evaluation to coincide with an IEP review date, or to ensure its completion in time for incorporation into the IEP for the upcoming year, when decisions about the child's placement and teacher assignments will be made. The same is true for home-based interventions. All too often, interventions are begun late in the academic year and there is insufficient information to inform the planning process. Thoughtful planning in initiating treatment and evaluating its efficacy can also provide the kind of hard data that managed care companies use to authorize continued treatment. Conducting an outcome evaluation using the suggested steps will make the evaluation as useful as possible to the child.

Step 7. Determine Efficacy of Treatment

With the evaluation data in hand, one can begin to analyze it. But more than just scores must be considered: In addition to a treatment's benefits, what are its costs? Cost–benefit analysis may require collecting more data. For example, for medication trials data must be collected on possible side effects. Cost is also considered when examining the efficacy of school- and home-based treatments: Is the treatment acceptable, or is it unacceptable in some way? Are the parents and teachers satisfied with it? A growing body of evidence links satisfaction and acceptability with willingness to implement the intervention, and in some cases, to the effectiveness and maintenance of interventions (e.g., Bresten et al., 1999; Reimers, Wacker, Cooper, & DeRaad, 1992). Cost–benefit data yield invaluable information about the factors that affect treatment fidelity and maintenance in the long run.

Step 8. Continue, Modify, or Replace Treatment

With the final step one comes full circle, to the reason for conducting the assessment in the first place. Was the intervention effective? If so, in which areas? Is there room for improvement? How then should it be modified? Should the treatment be continued? If not, when and with what should it be replaced? Only by carefully carrying out Steps 1–7 can one arrive at Step 8 with the data to make an informed decision.

EVALUATING PHARMACOLOGICAL TREATMENT

Medication, especially stimulant medication, can be an integral part of an empirically supported treatment package for many children with AD/HD. There is considerable evidence, particularly from the Multimodal Treatment Study of Children with AD/HD (MTA) funded by the National Institute of Mental Health, that stimulant medication is one of the most effective treatments for reducing AD/HD symptomatology. Part of its success in the comprehensive national study was the careful way in which it was prescribed and monitored. Unfortunately, such is often not the case in practice. There are still stories of children who are placed on Ritalin or other medications, sometimes at extremely high doses, without a thorough diagnostic evaluation. Thus, there may be children on stimulants whose difficulties relate not to AD/HD but rather to environmental conditions. Following the diagnostic procedure outlined in earlier chapters helps to avoid this problem.

Nevertheless, even when children are appropriately diagnosed, medication is not always prescribed based on the latest research findings. Physicians often rely solely on the child's weight as a guide. Although this is certainly a reasonable way to decide initial dosage, further evaluation is important for tailoring prescriptions. Because of the variability in medication responsiveness (e.g., Rapport, DuPaul, & Kelly, 1989), one should look at more than just weight to determine optimum dosage. Some children respond better as the level of medication increases; others show peak responsiveness at a moderate dose. Without additional data, it is impossible for physicians to determine such differences.

Once medication is prescribed, it is often inadequately monitored. Children may be placed on a medication dose at 8 years old and never have the dose reevaluated, even after entering adolescence. Furthermore, decisions about changing the dose can be quite subjective. An all too common scenario involves parents and teachers noticing a deterioration in the child's performance and the dose is increased with no investigation into the reason for the deterioration. The change could be due to things completely unrelated to the child's AD/HD, or at least to things better remedied by other interventions. Determining whether the increase helped is often done subjectively as well, using, for example, an informal discussion among parents, teachers, and physician as to whether "things are going better."

Sometimes the increase improves functioning but also brings on side effects. Without a systematic examination of the pros and cons of different doses, it is hard for a physician to weigh the benefits of the increased dose against the cost of the side effects.

Partially for these reasons, there remains considerable concern about the overmedication of children and the dangers of giving them drugs. Many parents are reluctant to even consider stimulant medication because of these potential drawbacks. Some physicians, wary of lawsuits, are reluctant to prescribe a high enough dose to be therapeutic, or even to prescribe the medication at all. Thus, a potentially helpful treatment for a particular child may be ruled out.

All of this argues for a more systematic evaluation of the effectiveness of a specific medication and a specific dose for a given child. One effective approach is to conduct a double-blind drug–placebo trial. Such a trial can be invaluable when determining whether to initiate medication, to change the dosage, or to remove a medication from the treatment package.

Stimulant Medication Trial

In the following discussion of medication trials, reference is made to Ritalin. This is because Ritalin is still the most widely used and studied medication for the treatment of AD/HD, but such trials can be conducted with any medication, including Adderall or Concerta, albeit with certain adaptations that must sometimes be made to accommodate that medication's characteristics (e.g., sustained release).

General Description

In many stimulant medication trials, the 1-month format consists of a 4-week double-blind drug–placebo trial comparing three active Ritalin dosages (i.e., low, medium, and high) against a placebo (10 mg lactose). Each condition is given twice daily for 1 week. Some trials, such as those at summer camp programs, inpatient settings, or research centers, involve daily dosage changes (e.g., Smith et al., 1998) or medication given three times a day (Greenhill et al., 1996).

In the weekly format, the order of active doses and placebo is generally random, with two constraints. First, the trial is not started with the highest dose, because side effects are more likely to occur on that dose. If a problematic dose is given early in the trial, it may be hard to convince the parents to examine the benefits of lower doses. Second, the high dose is preceded by the medium dose, because going directly from the low dose to the high dose may be too great a change for the child's system and thus may increase the risk of side effects. This results in six possible trial orders (see Table 8.3.).

The range of active doses varies with age. Commonly recommended levels for children 4–6 years old are 5, 7.5, and 10 mg. For children 6–12 years, dosages are usually 5, 10, and 15 mg. For children 13 years and older, 10, 15, and 20 mg are often employed. The ultimate dosage decision rests with the prescribing physician.

One of the advantages of a comprehensive trial is the blind evaluation. Although both the child and the raters of the child's behavior should be blind to the order of the dosages, obviously the prescribing physician as well as important contact individuals (e.g., the school nurse, the person coordinating the trial) should know the order.

TABLE 8.3. Possible Ordering of Dosages
for Double-Blind Drug–Placebo Stimulant Medication Trial

Ordering	Week 1	Week 2	Week 3	Week 4
A	Placebo	Low	Medium	High
B	Placebo	Medium	High	Low
C	Low	Placebo	Medium	High
D	Low	Medium	High	Placebo
E	Medium	High	Placebo	Low
F	Medium	High	Low	Placebo

Timing of Data Collection

Although stimulant trials can begin and end at any time, there are advantages to beginning each trial on a Saturday and ending on the following Friday. First, having the trial begin on the weekend gives the parent 2 full days to observe both benefits and side effects. Also, if there are significant side effects, the parent can more quickly notice them and, if necessary, have the trial stopped before the child goes to school. In addition, a Friday ending facilitates teacher ratings, because the child can be rated for the entire school week.

Using the Saturday–Friday schedule, weekly ratings are obtained for the child's AD/HD symptoms, level of functional competence and impairment, and any side effects or other costs. These data are obtained via rating scales from parents, teachers, and any other significant adults (e.g., after-school care providers). Children 9 years and older complete similar self-report ratings. If direct observation of the child seems critical to evaluating the outcome, then clinic-based child testing should also be conducted. As mentioned, some medication trials include daily dosage changes and ratings (e.g., Smith et al., 1998). Though helpful, this is more feasible in camp or inpatient settings. Weekly ratings still give useful results and are not so overwhelming for parents and teachers. A typical flow of events for a stimulant drug trial is outlined in Table 8.4.

What to Measure and How

Once the particulars of the drug trial are worked out, one must decide how to evaluate the medication's effectiveness. A first step could be to measure the behaviors that cause the most trouble, something probably known from the diagnostic assessment, particularly for the AD/HD symptoms and the functional impairment. However, if the diagnostic assessment was not recent, current information may not be available to guide the choice of measures. Similarly, the behaviors that cause the child the most difficulty may be too broad or not immediately sensitive to medication effects, so one should choose behaviors likely to be observable when the medication is most effective (e.g., 1½ to 2 hours

TABLE 8.4. Sequence of Medication Trial Events

Step	Procedure
1.	Referral is made for medication trial.
2.	Child is scheduled for medical exam.
3.	Physician receives medication-protocol ordering and school consent form.
4.	If trial is medically reasonable to pursue, physician forwards prescription to pharmacy.
5.	Child's family or health-care professional picks up medication from pharmacy.
6.	Health-care professional meets with parents and child to discuss trial format, answer questions, obtain written consent, give out Week 1 medication (if not already picked up by parents), distribute rating scales, and schedule subsequent appointments. (*Note*: If driving distance too great, all 4 weeks of medication and rating scales can be distributed at once.)
7.	Parent, teacher, and/or self-report rating scales are completed at each week's end and returned via self-addressed, stamped envelopes or during follow-up visits.
8.	After trial is completed, all ratings are scored and trial data summary sheets are filled out.
9.	Child health-care professional interprets findings, summarizes opinion in a brief letter to physician.
10.	Physician reviews findings, decides whether to continue medication and if so, at what dosage. If not, decides whether to try alternate stimulant medication or another type of medication.

postingestion). The behaviors also should be measurable during the time frame of the trial. Finally, as outlined earlier, one should assess the treatment integrity, that is, compliance with the medication regimen. Whether the medication was taken, how consistently it was taken, and at what time it was administered will be important to know, because it will shed light on the interpretation of data. This information can be gathered through an informal interview, or a checklist can be devised that will be completed along with the rating of potential side effects. In deciding which measures to use, one should consult the research literature for measures that have proven sensitive to medication effects. Even though such research relates to efficacy in groups versus individuals, it is a good place to begin evaluating responsiveness for a specific child. Some assessment procedures that meet these criteria are discussed below, followed by a sample case description.

The tools used to evaluate the effectiveness of a medication will yield data in three broad areas: AD/HD symptoms, functional domains, and side effects. This can then be used to answer the following questions. First, does the medication have any effect on the child's inattention, impulsivity, or hyperactivity? Second, does it result in any improvement in the areas where AD/HD is causing difficulties for the child (e.g., home, school, peers)? Third, are there any serious side effects? By examining results from all three areas, a more informed decision about the medication in general, and the dosage in particular, can be made. What follows is a brief description of measures for each of these three areas that have proven to be sensitive to drug effects (see Tables 8.5. and 8.6.). More-detailed information on most of these measures can be found in Chapter 4.

TABLE 8.5.   Possible Medication Trial Measures

Trial data		
Parent input about child	Teacher input about child	Direct input from child
AD/HD Rating Scale	AD/HD Rating Scale	Self-Report AD/HD Rating Scale
Home Situations	School Situations	Social Skills Rating Scale
Questionnaire-Revised	Questionnaire-Revised	Side Effects Rating Scale
SKAMP Rating Scale	SKAMP Rating Scale	Conners' CPT
Parenting Stress Index	Academic Performance	Behavioral observations during CPT
Social Skills Rating Scale	Rating Scale	Behavioral observations during
(short form)	Social Skills Rating Scale	Restricted Academic Situations
Side Effects Rating Scale	Side Effects Rating Scale	Task
Information on medication		BASC Structured Observation
compliance		System (SOS)
		Achenbach Direct Observation
		Form (DOF)

Note: AD/HD = Attention deficit/hyperactivity disorder; CPT = Continuous Performance Test.

AD/HD Symptomatology

To be an effective treatment, medication should reduce some of the core AD/HD symptoms. To determine whether inattention, impulsivity, or hyperactivity have been reduced, one can choose from one of the narrow-band rating scales described earlier. The AD/HD Rating Scale-IV (DuPaul et al., 1998) is an option, given its brevity and psychometric characteristics, especially test-retest reliability, limited practice effects, normative data, and the opportunity for parent, teacher, and child report. The total and subscale scores yield a rich data set. The CAP, the SNAP, and the ADDES have similar advantages.

Although diagnostic interviews can also provide information about inattention and hyperactivity-impulsivity, they are too long for this purpose. Likewise, some of the broad-band measures, though capturing the two definitive AD/HD factors, are too broad, unless one wants to use them to assess other areas related to functional impairment. The time frame for completing broad-band rating scales (e.g., 2 or 6 months) is also much longer than a typical trial (e.g., 1 week). One could give instructions to complete the form for only the past week, but the items may not capture the short-term behaviors that are sensitive to medication.

If weekly clinic-based assessments are possible, a way to examine inattention and impulsivity is through a continuous performance test. As mentioned earlier, the Conners' CPT seems the best candidate at this time because of its fidelity to current etiological conceptualizations of AD/HD and its broad normative data. Although the Conners' CPT does not assess the hyperactivity component, behavioral coding of the child's activity level during the task could add this information. Sometimes distance, time, and funding prohibit clinic testing. If so, the narrow-band rating scales do a good job of assessing this aspect of medication responsiveness.

TABLE 8.6. Outcome Indicators for Pharmacological Interventions

Target of intervention	Sample outcome indicators	Area of functioning	Possible measures
Increase attention to task	Task productivity: Number of problems/percentage of worksheet completed within time period; percentage of items completed relative to work assigned	School	Academic Performance Rating Scale; Academic Completion Rate
	Following through on parent requests	Home	BASC Parent Rating Scale; Conners' Parent Rating Scale; Home Situatinos Questionnaire; Parenting Stress Index
	On-task behavior: Percentage of time spent on-task playing sports; greater recall of game score	Social	Unstructured observations; AD/HD Rating Scale-IV, Social Skills Rating Scale
Decrease hyperactivity	Inappropriate vocalizations	School	AD/HD Rating Scale-IV; SKAMP Rating Scale; School Situations Questionnaire-Revised; BASC SOS or Achenbach DOF
	Inappropriate movements	Home	AD/HD Rating Scale-IV; SKAMP; Home Situations Questionnaire; ADDES
	Inappropriate movements	School	AD/HD Rating Scale-IV; SKAMP; School Situations Questionnaire; ADDES; Direct observation
	Feelings of restlessness	Self	Self-Report AD/HD Rating Scale-IV
Decrease impulsivity	Number of careless errors	School	Academic Performance Rating Scale; Academic Efficiency Score; SKAMP; School Situations Questionnaire-Revised

School Functioning

Stimulant medication can increase positive interactions with teachers (e.g., Swanson et al., 1998a; Whalen, Henker, & Dotemoto, 1980). Decreases in disruptive behavior in the classroom, increased compliance with teacher requests, and increased attention to academic tasks all serve to improve the overall relationship between a teacher and a child who has AD/HD. Although this improvement can be captured through any of the direct observational coding systems described earlier (e.g., the BASC SOS; the Achenbach DOF), such systems greatly increase the cost of the trial and thus make it unlikely to be completed.

However, one would not want to miss capturing these improvements. The AD/HD Rating Scale-IV and School Situations Questionnaire-Revised are helpful, as is the SKAMP rating scale. The SKAMP was developed by Swanson, Pelham, and their colleagues (Swanson, 1992) and modified by Greenhill and colleagues (Greenhill et al., 1996) for the MTA study. Respondents rate the child using a 7-point impairment scale (*normal, slight, mild, moderate, severe, very severe,* or *maximal*) on 10 different aspects of the child's daily routine, with an emphasis on classroom behavior (e.g., getting started, sticking with tasks, attending to topic, stopping for transition, interacting with students, interacting with staff, remaining quiet, staying seated). Scores can be averaged to obtained SKAMP Attention and SKAMP Deportment subscale scores. All three scores can be used to obtain quick, valid, and clinically useful data on how much and in which areas the medication is resulting in improvements.

One should sample other areas of academic functioning as well. Although there is limited evidence that medication affects a child's actual knowledge base in the short term, there is considerable support for short-term changes in the building blocks of learning (i.e., concentration, productivity, accuracy, and preparedness) (DuPaul, Barkley, & McMurray, 1994; Pelham & Milich, 1991; Rapport & Kelly, 1991; Smith, Pelham, Gnagy, & Yudell, 1998). There are several measures that effectively tap these dimensions.

The Academic Performance Rating Scale (APRS; DuPaul et al., 1991) screens for difficulties in school functioning. It asks the teacher to rate the child in terms of success, productivity, and accuracy in major subject areas. Norms are available and the measure has been useful in determining response to medication.

Another possible measure is a comparison of the amount of work completed with the amount of work assigned or with completion rates of typical classmates. This is the Academic Completion Rate (percentage of items completed relative to work assigned; Rapport, 1987). A corollary to the completion rate is not only the quantity of work, which can increase simply because of a child's impulsivity and eagerness to finish an unpleasant task, but the quality. That is, its accuracy, termed the Academic Efficiency Score (Rapport et al., 1987). To arrive at this score, the child's desk work is rated for both the daily percentage of work that is completed and daily percentage of work that is correct. The combined scores are the Academic Efficiency Score (AES), or percentage of correctly completed work. These measures have the advantages of ecological validity and sensitivity to both behavioral interventions and medication effects. One possible disadvantage is that the assignment must be gradable in terms of percentage complete and percentage accurate. Thus, math problems are best for this rating.

Although direct classroom observation is not always feasible, analog assessments sometimes are, especially when the child and family are coming to the clinic for weekly medication doses. When this is the case, procedures such as the Restricted Academic Situations Task—wherein observations of on-task behavior, AD/HD behavior, academic productivity, and academic accuracy are coded—can be helpful in determining medication responsiveness. Another approach is to have teachers rate the classroom behaviors related to academic success via rating scales such as the SKAMP (Greenhill et al., 1996).

Home Functioning

One might expect medication effects to generalize to the child's functioning at home. The Home Situations Questionnaire-Revised (HSQ-R) (Adams et al., 1995; Barkley, 1990) is a way to obtain information about the scope and severity of symptoms in common home situations, particularly noncompliance. The face-valid nature of the HSQ-R and its brevity make it particularly good for examining responsiveness to medication. It has been used successfully in this regard for many years and an upward extension for adolescents recently developed by Adams and colleagues makes it applicable for a wider age range. As previously described, the SKAMP (Greenhill et al., 1996) can also assess home functioning, although the items relate more to school.

In some cases, it is useful to obtain information about parent–child interaction. Because stimulant medications can increase compliance with parental requests and attention to interactions (e.g., Barkley & Cunningham, 1979; Barkley, Karlsson, Pollard, & Murphy, 1985; Humphries, Kinsbourne, & Swanson, 1978; Pelham, Walker, Sturges, & Hoza, 1989), one may see improvement in the quality of parent–child interaction. This is more likely to be seen first by the parents and thus it may be very important to obtain parent report on this dimension. The Parenting Stress Index (short form; Abidin, 1995) has been shown to be sensitive to these changes in the quality of the parent–child interaction.

Social Functioning

To some extent, medication also can improve a child's interactions with peers (e.g., Smith, Pelham, Evans, et al., 1998). There can be many reasons for this. By increasing attention and decreasing impulsivity and hyperactivity, medication can result in children engaging in fewer inappropriate social behaviors, being more attentive to the rules of a game at recess (e.g., Pelham et al., 1990; whose turn, score of the game), and being less irritating to others (e.g., inappropriate vocalizations in class, cutting in line, falling out of chair in class). Measuring this area of functioning adds considerable length to the assessment battery, but it may need to be done if these behaviors have been particularly problematic for the child. If so, a direct classroom observation can be used, as can the Social Skills Rating Scale (Gresham & Elliott, 1990) or other such rating scales. The SSRS is completed by parents and teachers and in some cases, via child self-report. Obtaining cross-informant data is a major advantage, and data from the SSRS also lends itself to the development of interventions that complement medication, should there be room for improvement following titration of the dose.

Side Effects

Although many children experience no side effects with AD/HD medications, a small percentage do. Some of the more common side effects of stimulants include appetite reduction, insomnia, irritability, headaches, and stomach aches. Several rating scales have been developed to evaluate these potential difficulties. One is the Side Effects Rating Scale (Barkley, 1981/1998). This scale lists 17 common side effects and has been used effectively in medication trials for years. The respondent (e.g., parent, teacher, or older child) rates whether the problem is present and if so, its severity on a 10-point scale (*0 = absent*; *9 = serious*).

Another tool is the Stimulant Side Effects rating scale (SSE; Greenhill et al., 1996) used in the MTA study. Respondents rate side effects on a 4-point scale (*not at all* to *very much*). Teachers rate the child on 10 behaviors (i.e., motor tics; buccal-lingual movements; picking at skin or fingers; worried or anxious; dull, tired, listless; headache; stomachache; crabby or irritable; tearful, sad, depressed; and appetite loss). Parents rate the same behaviors plus an additional item related to sleeping difficulties.

Both scales are sensitive to medication effects. Ratings of individual side effects can be averaged across raters to provide a summary severity score. In addition, one can tally the number of significant side effects to arrive at a frequency count.

Sometimes, a rebound effect occurs, consisting of increased disruptive and irritable behaviors in the late afternoon. If this is happening, any of the behavioral rating scales described in Chapter 4 that target the behavior in question can be used, along with the side effects rating scales. The rater should complete the scale at different times of the day (e.g., midmorning, late afternoon). Again, one needs *baseline* data from the different times of day as well to draw conclusions about a rebound effect as well as about the effectiveness of introducing a small late-afternoon dose to counteract it.

Modifications to the Standard Trial

Tailoring the above procedure to the child and family will maximize the quality of data on a medication's efficacy.

Timing of the Trial

The timing of the trial is critical. Because outcome indicators for the school environment are an essential part of the assessment, major holidays and vacations are poor times to schedule a trial. Consider the following example.

Suppose it has been decided the week before Spring Break that a trial should be initiated. Beginning a trial at that time would result in needing to take time off the following week. To start after the holiday may leave too few weeks for the trial to be completed before decisions are made regarding specialized educational services. One could wait until after the break, but waiting delays refinement of the treatment plan, and may result in a loss of momentum if the parents are already ambivalent about the trial. One option is to collect baseline data prior to the holiday, collect no data during the holiday, and then initiate an abbreviated 3-week trial using two doses and a placebo. The doses tried should be different enough to provide a range of responses.

Medication Holidays

Another consideration is whether the child will be taking the medication on weekends or holidays during the trial. It is sometimes the case that children who take stimulant medication do so only during the school week and not on weekends or during school breaks. Although this may be an appropriate choice for the child's long-term treatment protocol, there are several points to consider when using this approach during a medication trial. For one thing, parents or primary caregivers would never have a chance to observe the medication's potential benefits. They could still provide information on possible rebound effects and side effects, but given that the child is rarely on medication in their presence, it would be hard for them to assess its benefits firsthand. For parents with concerns about medication, teacher-reported improvement may not be sufficient justification to keep the child on medication, even in the absence of significant side effects. This is particularly problematic if the family–school relationship is strained and the school advocates more strongly for medication than do the parents. In these situations, it is better to have the child take the medication every day, with each week of the trial beginning on Saturday. Adjustments in regimen can take place after the trial has been completed. This affords the parents the opportunity to see potential benefits for themselves, and they can also comment on how the medication affects the child's neighborhood peer relationships, sibling relationships, and interactions in the home.

Frequency of Ratings

Drug trials vary in terms of the frequency with which respondents rate the child's behavior and potential side effects. Obviously, the more frequent the rating, the more information obtained. Frequent ratings (e.g., every few hours, every day) are better for estimating when the medication will be most effective (e.g., number of hours postingestion, time of day) and permit an examination of its effects on various tasks. But extremely frequent monitoring is usually impractical for teachers and families. It also results in large amounts of cumbersome data for clinicians and pediatricians to interpret. Weekly monitoring, though it loses some accuracy due to retrospective reporting, is more feasible, thus the raters are more likely to cooperate fully.

Lack of Available Placebo

Using a placebo is the best way to examine expectancy effects. Unfortunately, some pharmacies cannot provide one, but it is still important to initiate some type of formal evaluation of medication. If necessary, one can modify the standard trial by simply omitting the placebo condition. Teachers and parents then rate the child's behavior off medication for baseline, with additional ratings collected each week for a range of doses. As before, raters are blind to the dosage order. In interpreting any improvement on medication, one should keep in mind the results from previous medication trials, which show that ratings of the child's behavior can improve dramatically (e.g., as much as 35%) on a placebo.

Rebound Effects

A modification of the standard trial can help to determine if rebound effects can be reduced. In this case, the trial could include a third, smaller dose given in midafternoon. The medication for morning, noon, and afternoon would have to be in separate bottles and clearly labeled for time of day. The third dose would be the one that varies. It would include a placebo, a dose equivalent to the morning and noon doses, and a smaller dose. Although slightly more trouble, this variation can provide information that will make the parents feel comfortable with their ultimate decision about medication for their child.

Nonstimulant Medications

Stimulants are particularly well suited to the protocol described above. The short half-life, the ability to switch dosages quickly and safely, and the rapidity with which behavioral changes can be observed enable their effectiveness to be evaluated relatively quickly. However, other medications are sometimes used to treat AD/HD. Some, such as antidepressants, require more time to reach a therapeutic level and thus are not amenable to a short evaluation protocol. Although not as precise as the double blind trial, one should at least obtain baseline data on the child's behavior prior to the start of these medications, with periodic examination of symptoms and side effects once therapeutic levels are reached. Similar procedures should be followed when a change in medication is being considered. Side effects specific to the medication should be monitored. Medical tests, blood work, and EKGs, for example, may be needed in addition to the rating scales and observations described earlier.

Case Example

Jennifer is a 10-year-old, fifth grade girl referred for a psychological assessment because of parent and teacher concerns about her home and school performance and behavior. Her initial multimethod assessment revealed that she had a diagnosis of AD/HD, Predominantly Inattentive subtype. Jennifer's primary difficulties were at school. Jennifer's teacher reported that she was a good-natured girl but had to be redirected constantly. She had difficulty completing her work independently and often had to have directions repeated. Her teacher was concerned about Jennifer's academic progress and about her ability to handle next year's work in middle school.

Her inattention and distractibility also caused difficulties at home, primarily because of homework. These difficulties had worsened over the past year due to additional homework and increased expectations for independent work. Although her parents had developed a sticker system to help Jennifer get her homework done, they were worried about the amount of time she was spending on it each night. They commented that Jennifer was a very pleasant and loving child, and despite their concerns, they reported no significant levels of parenting stress and were generally in agreement about parenting practices.

Because her difficulties seemed to be confined to inattention and distractibility with no problems in other areas such as oppositional behavior, a trial of Ritalin was recommended. A 4-week double-blind drug–placebo trial was begun. During the first week Jennifer was placed on a low dose, which she took twice a day for the entire week. During Week 2 she received a placebo dose twice daily. During Weeks 3 and 4 she received medium and high doses, respectively. At the end of each week, her parents and teacher completed ratings of her behavior and of any side effects.

An outcome evaluation was designed using the 8-step program given earlier. Step 1 is choosing outcome indicators (Fig. 8.1.). In Jennifer's case, these were how inattention affected home and school functioning. Specifically, it was important to see if medication affected her parents' perceptions of her inattention, and the degree to which her homework difficulties continued. At school, where the majority of problems existed, outcome indicators included the teacher's overall assessment of inattention, the degree to which Jennifer worked productively and accurately, and her behavior with regard to academic tasks.

Step 2 is determining the criteria for success. For her parents to be comfortable putting Jennifer on medication, the criteria for success were defined as clinically significant change. On some measures (e.g., AD/HD Rating Scale-IV) this is defined as reliable change calculated from the Jacobson–Truax methodology (i.e., RCIs > 1.96). On others, success is defined as the scores falling below clinical cutoffs (e.g., below 1.5 standard deviations).

Given the outcome indicators and the need to calculate clinically significant change, the methods to choose for the evaluation in Step 3 became clear. Her parents would complete the AD/HD Rating Scale-IV, the Side Effects Rating Scale, and the Homework Problem Checklist. Her teacher would complete the AD/HD Rating Scale-IV, the Academic Performance Rating Scale, and the SKAMP. Although clinic-administered tests such as the Conners' CPT and direct classroom observation would be helpful, the family lived too far from the clinic for this to be practical.

Step 4 is collecting baseline data. This step is important in medication trials where repeated administrations of some measures can result in practice effects. Prior to the start of the trial, baseline data were obtained using all measures. Once the trial had begun, Jennifer's parents and the school nurse completed a daily checklist showing when medication was given and any missed doses. This informal checklist addressed Step 5 by examining the integrity of the intervention. In Jennifer's case, the medication was administered as prescribed with no missed doses.

Step 6 is collecting outcome data. Each new dose was begun on Saturday and parent and teacher ratings were collected on Friday. The ratings were scored and faxed to the clinic. Side effects ratings were immediately examined to ensure that the trial was proceeding safely.

Step 7 is determining intervention efficacy based on the criteria for success from Step 2. A summary of the results obtained during baseline and during the 4-week medication trial appears in Table 8.7.

With regard to an analysis of the AD/HD Rating Scale-IV, parent ratings showed no major changes during the placebo or low-dose phase. Her Inattention score during both weeks was only 2 points less than baseline. Using the Jacobson–Truax methodology for determining clinically significant change, one divides this difference by 2.88, which is the appropriate standard error of difference for a girl her age. This yields an RCI of .69 for Inattention during placebo and low dose phases. Similar calculations yielded placebo-week RCI scores of .33 for Hyperactivity-Impulsivity and .21 for the Total score. Likewise, the RCI calculations for the low-dose week yielded nonsignificant indices of −.49 for Hyperactivity-Impulsivity, and .48 for the Total score.

In contrast, the differences between Jennifer's baseline scores and those obtained during the medium- and high-dosage weeks were much larger, particularly for Inattention. The RCI calculations for the medium-dose week yielded scores of 2.08 for Inattention, .49 for Hyperactivity-Impulsivity, and 1.69 for the Total. The corresponding RCI scores for the high-dose week were 2.43, .49, and

TABLE 8.7.   Summary of Medication Trial Results

Outcome measure	Baseline	Placebo	Low	Medium	High
ADHD Rating Scale-IV—Home Version					
Inattention	16	14 (.69)	14 (.69)	10 (2.08)	9 (2.43)
Hyperactivity-Impulsivity	6	6 (.33)	7 (−.49)	5 (.49)	5 (.49)
Total	29	21 (.24)	20 (.48)	15 (1.69)	14 (1.94)
ADHD Rating Scale-IV—School Version					
Inattention	22	20 (.58)	21 (.29)	13 (2.63)	16 (1.75)
Hyperactivity-Impulsivity	7	8 (−.33)	6 (.33)	5 (.66)	6 (.33)
Total	29	28 (.18)	27 (.35)	18 (1.95)	22 (1.24)
Side Effects Rating Scale—Home					
Number of side effects	2	2	1	3	5
Mean severity	1.5	1.5	2.0	2.7	6.6
Side Effects Rating Scale—School					
Number of side effects	1	2	1	2	4
Mean severity	1.0	1.5	1.0	3.5	6.3
SKAMP—Home					
Attention	3	4	2	1	2
Deportment	3	3	2	1	2
SKAMP—School					
Attention	5	5	4	2	1
Deportment	4	4	3	2	1
Homework Problem Checklist					
Number of problem behaviors	6	5	5	3	2
Academic Performance Rating Scale					
Academic productivity	49	47	51	60	66

Note. Values in parentheses are Reliable Change Indices.

1.94, respectively. Reliable change is thought to occur when the RCIs exceed 1.96 ($p \leq .05$).

On the teacher AD/HD Rating Scale-IV a similar pattern emerged, with little change noted during placebo or low-dose weeks and greater change during medium- and high-dose weeks. To calculate change for the teacher ratings, one first finds the difference between the score in question and the baseline score, then divides it by 3.42 for Inattention, 3.01 for Hyperactivity-Impulsivity, and 5.64 for the Total score; these are the appropriate standard errors of difference for a girl her age. As can be seen from the RCIs for each week (Table 8.7.), there were negligible gains during the placebo and low-dose weeks. Similar to the parent report, RCIs for Inattention were significant for the medium-dose week (e.g., 2.63) and approached significance for the high-dose week (e.g., 1.75).

Looking only at raw scores, one might conclude that both the medium-dose and high-dose conditions produced acceptable improvements in AD/HD symptomatology. Upon closer inspection, important differences become evident. Although the RCI calculations for parent ratings were significant for both the medium and high doses, teacher ratings were significant only for the medium-dose week. Results of the other rating scales (e.g., SKAMP, Homework Problem Checklist, Academic Productivity on the APRS) corroborated this. Though less dramatic, improvements were noted for medium and high doses in both parent and teacher ratings.

Step 8 is using the findings to choose a course of action. For medication, this involves examining not only clinically significant change in AD/HD symptomatology and home and school functioning (benefits), but side effects as well (costs). Because fewer side effects were noted during the medium-dose week, it was suggested to Jennifer's pediatrician that she would be a good candidate for a longer-term trial of Ritalin at the medium dosage level (see sample letter, Table 8.8.). If her physician agreed and her parents gave consent, medication would start immediately, with the same measures to be readministered in 3 months. If at that time her school difficulties continued, we would look at Jennifer's medication level and at the possibility of adding a school-based intervention.

EVALUATING SCHOOL-BASED TREATMENT

Either in combination with other treatments, or as the only treatment, school-based interventions have proven extremely effective at ameliorating the difficulties that children with AD/HD experience in that setting (e.g., Abramowitz, Reid, & O'Toole, 1994; Barkley et al., 1996; Barkley, 1999; Braswell et al., 1997; Cunningham et al., 1998; DuPaul & Henningson, 1993; Pfiffner, 1996; Shapiro, DuPaul, Bradley, & Bailey, 1996; Webster-Stratton, 1998; Zentall, 1993). These interventions run the gamut from individual interventions (e.g., adjusting the amount and pace of work assigned), to group interventions (e.g., social skills training, student-mediated conflict resolution program), to class-wide token economy programs, to school-wide comprehensive consultations. The focus of the intervention also varies, from increasing the child's skills (e.g., self-

TABLE 8.8.   Sample Medication Trial Feedback Letter to Physician

---

Dear Dr. X:

As you know, Jennifer D. was evaluated in our clinic several months ago. At that time she was identified as having Attention-Deficit/Hyperactivity Disorder (AD/HD), Predominantly Inattentive subtype. One of the recommendations emerging from her evaluation was that she undergo a controlled stimulant medication trial to determine whether this form of treatment might be beneficial in her overall clinical management. We recently completed this trial and are now writing to provide you with a summary of its format and results.

A four-week double-blind drug–placebo Ritalin trail was employed. During the first week, Jennifer received an inert placebo b.i.d.; 5 mg of Ritalin b.i.d. were used during week two; 10 mg of Ritalin b.i.d. during week three; and 15 mg of Ritalin b.i.d. during week four. At the end of each week, Jennifer's mother and teacher completed ratings pertaining to academic performance, behavior, and potential side effects. Jennifer also completed self-report ratings pertaining to these same areas of psychosocial functioning. At no time during the trial were Jennifer, her mother, her teacher, or the clinician collecting the ratings aware of which dosage was being given.

Input from all three informants indicated a positive response to medication. According to her mother, the medium and high Ritalin doses produced behavioral improvements above and beyond those observed during the placebo and low-dose conditions. Mrs. D. observed significant improvements in Jennifer's inattention symptoms, reporting only 2 of 9 symptoms during the medium- and high-dose weeks as opposed to 6 of 9 symptoms at baseline. Mrs. D. also reported improvements in Jennifer's ability to complete homework during the medium- and high-dose weeks; homework has been an area of great difficulty for her.

The teacher ratings also showed that medium and high medication doses were superior to placebo and low doses. In contrast to the mother's ratings, the teacher ratings indicated that the 10-mg week was superior to the 15-mg week in terms of improving Jennifer's attention span, productivity, and classroom behavior. A similar pattern emerged from Jennifer's self-report ratings.

Although Jennifer tolerated all doses well, she had a greater number and severity of side effects on the high dose. This was mainly mild appetite suppression both at home and at school.

Overall, the results from this recently completed trial indicate that Jennifer responded positively to stimulant medication, with no serious side effects. Of the three doses examined, the 10-mg b.i.d. week seemed to produce the best results with the fewest side effects. Thus, we suggest a longer trial of stimulant medication. We recommend that Jennifer be started on a 10-mg b.i.d. Ritalin dosage, 7 days a week, if this is medically appropriate.

It is our understanding that you will assume the responsibility for Jennifer's follow-up medication management. Should you have questions about the trial, or should you need any additional assistance in managing Jennifer's AD/HD, please feel free to contact me.

Sincerely,

(Clinician)

---

monitoring, social skills) to increasing the goodness-of-fit through environmental adaptations (e.g., seating rearrangement, altering task characteristics). Whatever the form, school-based treatments have a demonstrated effect on many areas of a child's functioning.

What to Measure and How

In assessing the potential benefits of a school-based intervention, the same three areas mentioned in the pharmacological assessment should be tapped.

Specifically, what is the effect of the intervention on specific AD/HD symptoms? What is its effect on functional impairment? What, if any, are the costs or disadvantages of the intervention? A brief review of procedures that can assess treatment efficacy in these areas is presented below and summarized in Table 8.9. As with the medication trial, we are not recommending use of all measures in any one child's assessment, because this would result in a cumbersome battery. Rather, we describe them all to illustrate the available options so that outcome evaluations can be tailored to the child and family. Many of the mea-

TABLE 8.9.   Outcome Indicators for School-Based Interventions

Target of intervention	Sample outcome indicators	Area of functioning	Possible measures
Increase attention to task	Accuracy of work; productivity	School	Academic Performance Rating Scale; Academic Efficiency Score
Decrease hyperactivity	Inappropriate movements	School	AD/HD Rating Scale-IV, SNAP, ADDES
Decrease impulsivity	Number of times raises hand before speaking out in class; number of times cut in lunch, recess, or bus lines	School	BASC SOS or Achenbach DOF; School Situations Questionnaire-Revised
	Frequency/number of careless errors	School	Academic Performance Rating Scale; School Situations Questionnaire-Revised
Increase school competence	Compliance with rules and teacher requests; number of redirecting commands; percentage of positive adult attention; good work habits	School	School Situations Questionnaire-Revised; BASC SOS; Achenbach DOF; Teacher–Student Behavior Coding System; SKAMP; BASC Teacher Rating Scale (Study Skills subscale)
Increase social competence	Level of aggression in unstructured social interactions (e.g., lunch room, recess, bus)	Social	AD/HD Rating Scale IV; School Situations Questionnaire-Revised; BASC SOS or Achenbach DOF; Social Behavior Coding System; Social Skills Rating Scale; BASC Teacher Rating Scale (Adaptive subscale)
Generalize skills	Percentage of time target behavior learned in social skills training group is observed in regular classroom	Social	BASC Teacher Rating Scale; Social Skills Rating Scale, Social Behavior Coding System

sures mentioned are similar to those for assessing medication outcome, but incontrast to medication measures, which must be administered frequently, more options exist for measuring the outcome of school-based treatments, such as broad-band scales and direct observations.

AD/HD Symptomatology

As detailed in Chapter 4, many rating scales can be completed by teachers to assess the child's symptoms in the classroom (e.g., Conners' scales, Achenbach scales). To measure the number and severity of AD/HD symptoms, the AD/HD Rating Scale-IV (DuPaul et al., 1998), SNAP (Pelham et al., 1992), ADDES (McCarney, 1995), Conners' DSM IV scale or the Conners' Global Index (CGI) (Conners, 1997) have all proven to be sensitive to picking up school-based treatment effects.

School Functioning

Because children with AD/HD often do not work up to their academic potential, this is an area of primary interest when evaluating the success of school-based interventions. Although there are certainly tangible measures already in place, such as grades, they are infrequent, and they require such major behavioral improvements that they are not sensitive to small yet meaningful treatment responses. As mentioned, process behaviors that contribute to the larger, more obvious academic improvements are better assessment targets. There are several excellent, quick, and face-valid tools for evaluating school-based interventions, including academic productivity and accuracy measures such as the APRS and Rapport et al.'s (1987) Academic Completion Rate and Academic Efficiency Score. Classroom behaviors can be assessed via the SKAMP (Greenhill et al., 1996), which helps not only in targeting areas for intervention but in assessing improvement in those areas as well.

Another area that can be evaluated is the organization of the child's desk. Teachers frequently complain that children with AD/HD are "pack rats." Atkins, Pelham, and Licht (1985) suggest examining the neatness and preparedness of the child's desk on a regular basis over the course of 2 to 3 weeks. Although neatness may not be a specific target of intervention, a child's increased attention to detail and task requirements may be reflected in a neater, more organized desk. Furthermore, if this area irritates the teacher, targeting it or monitoring its progress should further a more positive, supportive teacher–child relationship.

Of course, long-term school functioning outcomes need to be measured. This could include goal-attainment scaling with respect to goals set and met on the child's IEP, if one exists. Placement in special classes, integration into regular education, and grade retention can also serve as long-term indices.

Of equal interest is the child's overall behavioral competence. When clinicians are interested in broader changes resulting from long-term school interventions (e.g., increased self-esteem, increased frustration tolerance, improved social interactions), they can include one of the broad-band measures of behavior in the evaluation. The BASC (Reynolds & Kamphaus, 1994) has particular advantages because of its sampling of behavioral competence, its broad range of examined behaviors, its consistency across a wide age range, and its accompanying intervention manual. The sampling of competence as well as difficulty is compatible with the newer strength-based approaches to treatment (e.g., wraparound or system of care).

To examine symptom pervasiveness and severity over time, the School Situations Questionnaire-Revised (SSQ-R; Adams et al., 1995; DuPaul & Barkley, 1992) is as useful here as it is in assessing medication responsiveness. This scale is particularly helpful in targeting areas of intervention, and it can also examine the effect of an intervention on the behavioral severity and pervasiveness of the difficulty in a single setting as well as generalization of effects from one setting to another.

Direct observation can be used in addition to rating scales to monitor behavioral change. Particularly helpful are the observational forms available with the Achenbach and the BASC, as well as specific behavioral observation coding systems that include measures of off-task behavior, excessive gross-motor activity, and negative vocalizations (e.g., the AD/HD Behavior Coding System; Barkley, 1990). These can yield important information about the success and scope of an intervention. The BASC SOS is especially suitable for this. Observers rate the degree to which problem behaviors are disruptive. The informal observation also encourages the observer to examine the antecedents as well as the consequences of target behaviors, useful not only in evaluating an intervention's success but in conducting a functional analysis to design and refine the intervention. Additional observational systems that tap the child's interpersonal behaviors include the Social Behavior Coding System (see DuPaul & Stoner, 1994, and Table 8.10. for description). In this system, four categories are used to code teacher and/or peer interactions as positive, negative/nonaggressive, aggressive, or noninteractive.

Home Functioning

Although one wouldn't necessarily expect to see changes at home as a result of school interventions, they do sometimes occur (e.g., Barkley et al., 1996, 1999). School-based interventions can include components that increase the likelihood of generalization from school to home. Home–school communication, either informal, such as alerting parents to social skills training target behaviors, or more formal, such as daily report cards, can be an intervention in and of itself (see Kelley, 1990, for a description of various home–school communication strategies). Positive school functioning can decrease parenting stress; so too can improved communication between home and school that sometimes results from home–school note exchanges. Such a system requires, and thus furthers, a good understanding and implementation of behavioral skills (Abramowitz & O'Leary, 1991), so it is reasonable to look for changes in home functioning as a result of school-based interventions.

The Parenting Stress Index-short form (Abidin, 1995) might reflect changes as a result of decreased difficulties in parent–child interaction around school

TABLE 8.10.   Criteria for the Teacher-Student Behavior Coding System

Initiator/ behavior	How interaction was initiated
TA/ON	Teacher Approaches Student Engaged in On-Task Behavior: Teacher verbally or physically initiates an interaction with the student, who at moment of contact is engaged in on-task behavior. Not coded if student has raised hand to get teacher's attention.
TA/OFF	Teacher Approaches Student Engaged in Off-Task Behavior: Teacher physically or verbally initiates an interaction with the student who is off-task at the moment (i.e., interrupts attention to the tasks to engage in another behavior for 3 consecutive seconds or longer such as breaking eye contact with task materials or counting on fingers)
CA/APP	Child Approaches Teacher in an Appropriate Manner: Student physically or verbally initiates an interaction with the teacher in an appropriate manner including the following: raising hand; asking questions without raising hand when classroom rules are specifically relaxed; approaching teacher at desk during independent seatwork
CA/INAPP	Child Approaches Teacher in an Inappropriate Manner: Student physically or verbally initiates an interaction with teacher in an inappropriate manner including the following: calling out without permission; getting out of seat (unless during independent seatwork or similar activity when that is acceptable in the classroom)

	Quality of the interaction
Positive	Interaction includes any type of positive verbal comment regarding appropriate social or academic behavior. May also include physical contact (e.g., pat on shoulder) as long as it is not for discipline. Positive comments may be directed at the target student or the group if student is part of it.
Negative	Interaction includes verbal comments of disapproval such as criticism, negative reprimands or if teacher threatens to punish the student. May include physical contact (e.g., leading student by hand to his or her desk) if it occurs in response to inappropriate behavior on the part of the student. Student may be either directly targeted by the teacher or part of a group to whom the teacher makes a negative statement.
Other	Any other teacher-student interaction that is not coded as positive or negative such as: instructing the class; answering questions (unless the teacher adds "good job" or other approval statement); conversing with student; giving directions to class (e.g., to change activities)

issues, especially homework. School improvement that results in fewer arguments about school problems, fewer calls from the principal, and fewer hours spent on unfinished school work can all decrease parenting stress.

One measure that targets homework specifically is the Homework Problem Checklist (Anesko, Shoiock, Ramirez, & Levine, 1987), which asks parents to indicate the frequency with which various homework problems occur (e.g., denies having homework, fails to complete it). This could be used to identify target areas for intervention, serve as a baseline measure, and assist in evaluating the success of school- and home-based interventions that target homework-related skills.

Social Functioning

Social skills training is often a component of school-based interventions. There are several options for measuring its success. Rating scales are one option. For a *general* assessment of social competence, relevant scales from the BASC (Reynolds & Kamphaus, 1992) or the CBCL (Achenbach, 1991) tap target behaviors likely change with social skills training. However, sometimes one wants to make a specific evaluation of social skills as they relate to a specific intervention. In this case, a more comprehensive social skills rating scale, such as the Social Skills Rating System (SSRS, Gresham & Elliott, 1990), could be used. The SSRS asks the respondent to indicate how often a behavior occurs and how important they consider certain social skills to be. The latter is particularly useful when targeting behaviors for intervention. There are seven subscales, including Assertion and Self-Control subscales, which are especially applicable to friendship skills. Its norms permit the SSRS to be a more-specific measure of significant change. Parents and teachers should both complete this scale. Although the intervention might take place at school, parents might also see improved social competence at home. Most children go to school with others from their neighborhood; thus, improved social relations at school can sometimes be evident in informal play at home. Improved social relations within the classroom may also translate into more invitations for play or sleepovers.

One rating scale that can be used as a quick, global measure is the Social and Occupational Functioning Assessment Scale (SOFAS) (Goldman, Skodo, & Lave, 1992). This is a new scale used to rate current functioning and is derived from the Global Assessment Scale of the *DSM-IV* (APA, 1994). Social functioning is rated on a scale of 0–100, ranging from *excellent* to *grossly impaired*. To be counted, impairment must relate to psychological problems, not to lack of opportunity. The advantages are that the SOFAS is quick to complete and score and can be used to document both initial changes and changes over time. The disadvantages are that its behavioral rating anchors are not clearly specified; more behavioral descriptors are needed to obtain consistency in its use.

A somewhat different approach to measuring social skills is the Problem-Solving Measure for Conflict (PSM-C; Lochman & Lampron, 1986). The PSM-C is a modification of Spivack and Shure's Means–Ends Test (Shure & Spivack, 1972). The child responds to hypothetical vignettes. Responses are coded by trained raters who decide whether solutions the child chooses as a conclusion to a story stem are relevant or irrelevant. Solutions are judged irrelevant when they do not lead to the stated conclusion. The six PSM-C vignette *story stems* describe social problems and the *conclusions* describe resolutions of the problems. This is much more time-consuming than the other rating scales, so it may be more appropriate for research studies.

If one chooses an interview instead of a rating scale to assess social skills, the Social Adjustment Inventory for Children and Adolescents (Walsh, Allis, & Orvaschel, 1986) is one measure of adaptive functioning. This is a semistructured interview covering four major areas: school behavior, spare time activities and problems, peer relations (problems, activities, boy–girl relationships, and problems with opposite sex), and home life (activity and problems with siblings, relationship and problems with parents).

There are several observational systems that tap the child's interpersonal behaviors. As described earlier, the Social Behavior Coding System (DuPaul & Stoner, 1994) can be used to code peer interactions as well as teacher interactions. Four categories of behavioral interactions are coded: *positive, negative/ nonaggressive, aggressive,* and *noninteractive.* A similar observational coding system examining rates of positive and negative peer interaction is found in the Code for Observing Social Activity (COSA; Sprafkin, Grayson, Gadow, Nolan, & Paolicelli, 1986).

Treatment Acceptability

As with medication, school-based treatment can have costs. An effective treatment may be too difficult or time-consuming for the teacher to implement, and thus it will not continue. Similarly, if a teacher perceives that a treatment runs counter to his or her philosophy with respect to teaching and interacting with students, the treatment will be less than successful.

Many measures can assess a teacher's acceptance of an intervention. One of them, Elliot and Treuting's BIRS (1991), is a 24-item scale that asks teachers to rate the acceptability and effectiveness of various interventions on a 6-point scale. Psychometric qualities are good, with the measure yielding three factors: Acceptability, Effectiveness, and Time of Effect.

Case Example

Jacob was a 9-year-old boy referred by his teacher, school counselor, and mother to an outpatient clinic because of escalating difficulties in school. Jacob had previously received a diagnosis of AD/HD, Combined subtype. Medication was recommended and Jacob did in fact participate in a double-blind trial. Though 15 mg b.i.d. resulted in significant improvements at home and at school, Jacob also experienced significant side effects. He began to show increased irritability, sleep problems, rebound effects, and evidence of motor and vocal tics. Because Jacob was adopted, it was not possible to determine whether there was a positive family history for tics or Tourette's Disorder. Lower doses did not reduce the side effects to any great degree, nor did they result in any significant improvement in school functioning. The tics caused his physician and his parents to be concerned about continuing the medication, and eventually it was discontinued.

Despite the negative medication outcome, there was improvement at home. Jacob's parents had participated in parent training, and many of the problems at home were lessening. They had successfully instituted a token economy system, and Jacob's noncompliance and need for parental reminders and redirection were dramatically reduced. What remained were significant difficulties at school.

The difficult areas were his interactions with others, his schoolwork, and his overall conduct in the classroom. Jacob had significant trouble completing work independently. His teacher would send the work home as a way of motivating him to complete it in class next time. However, there was so much of it that Jacob was increasingly unable to finish both his classwork and his homework consistently. This was leading to increased arguments at home, with Jacob lying about the work that needed to be done and thus falling even further behind. When he did complete the work, he often lost it. His desk was a disaster area, full of scraps of paper, notes to parents, partially chewed pencils—even an occasional piece of food.

His grades fluctuated dramatically. On some quizzes and chapter tests, Jacob earned As and Bs. On others, it seemed he had not mastered the material at all. There was no consistent pattern to his strengths or weaknesses across subject areas. His behavior in class fluctuated as well. There were good days, but Jacob was increasingly disruptive in class. He was often out of his seat, roaming around the room and disturbing the other children. When he was in his seat, he would tip his chair until he fell. When asked to answer a question or read out loud, Jacob did so reluctantly and then only in a high-pitched, odd-sounding voice.

These difficulties were causing more and more problems with his classmates, who were becoming intolerant of his disruptions. On several occasions, the class had to have "silent lunch" because of his misbehavior in the lunch room. Silliness that was tolerated, even enjoyed, in earlier grades was increasingly viewed as strange by his friends. He usually spent recess running around the school yard by himself, occasionally interrupting a game to steal the ball.

These continuing difficulties and the fact that medication was no longer an option led to school-based interventions. Because of the comprehensive nature of his difficulties, the intervention had a number of components (e.g., preferential seating, adjusting task characteristics and assignment length) that were written into a Section 504 Accommodation Plan. The primary component was a token economy program whereby Jacob earned points for on-task behavior and for compliance with teacher requests and classroom rules, and lost points for out-of-seat and disruptive behavior. Points translated into weekly rewards, such as extra computer time and homework holidays. Because of the limited availability of high-interest reinforcing activities at school and the difficulty in identifying activities that could be lost under the point system, a daily home–school report card was implemented. Jacob's daily and weekly point tally was incorporated into the ongoing, successful token program at home. Obviously, this program required a good deal of extra effort on the part of the teacher, so it was essential to learn how much the intervention had resulted in meaningful change. If Jacob's behavior was not significantly improved with this program and it became clear that the level of support he needed was more than could be provided in a regular classroom, it might be necessary to consider additional special educational resources.

In light of the 8-step evaluation process, the effect of the token economy component on school factors is now examined. Obviously, one would look at any carryover to home, as well as assess the integrity of all intervention components (e.g., daily home–school notes; adaptation of task characteristics). The specific outcome indicators considered (Step 1) were those variables likely to be changed by the intervention, highlighting areas of particular interest to the teacher. After examining these, and after a discussion with the teacher, the following indicators were selected: on-task behavior as evidenced by work productivity and accuracy; out-of-seat behavior; social difficulties resulting from disruptive behavior; noncompliance with class rules and teacher requests; and overall AD/HD symptoms.

The criteria for deciding whether the program was successful (Step 2) comprised two factors. One was the degree to which clinically significant change was noted and scores no longer fell into the elevated range (e.g., *T* scores greater than 70; scores more than 2 standard deviations above the mean). The other was how satisfied Jacob's teacher was with the change (at least enough to continue the intervention) and how acceptable the teacher found the token program. Without these data, it was unlikely that the intervention would continue even if Jacob's behavior improved significantly.

The methods chosen (Step 3) were comprehensive, designed to sample all the areas. A combination of rating scales and direct observation was chosen to determine program success. To measure Jacob's on-task behavior, the Academic Performance Rating Scale was chosen because it measures productivity, which should increase as a function of greater attention to task. Because classroom observations would be used to determine treatment integrity (see Step 5), the BASC SOS was chosen to examine both adaptive (e.g., on-task) and maladaptive (e.g., disruptive) behaviors. Jacob's compliance with instructions was measured using the School Situations Questionnaire-Revised, with social skills assessed via the Social Skills Rating Scale. To avoid making the battery too long, the AD/HD Rating Scale-IV was chosen as the best measure of overall symptoms in the classroom. Finally, the BIRS was chosen to examine teacher acceptability and satisfaction with the program.

Significant change was not expected at home, first because most of the home difficulties had already been addressed through parent training and secondly because the focus of the intervention was on school behaviors unlikely to generalize to the home. Nevertheless, to ensure that home behaviors did not deteriorate due to so much emphasis on school, Jacob's parents also completed the AD/HD Rating Scale-IV and the Home Situations Questionnaire-Revised.

Baseline data (Step 4) were collected 2 weeks before beginning the program, with follow-up data to be collected 1 month later. The BASC SOS was completed for a peer who was not having difficulty to provide a comparison with Jacob's behavior.

Step 5, determining intervention integrity, was essential for assessing whether the program was succeeding and for learning what, if anything, needed to be refined. Gresham's (1989) Intervention Integrity Checklist (Table 8.2.) was implemented. The components of the token system were listed and an outside observer checked off whether or not the intervention occurred.

Step 6, collecting outcome data, took place approximately 1 month after the start of the program. As with the baseline data and intervention integrity data, care was taken to conduct the classroom observation on a day representative of the class schedule and thus of Jacob's behavior, being sure to sample the settings and tasks most likely to be problematic.

The data were analyzed (Step 7) and the process of determining the efficacy of the intervention was begun. A summary of the data is presented in Table 8.11. The results, which were presented to Jacob's teacher and his parents, indicated that the token economy program did result in several significant improvements. On the APRS, academic productivity increased significantly, and the number and severity of problematic school situations was significantly decreased. Post-treatment scores fell below the clinical range for noncompliance. The remaining difficulties occurred at lunch, in the hallways, at recess, and on the bus.

These social difficulties were also reflected on the Social Skills Rating Scale (SSRS). The SSRS standard scores on both scales improved little; scores on the problem behaviors stayed in the clinical range (e.g., more than 2 standard deviations from the mean). Classroom observations showed that Jacob engaged in significantly less disruptive behavior and more adaptive behavior. His overall levels were still not commensurate with his classmate, but the change was in the right direction.

The teacher rated his overall symptoms as being significantly better on the AD/HD Rating Scale-IV. Using the Jacobson–Truax methodology, RCIs exceeded the significant change level of 1.96 for the Inattention, Hyperactivity-Impulsivity, and Total scores. Jacob's teacher also indicated that she was generally satisfied

TABLE 8.11.   Summary of School-Based Intervention Results

Outcome measure	Pretreatment	Posttreatment
ADHD Rating Scale-IV—Home Version		
Inattention	14	11 (.84)
Hyperactivity-Impulsivity	11	10 (.36)
Total	25	21 (.74)
ADHD Rating Scale-IV—School Version		
Inattention	27	19 (2.01)
Hyperactivity-Impulsivity	30	21 (2.28)
Total	57	40 (2.45)
Home Situations Questionnaire-Revised		
Number of problem situations	6 (<1.5 SD)	5 (<1 SD)
Mean severity	4.3 (>1.5 SD)	3.8 (<1.5 SD)
School Situations Questionnaire-Revised		
Number of problem situations	9 (>2 SD)	4 (<1 SD)
Mean severity	6.9 (>2 SD)	5.2 (<1.5 SD)
Social Skills Rating Scale (standard scores)		
Social Skills Scale	85 (−1 SD)	88 (approx. −1 SD)
Problem Behaviors Scale	136 (>2 SD)	124 (>1.5 SD)
BASC Structured Observation Scale		
% of time adaptive behaviors vs. % of time peer	25% vs. 80%	68% vs. 85%
% of time maladaptive behaviors vs. % of time peer	85% vs. 20%	50% vs. 26%
Academic Performance Rating Scale		
Academic productivity	42	66

with the program and found the interventions acceptable as measured on the BIRS. As expected, no major changes in home behavior were shown on parent ratings, but no deterioration was noted either.

Using the comprehensive evaluation procedure provided information on three areas: symptoms, functioning, and treatment acceptability and satisfaction, from which the following decisions were made (Step 8): The program would continue but with modifications. The frequency of feedback on school tasks would begin to be faded in 1 month. Adaptations would be made to specifically target recess and bus behavior, with the possibility of a social skills training group added to the intervention package.

EVALUATING HOME-BASED TREATMENT

As detailed in Chapter 6, parent training programs have empirical support (Pelham et al., 1998). Whether used alone as the primary treatment (e.g., Anastopoulos et al., 1993; Pisterman, Firestone, McGratta, Goodman, Webster, & Mallory, 1992) or in combination with other treatments such as stimulant medication (e.g., Horn et al., 1991; Pelham et al., 1988), parent training improves child, parent, and family systems outcome. Parent training seems to increase the goodness-of-fit between the child and the demands of the home environment. Increased parental understanding of AD/HD and of why behavior problems occur, along with knowledge of strategies to address these difficulties, increases child compliance, decreases parenting stress, and improves the parental sense of competence. Although these group data are encouraging, one still needs to examine the benefits of parent training for a given child and family.

What to Measure and How

Because of the potentially broad effects of parent training, outcome evaluations need to examine its effects on AD/HD symptoms; on functioning in home, in school, and with peers; and its satisfaction and acceptability for those involved as well. Many measures can examine treatment effectiveness in these areas. Some that were described in Chapter 4 and earlier in this chapter are essential components in the initial diagnosis, and have proven sensitive to treatment effects from pharmacological and school-based interventions. Others are more specific to behaviors typically targeted in parent training. A brief review of some of the procedures used successfully in determining the efficacy of home-based interventions is given next and summarized in Table 8.12. As before, we are not recommending that all measures be used in a single evaluation, because this would result in a cumbersome battery.

AD/HD Symptomatology

As with school-based treatments, it is helpful to examine the degree to which a home-based intervention addresses the core symptoms of AD/HD, that

TABLE 8.12. Outcome Indicators for Home-Based Interventions

Target of intervention	Sample outcome indicators	Area of functioning	Possible measures
Decrease oppositional behavior	Number of problematic home situations	Home	Home Situations Questionnaire-Revised
	Compliance with parental requests	Home	BASC or Conners' Parent Rating Scale; Disruptive Behavior Disorders Rating Scale
Decrease parental conflict	Parental agreement on behavior management techniques	Home	Parenting Alliance Inventory; Parenting Practices Scale
	Marital satisfaction	Home	Dyadic Adjustment Scale; Marital Satisfaction Inventory-Revised; Locke-Wallace
	Parenting stress	Home	Parenting Stress Index; Parenting Practices Scale
Improve parenting effectiveness	Parental agreement on management	Home	Parenting Alliance Scale
	Use of appropriate, nonphysical strategies	Home	Parenting Scale, Parenting Practices Scale
	Knowledge of AD/HD and behavior management principles	Home	Parenting Scale, Test of AD/HD Knowledge
	Parenting satisfaction	Home	Parenting Sense of Competence, Parenting Stress Index

is, inattention and hyperactivity-impulsivity. Although direct effects on these symptoms are more likely to be seen with medication, home-based interventions can also reduce their expression. Measures such as the AD/HD Rating Scale-IV, the SNAP, Conners' DSM-IV scale, the Connors' CGI, and the ADDES are just as effective when used with parents as when used with teachers. Because these procedures have strong psychometric qualities and norms, one can calculate clinically significant change using the Jacobson–Truax methodology. In addition, their brevity makes it possible to include them in a large multimethod assessment battery without adding much to its length. All have proven sensitive to home-based treatment effects.

Home Functioning

As the name implies, home-based interventions target child behaviors likely to be seen at home. They can also target areas affected by the child's AD/HD (e.g., parenting stress) and can be influential in determining symptom severity and the expression of comorbid conditions.

One of the primary targets of parent training programs is child noncompliance. This is true for several reasons (Barkley, 1987). First, it is one of the most frequent complaints of families who seek treatment. Second, it underlies many negative parent–child interactions, so if one improves a child's compliance, one will likely see other improvements as well (e.g., increased satisfaction in parenting role). Third, noncompliance may have to be addressed first to effect any positive change in other areas.

In evaluating parent training on noncompliance, a number of measures can be used. One can examine the global outcome, that is, whether the child is more compliant with parental requests. The Home Situations Questionnaire-Revised specifically asks the parent to rate how much of a problem noncompliance is in a number of typical home situations, and it has successfully monitored treatment efficacy. Broad-band rating scales (e.g., BASC, Conners', Achenbach), as well as narrow-band scales that tap oppositional and conduct behaviors (e.g., SNAP), are also useful.

One should examine as well any changes that may contribute to the child's increased compliance (or lack thereof). Increased positive parental attention and improved parent–child emotional climate are critical elements for increasing child compliance (Anastopoulos et al., 1993; Webster-Stratton, 1998). Measures such as the Parenting Stress Index (Abidin, 1995) are helpful for seeing whether such changes have taken place. The long form of the PSI contains many subscales that reflect positive change of all kinds. The major subscales of both the long and the short forms can demonstrate improved parent–child interaction and parent perceptions of a child's temperament.

Most parent training programs specifically include sessions on the causes of childhood misbehavior and the skills necessary to address them. Thus, one should determine (1) if the parents actually learned the information and (2) if they were able to use the new skills with their child. Two scales seem particularly well suited to measuring these areas. The Parenting Scale (PS; Arnold et al., 1993) assesses ineffective discipline practices, and the 34-item Parenting Practices Scale (PPS; Strayhorn & Weidman, 1988) measures how often parents use the parenting practices commonly taught in the training programs.

In addition to parent reports, informal observations can reveal how often parents actually use the strategies. During a clinic visit, parents and children can be asked to complete several tasks likely to produce noncompliance (e.g., picking up toys left on the floor by another child). Parent–child interactions are observed and behaviors coded for the parents' use of effective, nonpunitive strategies and for child compliance.

Another focus of parent training programs is increasing the consistency between parents in using these strategies. The child's compliance is likely to increase if both parents are using similar techniques in similar ways. To see if this is occurring, the Parenting Alliance Inventory (Abidin & Brunner, 1995) can be used.

One should also learn whether knowing and using the new strategies has improved the parents' perception of their own efficacy and competence as parents and reduced the overall stress in their parenting role. Regarding parenting efficacy, the Parenting Sense of Competence Scale (PSCS; Johnston & Mash, 1989) examines a parent's or caregiver's sense of competence or efficacy and the overall satisfaction with their parenting role. With regard to stress and satisfaction in parenting, the Parenting Stress Index (PSI; Abidin, 1995) is sensitive to changes resulting from parent training (Anastopoulos et al., 1992, 1993). The

long form provides subscale scores in areas such as the parent's sense of compe-
tence and how reinforcing the child is to the parent. When a battery is getting
lengthy, the short form (PSI-SF) still permits an evaluation of Total Stress,
Parental Distress, Parent–Child Dysfunctional Interaction, and Difficult Child.
For parents of adolescents, the Stress Index for Parents of Adolescents (SIPA;
Sheras & Abidin, 1998) examines changes in parenting stress as it relates to
Adolescent Characteristics, Parent Characteristics, Adolescent–Parent Interac-
tions, and Stressful Life Circumstances.

Because parents of children with AD/HD are often less satisfied in their
parenting role and disagree more often as well (e.g., Anastopoulos et al., 1992;
Barkley et al., 1996; Shelton et al., 1998), their marital relationship as well as
individual psychological functioning can suffer. The parents often report significant marital dissatisfaction and higher levels of depression and psychological
distress (e.g., Barkley, Anastopoulos et al., 1992; Barkley et al., 1996). Parent
training usually increases parenting satisfaction, efficacy, and consistency, so it
may also improve other areas of family functioning. Furthermore, some programs (e.g., Robin & Foster, 1989) specifically include a family therapy component in which discord and ineffective negotiation and communication patterns
are addressed directly. As a result, one might see positive changes in family
functioning.

Many measures can examine this aspect of parent training outcome. Some
may have been administered as part of the initial diagnostic battery. For marital
interaction, the Dyadic Adjustment Scale (Spanier, 1989), Locke-Wallace (Locke
& Wallace, 1959), and Marital Satisfaction Inventory-Revised (Snyder, 1981) all
work well. As described earlier, all have solid psychometric qualities and all
have been used in research (e.g., Anastopoulos et al., 1992, 1993; Barkley, Anastopoulos et al., 1992).

For evaluating individual psychological functioning, the SCL-90-R is a
quick, reliable measure of overall psychological distress. To assess depression
and anxiety, the Beck Depression Inventory-II and the Beck Anxiety Inventory
are valid and reliable.

Especially for parent training programs that include family therapy, one
might examine the behavioral competence of siblings, who could be at risk for
developing oppositional or other inappropriate behaviors. Any of the broad-
band measures described earlier (e.g., BASC, Conners', Achenbach) could be
used for this purpose. Finally, one may wish to assess the functioning of the
family as a unit. Measures that examine the family's emotional climate (e.g.,
Family Environment Scale; Moos & Moos, 1983), the degree to which family
members are perceived as supportive (e.g., Family Support Scale; Dunst, Trivette, & Deal, 1994), or other family characteristics (e.g., adaptability and cohesion; FACES-II, Olson & Portner, 1983) can reveal the degree to which parent
training has improved not only parenting, but family functioning as a whole.

School Functioning

One would not necessarily expect a large generalization from home-based
interventions to the child's behavior at school, but it is reasonable to see some

improvement in school-related areas of parent–child interactions, such as home-work. The tedious nature of homework makes it a common area of noncompli-ance. Parents and children frequently describe homework as a major battle-ground. Parent training programs can enable the parents to (1) understand how AD/HD makes it difficult for the child to complete the homework, (2) adapt the homework schedule to make it easier for the child to complete it successfully (e.g., breaking it down into smaller pieces; taking frequent breaks), and (3) re-ward the child's effort and compliance through a token economy system. Thus an examination of this is in order. The Home Situation Questionnaire-Revised can be used here as well, because one of the items asks how much of a problem it is when the child is asked to do homework. Another measure is the Homework Problem Checklist (Anesko, Schoiock, Ramirez, & Levine, 1987), which asks parents to indicate how often certain problems, such as denying having home-work or failing to complete it, occur.

Social Functioning

Although most home-based treatments do not target peer interaction specif-ically, increased compliance can also improve peer interactions. An increase in social skills or a decrease in fighting with friends and siblings can be targeted in a home token economy program. Giving the child positive attention when he or she is interacting appropriately with friends and siblings may also result in improvements. Many measures can tap these improvements in social function-ing. The HSQ-R already targets playing with other children and may have been included in the treatment planning phase to target social interactions as a focus of intervention. If necessary, one can add other social situations to the measure and use the same format to have parents rate the problem's severity both before and after treatment.

Sometimes social interaction is the focus of parent–child conflict. To the extent that parent training results in a more effective resolution of problems concerning dating, curfew, choice of friends (e.g., Robin & Foster, 1989), and so on, one can expect to see improvement here, too. The Issues Checklist for Parents and Teenagers (Barkley & Murphy, 1998; adapted from Robin & Foster, 1989) examines this type of change. This face-valid checklist measures 44 differ-ent situations and asks the respondent to list the dyads for whom the situation is or is not a problem. If it is a problem, the respondent indicates how frequent and how intense discussions over these topics are on a 5-point scale (1 = calm; 5 = angry). Of course, the measures mentioned earlier that assess the child's social skills (e.g., BASC, CBCL, SSRS) examine broader improvements in this area.

Treatment Acceptability

Parental satisfaction with and acceptance of treatments is key in conducting a cost–benefit analysis of parent training. Several measures of parent satisfac-tion can be used. One is the Parent's Consumer Satisfaction Questionnaire developed by Forehand and McMahon (1981) for use as part of their parenting program for children with oppositional behavior. This 47-item scale rates parent satisfaction with the overall program, with the teaching format, with the specific techniques, and with the therapists as well.

A similar measure is the Therapy Attitude Inventory (TAI; Eyberg, 1993), a 10-item multiple-choice questionnaire in which the parents rate how satisfied they are with the intervention and whether improvement occurred. Like the Forehand and McMahon measure, the TAI was developed to evaluate parent training. It has been used primarily with parents of preschoolers with disruptive behavior disorders. Internal consistency and test-retest reliability are high (Brestan et al., 1999). Changes in child compliance and parent behavior ratings have been shown to relate to parent satisfaction (Brestan et al., 1999). The Parent Satisfaction Questionnaire (Stallard, 1996) and the Family Satisfaction Survey (FSS; Measelle, Weinstein, & Martinez, 1998) assess similar constructs.

One must also examine the *satisfaction* of the child. A measure developed specifically for this purpose is the Youth Client Satisfaction Questionnaire (Shapiro et al., 1997) for 11–17 year olds. This measure has two factors: Relationship with Therapist and Benefits of Therapy. It has good test-retest reliability and internal consistency, and child satisfaction scores are associated with changes in parent-reported behavior problems, parent satisfaction, parental and therapist ratings of treatment progress, and the *DSM* Global Assessment of Functioning.

Many scales also rate the treatment *acceptability* to the child, parent, teacher, and even therapist. Although there is some natural overlap between acceptability and satisfaction with outcome, data suggest that examining acceptability goes beyond whether someone is satisfied with an outcome. For example, a parent might be quite happy with the results of a home incentive program addressing their child's oppositional behavior, but the time it takes to implement it may not be acceptable.

One of the most frequently used measures of acceptability is the Treatment Evaluation Inventory developed by Kazdin (1986). This 15-item rating scale can be used by staff and parents to rate the acceptability of various interventions (positive reinforcement of incompatible behavior, positive practice, medication, and time-out strategies). Originally designed for parents of children ages 6–17 years, it also works across a wider age range (e.g., 2–22 years, Miller & Kelley, 1992). A similar measure is the Abbreviated Acceptability Rating Profile, a shorter version of the Intervention Rating Profile (Tarnowski & Simonian, 1992). Both measures have good internal consistency and test-retest reliability, have been used successfully with culturally diverse populations, and can distinguish among psychosocial and pharmacological treatments. Although used less frequently, there are also rating scales that examine an intervention's acceptability to children (usually over age 10 or 11). One example is the Children's Intervention Profile (Witt & Elliott, 1986), which measures children's reactions to 12 different teacher strategies for oppositional and conduct behavior.

Case Example

Adam is an 8-year-old boy referred for an evaluation because of difficulty sitting still, following directions, and complying with parental requests. Academic and behavioral immaturity had resulted in Adam having to repeat the first grade and undergo school-based testing. No learning disabilities or other difficulties were identified. He is currently in a regular second grade classroom with no special-educational services. Adam and his 10-year-old brother live with their biological parents. There are no environmental stressors or recent major changes in the family. The evaluation resulted in a diagnosis of AD/HD, Combined subtype; and Oppositional Defiant Disorder. Because of significant oppositional behaviors at home and the parenting stress reported by his mother, parent training was recommended. Within 2 weeks of the evaluation, Adam's parents began a 10-session training program designed for parents of children with AD/HD (Anastopoulos & Barkley, 1990). To determine if the parent training was successful, the following outcome evaluation process was initiated.

In Step 1, several outcome indicators were chosen that addressed both child and parent factors. Noncompliance was the main target of the intervention, so the child outcome indicators were number of problematic home situations, degree of oppositional behavior, and improvement in attending to parental requests. Parent outcome indicators were evidence that behavior management strategies had been learned and used, had increased consistency between parents, and had decreased parenting stress. Because the difficulties were mainly at home and no school factors were targeted, no school indicators were selected.

In Step 2, criteria for success were defined. In this case, the success indicators were problem behavior that decreased below the clinical range (e.g., T scores less than 70), significant increase in parental knowledge and use of effective techniques, parenting stress that decreased below clinical levels (e.g., less than 85 percentile), and other behavioral indicators such as the overall level of AD/HD behaviors.

In Step 3, evaluation methods were chosen, informed by the outcome indicators and the success criteria. Rating scales with norms and strong psychometric qualities were chosen as the most efficient methods for collecting the pre- and posttreatment data. To examine the number of noncompliance situations, the HSQ-R was selected. Noncompliance being the main issue, it was important to have a broad-band measure that could tap oppositional and aggressive behaviors. Overall behavior was assessed using the BASC Parent Rating Scale, for two reasons. First, baseline levels from these measures were already available from the diagnostic evaluation. Second, the BASC allows examination of any child strengths resulting from the intervention.

To examine the impact of parent training on the parent outcome indicators, the Parenting Scale (Arnold et al., 1993) was chosen to assess the knowledge and use of appropriate parental disciplinary practices, and the Parenting Stress Index-short form (Abidin, 1995) was used to measure parenting stress. Because both parents were attending parent training and there was some disagreement on how to manage Adam's behavior, the Parenting Alliance Inventory (Abidin & Brunner, 1995) was also used to see how much Adam's parents were working together as parents. To assess the acceptability of the parent training, Kazdin's (1986) TEI was selected. The TEI samples acceptance of most parent training components (e.g., positive reinforcement, time-out).

In Step 4 baseline data were collected. Parent training was scheduled to begin shortly after the diagnostic evaluation, so almost all of the baseline data could be taken from the measures administered during the diagnostic process (e.g., BASC, AD/HD Rating Scale-IV, Parenting Stress Index). The remaining measures (e.g., Home Situations Questionnaire-Revised) were collected just prior to the first meeting of the parent training group.

In Step 5 the integrity of the parent training intervention was determined. The therapist kept a checklist of each training session's major points and the degree to which Adam's parents implemented them. They were very motivated to apply the strategies faithfully. With the exception of a brief delay in getting the home token economy system up and running, all components were implemented as designed.

In Step 6 outcome data were collected. When the parent training program was completed approximately 3 months later, posttreatment data were collected and scored.

In Step 7 the process of analyzing the success of the parent training was begun. A summary of the pre- and posttreatment outcome scores is presented in Table 8.13.

During Adam's initial evaluation his mother completed the AD/HD Rating Scale-IV. Adam's Inattention score was then 18, his Hyperactivity-Impulsivity score 21, and his Total score 39. His mother's posttreatment ratings placed Adam's Inattention score at 14, his Hyperactivity-Impulsivity score at 16, and his

TABLE 8.13. Summary of Parent Training Results

Outcome measures	Pretreatment	Posttreatment
ADHD Rating Scale-IV—Home Version		
Inattention	18	14 (1.13)
Hyperactivity-Impulsivity	21	16 (1.81)
Total	39	30 (1.68)
Home Situations Questionnaire-Revised		
Number of problem situations	12 (>2 SD)	3 (<1 SD)
Mean severity	5.3 (>2 SD)	4.8 (>1.5 SD)
BASC Parent Rating Scale (*T* scores)		
Aggression	71	66
Conduct	72	64
Internalizing	46	40
Adaptive Skills	46	51
Parenting Stress Index—Short Form		
Parental Distress	26	21
Parent/Child Interaction	32	22
Difficult Child	48	41
Total	108	84
Parenting Scale		
Overreactivity	4.4	2.1
Laxness	3.4	2.8
Verbosity	5.5	3.2
Total	4.2	2.6
Parenting Alliance Inventory	64	72

Total score at 30. Comparison of these scores with the initial assessment scores yielded RCIs of 1.13 (Inattention), 1.81 (Hyperactivity-Impulsivity), and 1.68 (Total). Inattention change was not statistically significant. However, Hyperactivity-Impulsivity change did approach significance, indicating a positive effect on this component.

The data were supported by an inspection of the pre- and posttreatment scores on the other measures collected at the 1-month follow-up. Many of Adam's problematic behaviors were reduced to subclinical levels. In particular, externalizing behaviors as measured on the BASC Aggression and Conduct Problems subscales were all well below *T* scores of 70. The number of problematic home situations was reduced as well. In addition, Adam's mother reported a total parenting stress score that fell below the at-risk range. The Parenting Scale indicated use of more-effective parenting strategies, and parental agreement, as measured on the Parenting Alliance Inventory, became stronger. Finally, on the Treatment Evaluation Inventory, both parents rated the behavior management strategies very positively and attributed much of the change in Adam to these techniques.

In Step 8 the three areas of outcome data (symptomatology, functioning, and treatment acceptability) were examined to determine future treatment directions. Although significant gains were noted following parent training, the evaluation indicated room for improvement. The number of problematic home situations was greatly reduced, but three situations remained where there was significant noncompliance, with average severity ratings still quite high. Coupled with the relatively high-stress subscale score for Difficult Child, it appeared that further follow-up was needed. Specific recommendations were made to target the three remaining home situations, with follow-up data to be collected 1 month later.

With regard to AD/HD symptomatology, there was little effect on inattention, and hyperactivity-impulsivity difficulties could be further reduced. Thus, a stimulant medication trial was recommended to address these symptoms.

CONCLUSION

As is evident from the preceding discussion, assessment plays a vital role in determining whether or not an intervention is effective. For ease of discussion, the examples in this chapter illustrated only single interventions, but multiple interventions often comprise a child's treatment package. In these instances, the outcome evaluation process becomes even more important as one attempts to determine if any change occurred, and what were the critical therapeutic components related to this improvement.

Coming full circle, outcome evaluation is the crucial link between problem and solution. The diagnostic assessment for any childhood disorder should never be an end unto itself. Rather, diagnosis is the first stop on a journey toward helping these children and their families reach their optimal potential, with the outcome evaluation as a guidepost along the way.

References

Abidin, R. R. (1995). *Parenting Stress Index* (3rd ed.). Odessa, FL: Psychological Assessment Resources.

Abidin, R. R., & Brunner, J. F. (1995). Development of a Parenting Alliance Inventory. *Journal of Clinical Child Psychology, 24*, 31–40.

Abikoff, M., & Gittelman, R. (1985). Hyperactive children treated with stimulants: Is cognitive training a useful adjunct? *Archives of General Psychiatry, 42*, 953–961.

Abikoff, H., Gittelman-Klein, R., & Klein, D. (1977). Validation of a classroom observation code for hyperactive children. *Journal of Consulting and Clinical Psychology, 45*, 772–783.

Abramowitz, A. J., & O'Leary, S. G. (1991). Behavioral interventions for the classroom: Implications for students with ADHD. *School Psychology Review, 20*, 220–234.

Abramowitz, A. J., Reid, M. J., & O'Toole, K. (1994). *The role of task timing in the treatment of ADHD.* Paper presented at the Association for the Advancement of Behavior Therapy, San Diego, CA.

Achenbach, T. M. (1985). *Assessment of taxonomy of child and adolescent psychopathology.* Burlington, VT: University of Vermont & State Agricultural College.

Achenbach, T. M. (1991a). *Manual for the Child Behavior Checklist/4–18 and 1991 Profile.* Burlington, VT: University of Vermont, Department of Psychiatry.

Achenbach, T. M. (1991b). *Manual for the Teacher's Report Form and 1991 Profile.* Burlington, VT: University of Vermont, Department of Psychiatry.

Achenbach, T. M. (1991c). *Manual for the Youth Self-Report and 1991 Profile.* Burlington, VT: University of Vermont, Department of Psychiatry.

Achenbach, T. M. (1992). *Manual for the Child Behavior Checklist/2–3 and 1992 Profile.* Burlington, VT: University of Vermont, Department of Psychiatry.

Achenbach, T. M. (1996). *ADHD Report, 4*(4), 5–9.

Achenbach, T. M. (1997a). *Manual for the Young Adult Self-Report and Young Adult Behavior Checklist.* Burlington, VT: University of Vermont, Department of Psychiatry.

Achenbach, T. M. (1997b). *Guide for the Caregiver–Teacher Report From for Ages 2–5.* Burlington, VT: University of Vermont, Department of Psychiatry.

Achenbach, T. M., & Edelbrock, C. S. (1983). *Manual for the Child Behavior Checklist and Revised Child Behavior Profile.* Burlington, VT: University of Vermont, Department of Psychiatry.

Achenbach, T. M., & Edelbrock, C. S. (1987). Empirically based assessment of the behavioral/emotional problems of 2– and 3–year-old children. *Journal of Abnormal Child Psychology, 15*, 629–650.

Achenbach, T. M., Edelbrock, C., & Howell, C. T. (1987). Empirically based assessment of the behavioral/emotional problems of 2- and 3-year-old children. *Journal of Abnormal Child Psychology, 15*(4), 629–650.

Achenbach, T. M., & Rescorla, L. A. (2000). *Manual for the ASEBA Preschool Forms and Profiles.* Burlington, VT: University of Vermont, Department of Psychiatry.

Adams, C. A., & Drabman, R. C. (1994). BASC: A critical review. *Child Assessment News, 4,* 1–5.

Adams, C. D., Kelley, M. L., & McCarthy, M. (1997). The Adolescent Behavior Checklist: Development and initial psychometric properties of a self-report measure for adolescents with ADHD. *Journal of Clinical Child Psychology, 26,* 77–86,

Adams, C. D., McCarthy, M., & Kelley, M. L. (1995). Adolescent versions of the Home and School Situations Questionnaires: Initial psychometric properties. *Journal of Clinical Child Psychology, 24,* 377–385.

Adams, C. D., Reynolds, L. K., Perez, R. A., Powers, D., & Kelley, M. L. (1998). The Adolescent Behavior Checklist: Validation using structured diagnostic interviews. *Journal of Psychopathology and Behavioral Assessment, 20,* 103–125.

Alessandri, S. M. (1992). Attention, play, and social behavior in ADHD preschoolers. *Journal of Abnormal Child Psychology, 20,* 289–302.

Aman, M. G., & Werry, J. S. (1984). The Revised Behavior Problem Checklist in clinical attenders and nonattenders: Age and sex effects. *Journal of Clinical Child Psychology, 13,* 237–242.

American Psychiatric Association. (1952). *Diagnostic and statistical manual of mental disorders.* Washington, DC: Author.

American Psychiatric Association. (1968). *Diagnostic and statistical manual of mental disorders* (2nd ed.). Washington, DC: Author.

American Psychiatric Association. (1980). *Diagnostic and statistical manual of mental disorders* (3rd ed.). Washington, DC: Author.

American Psychiatric Association. (1987). *Diagnostic and statistical manual of mental disorders* (3rd ed., revised). Washington, DC: Author.

American Psychiatric Association. (1994). *Diagnostic and statistical manual of mental disorders* (4th ed.). Washington, DC: Author.

Anastopoulos, A. D., & Barkley, R. A. (1990). Counseling and training parents. In R. A. Barkley, *Attention Deficit Hyperactivity Disorder: A handbook for diagnosis and treatment.* New York: Guilford Press.

Anastopoulos, A. D., Guevremont, D. C., Shelton, T. L., & DuPaul, G. J. (1992). Parenting stress among families of children with Attention-deficit hyperactivity disorder. *Journal of Abnormal Child Psychology, 20,* 503–520.

Anastopoulos, A. D., Shelton, T. L., DuPaul, G. J., & Guevremont, D. C. (1993). Parent training for attention-deficit hyperactivity disorder: Its impact on parent functioning. *Journal of Abnormal Child Psychology, 21,* 581–596.

Anastopoulos, A. D., Spisto, M. A., & Maher, M. (1994). The WISC-III Freedom From Distractibility factor: Its utility in identifying children with Attention Deficit Hyperactivity Disorder. *Psychological Assessment, 6,* 368–371.

Anderson, J. C., Williams, S., McGee, R., & Silva, P. A. (1987). DSM-III disorders in preadolescent children. Prevalence in a large sample from the general population. *Archives of General Psychiatry, 44*(1), 69–76.

Anesko, K. M., Schoiock, G., Ramirez, R., & Levine, F. M. (1987). The Homework Problem Checklist: Assessing children's homework difficulties. *Behavioral Assessment, 9,* 179–185.

Angold, A., & Costello, E. J. (1995). A test-retest reliability study of child-reported psychiatric symptoms and diagnoses using the Child and Adolescent Psychiatric Assessment (CAPA-C). *Psychological Medicine, 25,* 755–762.

Angold, A., Prendergast, M., Cox, A., Harrington, R., Simonoff, E., & Rutter, M. (1995). The Child and Adolescent Psychiatric Assessment (CAPA). *Psychological Medicine, 25,* 739–753.

Applegate, B., Lahey, B. B., Hart, E. L., Waldman, I., Biederman, J., Hynd, G. W., Barkley, R. A., Ollendick, T., Frick, P. J., Greenhill, L., McBurnett, K., Newcorn, J., Kerdyk, L., Garfinkel, B., & Shaffer, D. (1997). Validity of the age of onset criterion for ADHD: A report from the *DSM-IV* field trials. *Journal of the American Academy of Child and Adolescent Psychiatry, 36,* 1211–1221.

Arnold, D. S., O'Leary, S. G., Wolff, L. S., & Acker, M. M. (1993). The Parenting Scale: A measure of dysfunctional parenting in discipline situations. *Psychological Assessment, 5,* 137–144.

Arnold, L. E. (1996). Sex differences in ADHD: Conference summary. *Journal of Abnormal Child Psychology, 24,* 555–570.

Arnsten, A. F. T., Steere, J. C., & Hunt, R. D. (1996). The contribution of α2 noradrenergic mechanism to prefrontal cortical cognitive function. *Archives of General Psychiatry, 53,* 448–455.

Atchley, R. C. (1975). The life course, age grading, and age-linked demands for decision making. In N. Datan & L. H. Ginsberg (Eds.), *Life-span developmental psychology: Normative life crises.* New York: Academic Press.

Atkins, M. S., Pelham, W. E., & Licht, M. H. (1985). A comparison of objective classroom measures and teacher ratings of attention deficit disorder. *Journal of Abnormal Child Psychology, 13*(1), 155–167.

August, G. H., & Garfinkel, G. D. (1990). Comorbidity of ADHD and reading disability among clinic-referred children. *Journal of Abnormal Child Psychology, 18,* 29–45.

August, G. J., Realmuto, G. M., MacDonald, A. W., Nugent, S. M., & Crosby, R. (1996). Prevalence of ADHD and comorbid disorders among elementary school children screened for disruptive behavior. *Journal of Abnormal Child Psychology, 24,* 571–595.

August, G. J., & Stewart, M. A. (1983). Family subtypes of childhood hyperactivity. *Journal of Nervous and Mental Disease, 171,* 362–368.

Barkley, R. A. (1977). The effects of methylphenidate on various measures of activity level and attention in hyperkinetic children. *Journal of Abnormal Child Psychology, 5,* 351–369.

Barkley, R. A. (1981). *Hyperactive children: A handbook for diagnosis and treatment.* New York: Guilford Press.

Barkley, R. A. (1987). A review of child behavior rating scales and checklists for research in child psychopathology. In M. Rutter, A. H. Tuma, & I. Lann (Eds.), *Assessment and diagnosis in child psychopathology.* New York: Guilford Press.

Barkley, R. A. (1990). *Attention-deficit hyperactivity disorder: A handbook for diagnosis and treatment.* New York: Guilford Press.

Barkley, R. A. (1991). The ecological validity of laboratory and analogue assessment methods of ADHD symptoms. *Journal of Abnormal Child Psychology, 19,* 149–178.

Barkley, R. A. (1997). *ADHD and the nature of self-control.* New York: Guilford Press.

Barkley, R. A. (1998). *Attention-deficit hyperactivity disorder—A handbook for diagnosis and treatment* (2nd ed.). New York: Guilford Press.

Barkley, R. A., & Biederman, J. (1997). Toward a broader definition of the age of onset criterion for attention-deficit hyperactivity disorder. *Journal of the American Academy of Child and Adolescent Psychiatry, 36,* 1204–1210.

Barkley, R. A., & Cunningham, C. E. (1979). The effects of methylphenidate on the mother–child interactions of hyperactive children. *Archives of General Psychiatry, 36,* 201–208.

Barkley, R. A., & Edelbrock, C. S. (1987). Assessing situational variation in children's behavior problems: The Home and School Situations Questionnaires. In R. Prinz (Ed.), *Advances in behavioral assessment of children and families* (Vol. 3, pp. 157–176). Greenwich, CT: JAI Press.

Barkley, R. A., & Grodzinsky, G. (1994). Are neuropsychological tests of frontal lobe functions useful in the diagnosis of attention deficit disorders? *Clinical Neuropsychologist, 8,* 121–139.

Barkley, R. A., & Murphy, K. R. (1995). *An examination of ADHD symptomatology in an adult community sample.* Unpublished manuscript.

Barkley, R. A., & Murphy, K. R. (1998). *Attention-deficit/hyperactivity disorder: A clinical workbook* (2nd ed.). New York: Guilford Press.

Barkley, R. A., Copeland, A. P., & Sivage, C. (1980). A self-control classroom for hyperactive children. *Journal of Autism and Developmental Disorders, 10,* 75–89.

Barkley, R. A., Karlsson, J., Pollard, S., & Murphy, J. (1985). Developmental changes in the mother-child interactions of hyperactive boys: Effects of two doses of Ritalin. *Journal of Child Psychology and Psychiatry, 26,* 705–715.

Barkley, R. A., Fisher, M., Newby, R., & Breen, M. (1988). Development of a multi-method clinical protocol for assessing stimulant drug responses in ADHD children. *Journal of Clinical Child Psychology, 17,* 14–24.

Barkley, R. A., Fischer, M., Edelbrock, C. S., & Smallish, L. (1990). The adolescent outcome of hyperactive children diagnosed by research criteria: I. An 8-year prospective follow-up study. *Journal of the American Academy of Child and Adolescent Psychiatry, 29,* 546–557.

Barkley, R. A., Anastopoulos, A. D., Guevremont, D. C., & Fletcher, K. E. (1991). Adolescents with attention-deficit hyperactivity disorder: Patterns of behavioral adjustment, academic functioning, and treatment utilization. *Journal of the American Academy of Child and Adolescent Psychiatry, 30,* 752– 761.

Barkley, R. A., DuPaul, G. J., & McMurray, M. D. (1991). Attention deficit disorder with and without hyperactivity: Clinical response to three dose levels of methylphenidate. *Pediatrics, 87*(4), 519–531.

Barkley, R. A., Anastopoulos, A. D., Guevremont, D. C., & Fletcher, K. E. (1992). Adolescents with attention-deficit hyperactivity disorder: Mother–adolescent interactions, family beliefs and conflicts, and maternal psychopathology. *Journal of Abnormal Child Psychology, 20,* 263–288.

Barkley, R. A., Guevremont, D. C., Anastopoulos, A. D., & Fletcher, K. E. (1992). A comparison of three family therapy programs for treating family conflicts in adolescents with attention-deficit hyperactivity disorder. *Journal of Consulting and Clinical Psychology, 60,* 450–462.

Barkley, R. A., Guevremont, D. C., Anastopoulos, A. D., DuPaul, G. D., & Shelton, T. L. (1993). Driving-related risks and outcomes of attention-deficit hyperactivity disorder in adolescents and young adults: A 3– to 5–year follow-up survey. *Pediatrics, 92,* 212–218.

Barkley, R. A., Shelton, T. L., Crosswait, C. R., Moorehouse, M., Fletcher, K., Barrett, S., Jenkins, L., & Metevia, L. (1996). Preliminary findings of an early intervention program with aggressive hyperactive children. In C. F. Ferris & T. Grisso (Eds.), *Annals of the New York Academy of Sciences* (Vol. 794—Special Issue, Understanding aggressive behavior in children; pp. 277–289).

Barkley, R. A., Shelton, T. L., Crosswait, C. R., Moorehouse, M., Fletcher, K., Barrett, S., Jenkins, L., & Metevia, L. (1999). Multimethod psycho-educational intervention for preschool children with aggressive and hyperactive-impulsive behavior. *Child Psychology and Psychiatry, 20*(2), 117–129.

Bauermeister, J. J., Berrios, V., Jimenez, A. L., Acevedo, L., & Gordon, M. (1990). Some issues and instruments for the assessment of attention-deficit hyperactivity disorder in Puerto Rican children. *Journal of Clinical Child Psychology, 19,* 9–16.

Bauermeister, J. J., Alegria, M., Bird, H. R., Rubio-Stipec, M., & Canino (1992). Are attentional-hyperactivity deficits unidimensional or multidimensional syndromes? Empirical findings from a community survey. *Journal of the American Academy of Child and Adolescent Psychiatry, 31,* 423–431.

Baumgardner, T. L., Singer, H. S., Denckla, M. B., Rubin, M. A., Abrams, M. T., Colli, M. J., & Reiss, A. L. (1996). Corpus callosum morphology in children with Tourette syndrome and attention-deficit hyperactivity disorder. *Neurology, 47,* 477–482.

Baumgaertel, A., Wolraich, M. L., & Dietrich, M. (1995). Attention deficit disorders in a German elementary school-aged sample. *Journal of the American Academy of Child and Adolescent Psychiatry, 34,* 629–638

Beck, A. T., & Steer, R. A. (1993). *The Beck Anxiety Inventory—1993 Edition.* San Antonio, TX: Psychological Corporation.

Beck, A. T., Steer, R. A., & Brown, G. K. (1996). *Beck Depression Inventory—II.* San Antonio, TX: Psychological Corporation.

Bennett, D. S., Power, T. J., Rostain, A. L., & Carr, D. E. (1996). Parent acceptability and feasibility of ADHD interventions: Assessment, correlates, and predictive validity. *Journal of Pediatric Psychology, 21,* 643–657.

Bennett, L. A., Wolin, S. J., & Reiss, D. (1988). Cognitive, behavioral, and emotional problems among school-age children of alcoholic parents. *American Journal of Psychiatry, 145,* 185–190.

Bhatia, M. S., Nigam, V. R., Bohra, N., & Malik, S. C. (1991). Attention deficit disorder with hyperactivity among paediatric outpatients. *Journal of Child Psychology and Psychiatry, 32,* 297–306.

Biederman, J., Munir, K., Knee, D., Armentano, M., Autor, S., Waternaux, C., & Tsuang, M. (1987). High rate of affective disorders in probands with attention deficit disorders and in their relatives: A controlled family study. *American Journal of Psychiatry, 144,* 330–333.

Biederman, J., Newcorn, J., & Sprich, S. (1991). Comorbidity of attention deficit hyperactivity disorder with conduct, depressive, anxiety, and other disorders. *American Journal of Psychiatry, 152,* 1652–1658.

Biederman, J., Faraone, S. V., Keenan, K., Benjaminm, J., Krifcher, B., Moore, C., Sprich-Buckminster,

S., Vgeglia, K., Jellinek, M. S., & Steingold, R. (1992). Further evidence for family-genetic risk factors in attention-deficit hyperactivity disorder: Patterns of comorbidity in probands and relatives in psychiatrically and pediatrically referred samples. *Archives of General Psychiatry, 49*, 728–738.

Biederman, J., Faraone, S. V., Spencer, T., Wilens, T., Norman, D., Lapey, K. A., Mick, E., Lehman, B. K., & Doyle, A. (1993). Patterns of psychiatric comorbidity, cognition, and psychosocial functioning in adults with attention-deficit hyperactivity disorder. *American Journal of Psychiatry, 150*, 1792–1798.

Biederman, J., Faraone, S. V., Mick, E., Spencer, T., Wilens, T., Kiely, K., Guite, J., Ablon, J. S., Reed, E., & Warburton, R. (1995). High risk for attention-deficit hyperactivity disorder among children of parents with childhood onset of the disorder: A pilot study. *American Journal of Psychiatry, 152*, 431–435.

Biederman, J., Faraone, S. V., Milberger, S., Curtis, S., Chen, L., Marrs, A., Ouellette, C., Moore, P., & Spencer, T. (1996). Predictors of persistence and remission of ADHD into adolescence: Results from a four-year prospective follow-up study. *Journal of the American Academy of Child and Adolescent Psychiatry, 35*, 343–351.

Biederman, J., Wilens, T. E., Mick, E., Faraone, S. V., Weber, W., Curtis, S., Thornell, A., Pfister, K., Jetton, J. G., & Soriano, J. (1997). Is ADHD a risk for psychoactive substance use disorders? Findings from a four-year prospective follow-up study. *Journal of the American Academy of Child and Adolescent Psychiatry, 36*, 21–29.

Birch, H. G. (1964). *Brain damage in children: The biological and social aspects.* Baltimore: Williams & Wilkins.

Block, G. H. (1977). Hyperactivity: A cultural perspective. *Journal of Learning Disabilities, 110*, 236–240.

Boggs, S. R., Eyberg, S., & Reynolds, L. A. (1990). Concurrent validity of the Eyberg Child Behavior Inventory. *Journal of Clinical Child Psychology, 19*, 75–78.

Bornstein, P. H., & Quevillon, R. P. (1976). The effects of a self-instructional package on overactive preschool boys. *Journal of Applied Behavior Analysis, 9*, 179-188.

Braswell, L., August, G. J., Bloomquist, M. L., Realmuto, G. M., Skare, R., & Crosby, D. (1997). School-based secondary prevention for children with disruptive behavior: Initial outcomes. *Journal of Abnormal Child Psychology, 25*(3), 197–208.

Breen, M. J. (1989). Cognitive and behavioral differences in ADHD boys and girls. *Journal of Child Psychology and Psychiatry and Allied Disciplines, 30*(5), 711–716.

Breen, M. J., & Altepeter, T. S. (1991). Factor structures of the Home Situations Questionnaire and the School Situations Questionnaire. *Journal of Pediatric Psychology, 16*, 59–67.

Breen, M. J., & Barkley, R. A. (1983). The Personality Inventory for Children (PIC): Its clinical utility with hyperactive children. *Journal of Pediatric Psychology, 8*(4), 359–366.

Breslau, N. (1987). Inquiring about the bizarre: False positive in Diagnostic Interview Schedule for Children (DISC) ascertainment of obsessions, compulsions, and psychotic symptoms. *Journal of the American Academy of Child and Adolescent Psychiatry, 26*(5), 639–644.

Brestan, E. V., Jacobs, J. R., Rayfield, A. D., & Eyberg, S. M. (1999). A consumer satisfaction measure for parent-child treatments and its relation to measures of child behavior change. *Behavior Therapy, 30*, 17–30.

Brown, R. T., & Quay, L. C. (1977). Reflection-impulsivity of normal and behavior disordered children. *Journal of Abnormal Child Psychology, 5*, 457–462.

Burns, B. J., Goldman, S. K., Faw, L., & Burchard, J. (1999). The wraparound evidence base. In B. J. Burns & S. K. Goldman (Eds.), Promising practices in wraparound for children with serious emotional disturbance and their families. *Systems of Care: Promising Practices in Children's Mental Health, 1998 Series, Vol. IV* (pp. 77–100). Washington, DC: Center for Effective Collaboration and Practice, American Institutes for Research.

Burns, G. L., & Owen, S. M. (1990). Disruptive behaviors in the classroom: Initial standardization data on a new teacher rating scale. *Journal of Abnormal Child Psychology, 18*, 515–525.

Burns, G. L., Sosna, T. D., & Ladish, C. (1992). Distinction between well-standardized norms and the psychometric properties of a measure: Measurement of disruptive behaviors with the Sutter-Eyberg Student Behavior Inventory. *Child and Family Behavior Therapy, 14*, 43–54.

Burns, G. L., Walsh, J. A., & Owen, S. M. (1995). Twelve-month stability of disruptive classroom behavior as measured by the Sutter-Eyberg Student Behavior Inventory. *Journal of Clinical Child Psychology, 24,* 453–462.

Burns, G. L., Walsh, J. A., Owen, S. M., & Snell, J. (1997). Internal validity of attention-deficit hyperactivity disorder, oppositional defiant disorder, and overt conduct disorder symptoms in young children: Implications from teacher ratings for a dimensional approach to symptom validity. *Journal of Clinical Child Psychology, 26,* 266–275.

Byrne, J. M., Bawden, H. N., DeWolfe, N. A., & Beattie, T. L. (1998). Clinical assessment of psychopharmacological treatment of preschoolers with ADHD. *Journal of Clinical and Experimental Neuropsychology, 20*(5), 613–627.

Cadman, D., Shurvell, B., Davies, P., & Bradfield, S. (1984). Compliance in the community with consultants' recommendations for the developmentally handicapped children. *Developmental Medicine and Child Neurology, 26,* 40–46.

Cahn, D. A., & Marcotte, A. C. (1995). Rates of forgetting in attention-deficit hyperactivity disorder. *Child Neuropsychology, 1,* 158–163.

Campbell, S. B. (1987). Parent-referred problem three-year-olds: Developmental changes in symptoms. *Journal of Child Psychology and Psychiatry, 28,* 835–846.

Campbell, S. B. (1990). *Behavior problems in preschoolers: Clinical and developmental issues.* New York: Guilford Press.

Campbell, S. B. (1995). Behavior problems in preschool children: A review of recent research. *Journal of Child Psychology and Psychiatry, 36,* 113–149.

Campbell, S. B., & Cluss, P. (1982). Peer relations of young children with behavior problems. In K. H. Rubin & H. S. Ross (Eds.), *Peer relations of young children with behavior problems.* New York: Springer-Verlag.

Campbell, S. B., Douglas, V. I., & Morganstern, G. (1971). Cognitive styles in hyperactive children and the effect of methylphenidate. *Journal of Child Psychology and Psychiatry, 12,* 55–67.

Campbell, S. B., Breaux, A. M., Ewing, L. J., & Szumowski, E. K. (1984). A one-year follow-up of parent-identified "hyperactive" preschoolers. *Journal of the American Academy of Child Psychiatry, 23,* 243–249.

Campbell, S. B., Breaux, A. M., Ewing, L. J., & Szumowski, E. K. (1986). Correlates and predictors of hyperactivity and aggression: A longitudinal study of parent-referred problem preschoolers. *Journal of Abnormal Child Psychology, 14*(2), 217–234.

Cantwell, D., & Carlson, G. (1978). Stimulants. In J. Werry (Ed.), *Pediatric psychopharmacology* (pp. 171–207). New York: Brunner/Mazel.

Cardon, L. R., Smith, S. D., Fulker, D. W., Kimberling, W. J., Pennington, B. F., & DeFries, J. C. (1994). Quantitative trait locus for reading disability in chromosome 6. *Science, 266,* 276–279.

Carlson, C. (1986). Attention deficit disorder without hyperactivity: A review of preliminary experimental evidence. In B. Lahey & A. Kazdin (Eds.), *Advances in clinical child psychology* (Vol. 9, pp. 153–176). New York: Plenum Press.

Casey, B. J., Castellanos, F. X., Giedd, J. N., Marsh, W. L., Hamburger, S. D., Schubert, A. B., Vauss, Y. C., Vaituzis, A. C., Dickstein, D. P., Sarfatti, S. E., & Rapoport, J. L. (1997). Implication of right frontostriatial circuitry in response inhibition and attention-deficit/hyperactivity disorder. *Journal of the American Academy of Child and Adolescent Psychiatry, 36,* 374–383.

Castellanos, F. X., Giedd, J. N., Marsh, W. L., Hamburger, S. D., Vaituzis, A. D., Dickstein, D. P., Sarfatti, S. E., Vauss, Y. C., Snell, J. W., Lange, N., Kaysen, D., Krain, A. L., Ritchhie, G. F., Rajapakse, J. C., & Rapoport, J. L. (1996). Quantitative brain magnetic resonance imaging in attention-deficit hyperactivity disorder. *Archives of General Psychiatry, 53,* 607–616.

Chess, S. (1960). Diagnosis and treatment of the hyperactive child. *New York State Journal of Medicine, 60,* 2379–2385.

Chelune, G. J., Ferguson, W., Koon, R., & Dickey, T. O. (1986). Frontal lobe disinhibition in attention deficit disorder. *Child Psychiatry and Human Development, 16,* 221–234.

Childers, A. T. (1935). Hyperactivity in children having behavior disorders. *American Journal of Orthopsychiatry, 5,* 227–243.

Clements, S. D., & Peters, J. E. (1962). Minimal brain dysfunctions in the school-age child. *Archives of General Psychiatry, 6,* 185–197.

Cohen, M., Becker, M. G., & Campbell, R. (1990). Relationships among four methods of assessment of children with attention-deficit hyperactivity disorder. *Journal of School Psychology, 28*, 189–202.

Cohen, P., Velez, N., Kohn, M., Schwab-Stone, M., & Johnson, J. (1987). Child psychiatric diagnosis by computer algorithm: Theoretical issues and empirical tests. *Journal of the American Academy of Child and Adolescent Psychiatry, 26*(5), 631–638.

Conners, C. K. (1994, August). *The Continuous Performance Test (CPT): Use as a diagnostic tool and measure of treatment outcome.* Paper presented at the annual meeting of the American Psychological Association, Los Angeles, CA.

Conners, C. K. (1997). *Conners' Rating Scales—Revised; technical manual.* North Tonawanda, NY: Multi-Health Systems.

Conners, C. K., March, J. S., Fiore, C., & Butcher, T. (1993, December). *Information processing deficits in ADHD: Effects of stimulus rate and methylphenidate.* Presented at the 32nd annual meeting of the American College of Neuropsychopharmacology, Honolulu, HI.

Conners, C. K., Sitarenios, G., Parker, J. D. A., & Epstein, J. N. (1998a). The Revised Conners' Parent Rating Scale (CPRS-R): Factor structure, reliability, and criterion validity. *Journal of Abnormal Child Psychology, 26*, 257–268.

Conners, C. K., Sitarenios, G., Parker, J. D. A., & Epstein, J. N. (1998b). Revision and restandardization of the Conners' Teacher Rating Scale: Factor structure, reliability, and criterion validity. *Journal of Abnormal Child Psychology, 26*, 257–268.

Cook, E. H., Stein, M. A., Krasowski, M. D., Cox, N. J., Olkon, D. M., Kieffer, J. E., & Leventhal, B. L. (1995). Association of attention deficit disorder and the dopamine transporter gene. *American Journal of Human Genetics, 56*, 993–998.

Costello, E. J. (1986). Assessment and diagnosis of affective disorders in children. *Journal of Child Psychology and Psychiatry and Allied Disciplines, 27*(5), 565–574.

Costello, E. J., & Edelbrock, C. S. (1985). Detection of psychiatric disorders in pediatric primary care: A preliminary report. *Journal of the American Academy of Child and Adolescent Psychiatry, 24*(6), 771–774.

Costello, E. J., Edelbrock, C. S., & Costello, A. J. (1985). Validity of the NIMH Diagnostic Interview Schedule for Children: A comparison between psychiatric and pediatric referrals. *Journal of Abnormal Child Psychology, 13*(4), 579–595.

Cunningham, C. E., & Barkley, R. A. (1979). The interactions of hyperactive and normal children with their mothers during free play and structured task. *Child Development, 50*, 217–224.

Cunningham, C. E., & Siegel, L. S. (1987). Peer interactions of normal and attention-deficit-disordered boys during free-play, cooperative task, and simulated classroom situations. *Journal of Abnormal Child Psychology, 15*, 247–268.

Cunningham, C., Morgan, P., & McGucken, R. (1984). Down's syndrome: Is dissatisfaction with disclosure of diagnosis inevitable? *Developmental Medicine and Child Neurology, 26*, 33–39.

Cunningham, C. E., Benness, B. B., & Siegel, L. S. (1988). Famiy functioning, time allocation, and prenatal depression in the families of normal and ADHD children. *Journal of Clinical Child Psychology, 17*, 169–177.

Cunningham, C. E., Bremner, R. B., & Boyle, M. (1995). Large group community-based parenting programs for families of preschoolers at risk for disruptive behaviour disorders: Utilization, cost effectiveness, and outcome. *Journal of Child Psychology and Psychiatry, 36*, 1141–1159.

Cunningham, C. E., Bremner, R. B., & Secord-Gilbert, M. (1997). *COPE (The Community Parent Education Program): A school-based family systems oriented workshop for parents of children with disruptive behavior disorders (leader's manual).* Hamilton, Ontario, Canada: COPE Works.

Cunningham, C. E., Cunningham, L. J., & Matorelli, V. (1998). *Coping with conflict at school: The student-mediated conflict resolution program.* Hamilton, Ontario, Canada: COPE Works.

Danforth, J. S., & DuPaul, G. J. (1996). Interrater reliability of teacher rating scales for children with attention-deficit hyperactivity disorder. *Journal of Psychopathology and Behavioral Assessment, 18*, 227–237.

David, R. (1989). *Pediatric neurology for the clinician.* New York: Raven Press.

DeChillo, N. (1993, February). Collaboration between social workers and families of patients with mental illness. *Families in Society: The Journal of Contemporary Human Services*, 104–115.

DeChillo, N., Koren, P. E., & Schultze, K. H. (1994). From paternalism to partnership: Family and professional collaboration in children's mental health. *American Journal of Orthopsychiatry, 64*, 564–576.

DeChillo, N., Koren, P. E., & Mezera, M. (1996). Families and professionals in partnership. In B. A. Stroul (Ed.), *Children's mental health: Creating systems of care in a changing society*. Baltimore: Paul H. Brookes.

Derogatis, L. R. (1983). *Symptom Checklist-90—Revised Manual*. Minnetonka, MN: NCS Assessments.

Derogatis, L. R., & Cleary, P. A. (1977a). Confirmation of the dimensional structure of the SCL-90: A study in construct validation. *Journal of Clinical Psychology, 33*, 981–989.

Derogatis, L. R., & Cleary, P. A. (1977b). Factorial invariance across gender for the primary symptom dimensions of the SCL-90. *British Journal of Social and Clinical Psychology, 16*, 347–356.

Deutsch, K. (1987). *Genetic factors in attention-deficit disorders*. Paper presented at symposium on Disorders of Brain and Development and Cognition. Boston.

Dodge, K. A., McClaskey, C. L., & Feldman, E. (1985). A situational approach to the assessment of social competence in children. *Journal of Consulting and Clinical Psychology, 53*, 344–353.

Douglas, V. I. (1972). Stop, look, and listen: The problem of sustained attention and impulse control in hyperactive and normal children. *Canadian Journal of Behavioral Science, 4*, 259–282.

Douglas, V. I. (1983). Attention and cognitive problems. In M. Rutter (Ed.), *Developmental neuropsychiatry* (pp. 280–329). New York: Guilford Press.

Douglas, V. I., & Benezra, E. (1990). Supraspan verbal memory in attention deficit disorder with hyperactivity-, normal, and reading-disabled boys. *Journal of Abnormal Child Psychology, 18*, 617–638.

Duchnowski, A. J., & Kutash, K. (1993, October). *Developing comprehensive systems for troubled youth: Issues in mental health*. Paper presented at Symposium II: Developing Comprehensive Systems for Troubled Youth, Shakertown, KY.

Dunst, C. J., Trivette, C., & Deal, A. (1988). *Enabling and empowering families: Principles and guidelines for practice*. Cambridge, MA: Brookline Books.

Dunst, C. J., Trivette, C. M., Davis, M., & Cornwell, J. (1988). Enabling and empowering families of children with health impairments. *Children's Health Care, 17*(2), 71–81.

Dunst, C. J., Johanson, C., Trivette, C., & Hamby, D. (1991). Family-oriented early intervention policies and practices: Family-centered or not? *Exceptional Children, 3*, 115–126.

Dunst, C. J., Trivette, C., & Deal, A. (1994). *Supporting and strengthening families: Vol. 1. Methods, Strategies, and Practices*. Cambridge, MA: Brookline Books.

DuPaul, G. J. (1991). Parent and teacher ratings of ADHD symptoms: Psychometric properties in a community-based sample. *Journal of Clinical Child Psychology, 20*, 245–253.

DuPaul, G. J., & Barkley, R. A. (1992). Situational variability of attention problems: Psychometric properties of the Revised Home and School Situations Questionnaires. *Journal of Clinical Child Psychology, 21*, 178–188.

DuPaul, G. J., & Henningson, P. N. (1993). Peer tutoring effects on the classroom performance of children with attention-deficit hyperactivity disorder. *School Psychology Review, 22*, 134–143.

DuPaul, G. J., & Stoner, G. (1994). *ADHD in the schools: Assessment and intervention strategies*. New York: Guilford Press.

DuPaul, G. J., Rapport, M. D., & Perriello, L. M. (1991). Teacher ratings of academic skills: The development of the Academic Performance Rating Scale. *School Psychology Review, 20*, 284–300.

DuPaul, G. J., Anastopoulos, A. D., Shelton, T. L., Guevremont, D. C., & Metevia, L. (1992). Multimethod assessment of attention deficit hyperactivity disorder: The diagnostic utility of clinic-based tests. *Journal of Clinical Child Psychology, 21*, 394–402.

DuPaul, G. J., Kwasnik, D., Anastopoulos, A. D., & McMurray, M. B. (1993). *The effects of methylphenidate on self-report ratings of attention deficit hyperactivity disorder symptoms*. Unpublished manuscript, Lehigh University, Bethlehem, PA.

DuPaul, G. J., Barkley, R. A., & McMurray, M. B. (1994). Response of children with ADHD to methylphenidate: Interaction with internalizing symptoms. *Journal of the American Academy of Child and Adolescent Psychiatry, 33*, 894–903.

DuPaul, G. J., Power, T. J., Anastopoulos, A. D., Reid, R., McGoey, K. E. & Ikeda, M. J. (1997). Teacher ratings of attention-deficit/hyperactivity disorder symptoms: Factor structure and normative data. *Psychological Assessment, 9,* 436–444.

DuPaul, G. J., Anastopoulos, A. D., Power, T. J., Reid, R., Ikeda, M. J., & McGoey, K. E. (1998). Parent ratings of attention-deficit/hyperactivity disorder symptoms: Factor structure and normative data. *Journal of Psychopathology and Behavioral Assessment, 20,* 83–102.

DuPaul, G. J., Ervin, R. A., Hook, C. L., & McGoey, K. E. (1998). Peer tutoring for children with attention deficit hyperactivity disorder: Effects on classroom behavior and academic performance. *Journal of Applied Behavior Analysis, 31,* 579–592.

DuPaul, G. J., Power, T. J., Anastopoulos, A. D., & Reid, R. (1998). *Manual for the AD/HD Rating Scale-IV.* New York: Guilford Press.

DuPaul, G. J., Power, T. J., McGoey, K. E., Ikeda, M. J., & Anastopoulos, A. D. (1998). Reliability and validity of parent and teacher ratings of Attention-Deficit/Hyperactivity Disorder symptoms. *Journal of Psychoeducational Assessment, 16,* 55–68.

Ebaugh, F. G. (1923). Neuropsychiatric sequelae of acute epidemic encephalitis in children. *American Journal of Diseases of Children, 25,* 89–97.

Edelbrock, C. S. (1991). The Child Attention Problem Rating Scale. In R. A. Barkley, *Attention deficit hyperactivity disorder: A clinical workbook* (pp. 49–51). New York: Guilford Press.

Edelbrock, C., Costello, A. J., Duncan, M. K., Kalas, R., & Conover, N. C. (1985). Age differences in the reliability of the psychiatric interview of the child. *Child Development, 56*(1), 265–275.

Edelbrock, C. S., Rende, R., Plomin, R., & Thompson, L. (1995). A twin study of competence and problem behavior in childhood and early adolescence. *Journal of Child Psychology and Psychiatry, 36,* 775–786.

Eiraldi, R. B., Power, T. J., & Nezu, C. M. (1997). Patterns of comorbidity associated with subtypes of attention-deficit/hyperactivity disorder among 6- to 12-year-old children. *Journal of the American Academy of Child and Adolescent Psychiatry, 36,* 503–514.

Eisenstadt, T. H., Eyberg, S., McNeil, C. B., Newcomb, K., & Funderburk, B. (1993). Parent–child interaction therapy with behavior-problem children: Relative effectiveness of two stages and overall treatment. *Journal of Clinical Child Psychology, 22,* 42–51.

Elliott, S. N., & Treuting, M. V. (1991). The Behavior Intervention Rating Scale: Development and validation of a pretreatment acceptability and effectiveness measure. *Journal of School Psychology, 29,* 43–51.

Endicott, J., & Spitzer, R. L. (1978). A diagnostic interview: The Schedule for Affective Disorders and Schizophrenia. *Archives of General Psychiatry, 35*(7), 837–844.

Epstein, M. H., Cullinan, D., & Polloway, E. A. (1986). Patterns of maladjustment among mentally retarded children and youth. *American Journal of Mental Deficiency, 91,* 127–134.

Ernst, M., Cohen, R. M., Liebenauer, L. L., Jons, P. H., & Zametkin, A. J. (1997). Cerebral glucose metabolism in adolescent girls with attention-deficit/hyperactivity disorder. *Journal of the American Academy of Child and Adolescent Psychiatry, 36,* 1399–1406.

Ernst, M., Liebenauer, L. L., King, A. C., Fitzgerald, G. A., Cohen, R. M., & Zametkin, A. J. (1994). Reduced brain metabolism in hyperactive girls. *Journal of the American Academy of Child and Adolescent Psychiatry, 33,* 858–868.

Eyberg, S. (1993). Therapy Attitude Inventory (TAI). In L. VandeCreek (Ed.). *Innovations in clinical practice: A source book* (Vol. 12, pp. 337–362). Sarasota, FL: Professional Resource Press/ Professional Resource Exchange, Inc.

Eyberg, S. M., & Ross, A. W. (1978). Assessment of child behavior problems: The validation of a new inventory. *Journal of Clinical Child Psychology, 7*(2), 113–116.

Eyberg, S. M., & Robinson, E. A. (1982). Parent–child interaction training: Effects on family functioning. *Journal of Clinical Child Psychology, 11*(2), 130–137.

Eyberg, S. M., & Robinson, E. A. (1983). Conduct problem behavior: Standardization of a behavioral rating scale with adolescents. *Journal of Clinical Child Psychology, 12*(3), 347–354.

Fairbanks, L. D., & Stinnett, T. A. (1997). Effects of professional group membership, intervention type, and diagnostic label on treatment acceptability. *Psychology in the Schools, 34,* 329–335.

Faraone, S. V., Biederman, J., Chen, W. J., Krifcher, B., Keenan, K., Moore, C., Sprich, S., & Tsuang, M. T. (1992). Segregation analysis of attention-deficit hyperactivity disorder. *Psychiatric Genetics, 2,* 257–275.

Feighner, J. P., Robins, E., Guze, S. B., Woodruff, R. A., Jr., Winokur, G., & Munoz, R. (1972). Diagnostic criteria for use in psychiatric research. *Archives of General Psychiatry, 26*(1), 57–63.

Feingold, B. (1975). *Why your child is hyperactive*. New York: Random House.

Filipek, P. A., Semrud-Clikeman, M., Steingrad, R. J., Renshaw, P. F., Kennedy, D. N., & Biederman, J. (1997). Volumetric MRI analysis comparing subjects having attention-deficit hyperactivity disorder with normal controls. *Neurology, 48*, 589–601.

Fischer, M., Newby, R. F., & Gordon, M. (1995). Who are the false negatives on Continuous Performance Tests? *Journal of Clinical Child Psychology, 24*, 427–433.

Fisher, P., Lucas, C., Shaffer, D., Schwab-Stone, M., Dulcan, M., Graae, F., Lichtman, J., Willoughby, S., & Gerald, J. (1997). *Diagnostic Interview Schedule for Children, Version IV (DISC-IV): Test–retest reliability in a clinical sample*. Poster presentation at the 44th annual meeting of the American Academy of Child and Adolescent Psychiatry. Toronto, Canada.

Forehand, R. L., & McMahon, R. J. (1981). *Helping the noncompliant child: A clinician's guide to parent training*. New York: Guilford Press.

Frankenburg, W. K., Dodds, J. B., Archer, P., Bresnick, B., Maschka, P., Edelman, N., & Shapiro, H. (1990). *Denver II Screening manual*. Denver, CO: Denver Developmental Materials.

Frick, P. J., Lahey, B. B., Kamphaus, R. W., Lahey, B. B., Loeber, R., Christ, M. A., Hart, E. L., & Tannenbaum, L. E. (1991). Academic underachievement and the disruptive behavior disorders. *Journal of Consulting and Clinical Psychology, 59*, 289–294.

Friedman, D., Vaughan, H. G., & Erlenmeyer-Kimling, K. L. (1978). Stimulus and response related components of the late positive complex in visual discrimination tasks. *Electroencephalography and Clinical Neurophysiology, 45*(3), 319–330.

Friesen, B. J. (1993). Overview: Advances in child mental health. In H. C. Johnson (Ed.), *Child mental health in the 1990s* (pp. 12–19). (DHHS Publication No. SMA 93–2003). Rockville, MD: U.S. Department of Health and Human Services, Public Health Services, Substance Abuse and Mental Health Services Administration, Center for Mental Health Services.

Gadow, K. D. (1985). Relative efficacy of pharmacological, behavioral, and combination treatments for enhancing academic performance. *Clinical Psychology Review, 5*, 513–533.

Gadow, K., & Sprafkin, J. (1995). *Child Symptom Inventories*. Stony Brook, NY: Checkmate Plus.

Gaub, M., & Carlson, C. (1997a). Behavioral characteristics of *DSM-IV* AD/HD subtypes in a school-based population. *Journal of Abnormal Child Psychology, 25*, 103–111.

Gaub, M., & Carlson, C. (1997b). Gender differences in ADHD: a meta-analysis and critical review. *Journal of the American Academy of Child and Adolescent Psychiatry, 36*, 1036–1045.

Gilger, J. W., Pennington, B. F., & DeFries, J. C. (1992). A twin study of the etiology of comorbidity: Attention-deficit hyperactivity disorder and dyslexia. *Journal of the American Academy of Child and Adolescent Psychiatry, 31*, 343–348.

Gillis, J. J., Gilger, J. W., Pennington, B. F., & DeFries, J. C. (1992). Attention deficit disorder in reading-disabled twins: Evidence for a genetic etiology. *Journal of Abnormal Child Psychology, 20*, 303–315.

Gittelman, R., & Eskinazi, B. (1983). Lead and hyperactivity revisited. *Archives of General Psychiatry, 40*, 827–833.

Gittelman, R., Mannuzza, S., Shenker, R., & Bonagura, N. (1985). Hyperactive boys almost grown up: I. Psychiatric status. *Archives of General Psychiatry, 42*, 937–947.

Goldman, H. H., Skodol, A. E., & Lave, T. R. (1992). Revising Axis V for DSM-IV: A review of measures of social functioning. *American Journal of Psychiatry, 149*(9), 1148–1156.

Goodman, J. R., & Stevenson, J. (1989). A twin study of hyperactivity: II. The aetiological role of genes, family relationships, and perinatal adversity. *Journal of Child Psychology and Psychiatry, 30*, 691–709.

Gordon, M. (1979). The assessment of impulsivity and mediating behaviors in hyperactive and nonhyperactive children. *Journal of Abnormal Child Psychology, 7*, 317–326.

Gordon, M. (1983). *The Gordon Diagnostic System*. DeWitt, NY: Gordon Systems.

Gordon, M. (1995). *How to operate on ADHD clinic or subspecialty practice*. Syracuse, NY: GSI Publications.

Gordon, M., & Mettelman, B. B. (1988). The assessment of attention: I. Standardization and reliability of a behavior-based measure. *Journal of Clinical Psychology, 44*, 682–690.

Gordon, M., Mettelman, B. B., & DiNiro, D. (1989). Are continuous performance tests valid in the diagnosis of ADHD-hyperactivity? Paper presented at the 97th annual convention of the American Psychological Association, New Orleans, LA.

Gotlib, I. H. (1984). Depression and general psychopathology in university students. *Journal of Abnormal Psychology, 93,* 19–30.

Goyette, C. H., Conners, C. K., & Ulrich, R. F. (1978). Normative data for Revised Conners Parent and Teacher Rating Scales. *Journal of Abnormal Child Psychology, 6,* 221–236.

Green, S. M., Loeber, R., & Lahey, B. B. (1991). Stability of mothers' recall of the age of onset of their child's attention and hyperactivity problems. *Journal of the American Academy of Child and Adolescent Psychiatry, 30,* 131– 137.

Greenberg, L. M. (1987). An objective measure of methylphenidate response: Clinical use of the MCA. *Psychopharmacological Bulletin, 23,* 279–282.

Greenberg, L. M., & Crosby, R. D. (1992). Specificity and sensitivity of the Test of Variables of Attention (T.O.V.A.). Unpublished manuscript.

Greenberg, L. M., & Waldman, I. D. (1993). Developmental normative data on the Test of Variables of Attention (T.O.V.A.). *Journal of Child Psychology and Psychiatry and Allied Disciplines, 34,* 1019–1030.

Greenhill, L. L., Abikoff, H. B., Arnold, L. E., Cantwell, D. P., Conners, C. K., Elliott, G., Hechtman, L., Hinshaw, S. P., Hoza, B., Jensen, P. S., March, J. S., Newcorn, J., Pelham, W. E., Severe, J. B., Swanson, J. M., Vitiello, B., & Wells, K. (1996). Medication treatment strategies in the MTA study: Relevance to clinicians and researchers. *Journal of the American Academy of Child and Adolescent Psychiatry, 35,* 1304–1313.

Greenhill, L. L., Halperin, J. M., & Abikoff, H. (1999). Stimulant medications. *Journal of the American Academy of Child and Adolescent Psychiatry, 38*(5), 503–512.

Grenell, M. M., Glass, C. R., & Katz, K. S. (1987). Hyperactive children and peer interaction: Knowledge and performance of social skills. *Journal of Abnormal Child Psychology, 15,* 1–13.

Gresham, F. M. (1989). Assessment of treatment integrity in school consultation and referral intervention. *School Psychology Review, 18*(1), 37–50.

Gresham, F. M., & Elliott, S. N. (1990). *Social Skills Rating System: Manual.* Circle Pines, MN: American Guidance Service.

Grodzinsky, G. M., & Barkley, R. A. (February, 1996). *The predictive power of executive function tests for the diagnosis of attention-deficit hyperactivity disorder.* Paper presented at the annual meeting of the International Neuropsychological Society, Chicago.

Halperin, J. M., Newcorn, J. H., Koda, V. H., Pick. L., McKay, K. E., & Knott, P. (1997a). Noradrenergic mechanisms in ADHD children with and without reading disabilities: A replication and extension. *Journal of the American Academy of Child and Adolescent Psychiatry, 36,* 1688–1697.

Halperin, J. M., Newcorn, J. H., Kopstein, I., McKay, K. E., Schwartz, S. T., Siever, L. J., & Sharma, V. (1997b). Serotonin, aggression, and parental psychopathology in children with attention-deficit hyperactivity disorder. *Journal of the American Academy of Child and Adolescent Psychiatry, 36,* 1391–1398.

Hart, E. L., Lahey, B. B., Loeber, R., Applegate, B., & Frick, P. J. (1995). Developmental changes in attention-deficit hyperactivity disorder in boys: A four-year longitudinal study. *Journal of Abnormal Child Psychology, 23,* 729–750.

Hartsough, C. S., & Lambert, N. M. (1985). Medical factors in hyperactive and normal children: Prenatal, developmental, and health history findings. *American Journal of Orthopsychiatry, 55,* 190–201.

Healey, J. M., Newcorn, J. H., Halperin, J. M., Wolf, L. E., Pascualvaca, D. M., Schmeiderler, J., & O'Brien, J. D. (1993). The factor structure of ADHD items in *DSM-III-R*: Internal consistency and external validation. *Journal of Abnormal Child Psychology, 21,* 441–453.

Heaton, R. K., Chelune, G. J., Talley, J. L., Kay, G. G., & Curtiss-Glenn, R. (1993). *Wisconsin Card Sorting Test Revised and Expanded.* Odessa, FL: Psychological Assessment Resources.

Heflinger, C. A. (1995). Studying family empowerment and parental involvement in their child's mental health treatment. *Focal Point, 9*(1), 6–8.

Heilman, K. M., & Valenstein, E. (1979). *Clinical neuropsychology.* New York: Oxford University Press.

Helzer, J. E., Robins, L. N., Croughan, J. L., & Welner, A. (1981). Renard Diagnostic Interview: Its reliability and procedural validity with physicians and lay interviewers. *Archives of General Psychiatry, 38*(4), 393–398.

Hernandez, M., Isaacs, M. R., Nesman, T., & Burns, D. (1998). Perspectives on culturally competent systems of care. In M. Hernandez & M. R. Isaacs (Eds.), *Promoting cultural competence in children's mental health services* (pp. 1–25). Baltimore: Brookes.

Hewitt, P. L., & Norton, G. R. (1993). The Beck Anxiety Inventory: A psychometric analysis. *Psychological Assessment, 5*, 408–412.

Hinshaw, S. P. (1987). On the distinction between attentional deficits/hyperactivity and conduct problems/aggression in child psychopathology. *Psychological Bulletin, 111*, 127–155.

Hinshaw, S. P., Henker, B., & Whalen, C. K. (1984). Self-control in hyperactive boys in anger-inducing situations: Effects of cognitive-behavioral training and of methylphenidate. *Journal of Abnormal Child Psychology, 12*, 55–77.

Hodges, K., Kline, L., Stern, L., Cytryn, L., & McKnew, D. (1982). The development of a child assessment interview for research and clinical use. *Journal of Abnormal Child Psychology, 10*, 173–189.

Hodges, S., Nesman, T., & Hernandez, M. (1999). Promising practices: Building collaboration in systems of care. *Systems of Care: Promising Practices in Children's Mental Health, 1998 Series, Volume VI* (pp. xi–18).

Hohman, L. B. (1922). Postencephalitic behavior disorders in children. *Johns Hopkins Hospital Bulletin, 33*, 372–375.

Hooks, K., Milich, R., & Lorch, E. P. (1994). Sustained and selective attention in boys with attention-deficit hyperactivity disorder. *Journal of Clinical Child Psychology, 23*, 69–77.

Horn, W. F., Ialongo, N., Pacoe, J. M., Greenberg, G., Packard, T., Lopez, M., Wagner, A., & Puttler, L. (1991). Additive effects of psychostimulants, parent training, and self-control therapy with ADHD children: A 9-month follow-up. *Journal of the American Academy of Child and Adolescent Psychiatry, 32*, 182–189.

Hoza, B. (1994). Review of the Behavior Assessment System for Children. *Child Assessment News, 4*, 5, 8–10.

Humphries, T., Kinsbourne, M., & Swanson, J. (1978). Stimulant effects on cooperation and social interaction between hyperactive children and their mothers. *Journal of Child Psychology and Psychiatry, 19*, 13–22.

Hynd, G. W., Semrud-Clikeman, M., Lorys, A. R., Novey, E. S., Eliopulos, D., & Lytinen, H. (1991). Corpus callosum morphology in attention-deficit-hyperactivity disorder: Morphometric analysis of MRI. *Journal of Learning Disabilities, 24*, 141–146.

Hynd, G. W., Hern, K. L., Novey, E. S., Eliopulos, D., Marshall, R., Gonzalez, J. J., & Voeller, K. K. (1993). Attention-deficit hyperactivity disorder and asymmetry of the caudate nucleus. *Journal of Child Neurology, 8*, 339–347.

Irvine, A. B., Biglan, A., Smolkowski, K., & Ary, D. V. (1999). The value of the Parenting Scale for measuring the discipline practices of parents of middle school children. *Behaviour Research and Therapy, 37*, 127–142.

Jacobson, N. S., & Truax, P. (1991). Clinical significance: A statistical approach to defining meaningful change in psychotherapy research. *Journal of Consulting and Clinical Psychology, 59*, 12–19.

Jacobvitz, D., & Sroufe, L. A. (1987). The early caregiver–child relationship and attention-deficit disorder with hyperactivity in kindergarten: A prospective study. *Child Development, 58*, 1488–1495.

Jensen, P. S., Martin, D., & Cantwell, D. P. (1997). Comorbidity of ADHD: Implications for research, practice, and *DSM-V*. *Journal of the American Academy of Child and Adolescent Psychiatry, 36*, 1065–1079.

Johnston, C. (1996). Parent characteristics and parent–child interactions in families of nonproblem children and ADHD children with higher and lower levels of oppositional–defiant behavior. *Journal of Abnormal Child Psychology, 24*, 85–104.

Johnston, C., & Mash, E. J. (1989) A measure of parenting satisfaction and efficacy. *Journal of Clinical Child Psychology, 18*, 167–175.

Jones, M. L., Eyberg, S. M., Adams, C. D., & Boggs, S. R. (1998). Treatment acceptability of behavioral interventions for children: An assessment by mothers of children with disruptive behavior disorders. *Child and Family Behavior Therapy, 20*, 15–26.

Kagan, J. (1966). Reflection-impulsivity: The generality and dynamics of conceptual tempo. *Journal of Abnormal Psychology, 71*, 17–24.

Kahn, E., & Cohen, L. H. (1934). Organic driveness: A brain stem syndrome and an experience. *New England Journal of Medicine, 210*, 748–756.

Kaufman, J., Birmaher, B., Brent, D., Rao, U., Flynn, C., Moreci, P., Williamson, D., & Ryan, N. (1997). Schedule for Affective Disorders and Schizophrenia for School-Age Children—Present and Lifetime Version (K-SADS-PL): Initial reliability and validity data. *Journal of the American Academy of Child and Adolescent Psychiatry, 36*, 980–988.

Kazdin, A. E. (1986). Treatment Evaluation Inventory. *Journal of School Psychology, 24*, 23–35.

Keith, R. W. (1994). *Auditory Continuous Performance Test.* San Antonio, TX: The Psychological Corporation.

Kelley, M. L. (1990). *School–home notes: Promoting children's classroom success.* New York: Guilford Press.

Kendall, P. C., & Braswell, L. (1985). *Cognitive-behavioral therapy for impulsive children.* New York: Guilford Press.

Kendall, P. C., & Wilcox, L. E. (1979). Self-control in children: Development of a rating scale. *Journal of Consulting and Clinical Psychology, 47*, 1020–1029.

Kent, J. D., Blader, J. C., Koplewicz, H. S., Abikoff, H., & Foley, C. A. (1995). Effects of late-afternoon methylphenidate administration on behavior and sleep in attention-deficit hyperactivity disorder. *Pediatrics, 96*(2), 320–325.

Kinsbourne, M. (1977). The mechanism of hyperactivity. In M. Blau, I. Rapin, & M. Kinsbourne (Eds.), *Topics in child neurology.* New York: Spectrum.

Klein, R. (1993). *Schedule for Affective Disorders and Schizophrenia for School-Aged Children: Lifetime Version.* Unpublished manuscript, New York State Psychiatric Institute.

Klein, R. G., & Mannuzza, S. (1991). Long-term outcome of hyperactive children: A review. *Journal of American Academy of Child and Adolescent Psychiatry, 30*, 383–387.

Knitzer, J. (1993). Children's mental health policy: Challenging the future. *Journal of Emotional and Behavioral Disorders, 1*(1), 8–16.

Koren, P. E., Paulson, R. I., Kinney, R. F., Yatchmenoff, D. K., Gordon, L. J., & DeChillo, N. (1997). Service coordination in children's mental health: An empirical study from the caregiver's perspective. *Journal of Emotional and Behavioral Disorders, 5*(3), 162–172.

Kovacs, M. (1982). *The longitudinal study of child and adolescent psychopathology: I. The semi-structure psychiatric Interview Schedule for Children (ISC).* Unpublished manuscript, Western Psychiatric Institute.

Lachar, D. (1982). *Personality Inventory for Children (PIC): Reviewed format manual supplement.* Los Angeles: Western Psychological Services.

Lahey, B. B., Applegate, B., McBurnett, K., Biederman, J., Greenhill, L., Hynd, G. W., Barkley, R. A., Newcorn, J., Jensen, P., Richters, J. Garfinkel, B., Kerdyk, L., Frick, P. J., Ollendick, T., Perez, D., Hart, E. L., Waldman, I., & Shaffer, D. (1994). *DSM-IV* field trials for attention-deficit/ hyperactivity disorder in children and adolescents. *American Journal of Psychiatry, 151*, 1673–1685.

Lahey, B. B., Carlson, C. L., & Frick, P. J. (1997). Attention deficit disorder without hyperactivity: A review of research relevant to *DSM-IV.* In T. A. Wideger, A. J. Frances, H. A. Pincus, R. Ross, M. B. First, W. Davis, & M. Kline (Eds.), *DSM-IV Sourcebook* (Vol. 3, pp. 189–209). Washington, DC: American Psychiatric Association.

Lahey, B. B., Pelham, W. E., Schaughency, E. A., Atkins, M. S., Murphy, H. A., Hynd, G. W., Russo, M., Hartdagen, S., & Lorys-Vernon, A. (1988). Dimensions and types of attention deficit disorder with hyperactivity in children: A factor and cluster-analytic approach. *Journal of the American Academy of Child and Adolescent Psychiatry, 27*, 330–335.

Lahey, B. B., Schaughency, E., Strauss, C., & Frame, C. (1984). Are attention deficit disorders with and without hyperactivity similar or dissimilar disorders? *Journal of the American Academy of Child Psychiatry, 23*, 302–309.

Lahoste, G. J., Swanson, J. M., Wigal, S. B., Glabe, C., Wigal, T., King, N., & Kennedy, J. L. (1996).

Dopamine D4 receptor gene polymorphism is associated with attention-deficit hyperactivity disorder. *Molecular Psychiatry, 1*, 121–124.

Laufer, M., & Denhoff, E. (1957). Hyperkinetic behavior syndrome in children. *Journal of Pediatrics, 50*, 463–474.

Laufer, M., Denhoff, E., & Solomons, G. (1957). Hyperkinetic impulse disorder in children's behavior problems. *Psychosomatic Medicine, 19*, 38–49.

Lee, C. L., & Bates, J. E. (1985). Mother–child interaction at age two years and perceived difficult temperament. *Child Development, 56*, 1314–1325.

Levin, P. M. (1938). Restlessness in children. *Archives of Neurology and Psychiatry, 39*, 764–770.

Levine, M. (1985). *Manual for the Pediatric Examination of Educational Readiness.* Cambridge, MA: Educators Publishing Service.

Levy, F., Hay, D. A., McStephen, M., Wood, C., & Waldman, I. (1997). Attention-deficit hyperactivity disorder: A category or a continuum? Genetic analysis of a large-scale twin study. *Journal of the American Academy of Child and Adolescent Psychiatry, 36*, 737–744.

Lindsley, O. R. (1991). From technical jargon to plain English for application. *Journal of Applied Behavior Analysis, 24*, 449–458.

Lochman, J. E., & Lampron, L. B. (1986). Situational social problem-solving skills and self-esteem of aggressive and nonaggressive boys. *Journal of Abnormal Child Psychology, 14*, 605–617.

Locke, H. J., & Wallace, K. M. (1959). Short marital-adjustment and prediction tests: Their reliability and validity. *Marriage and Family Living, 21*, 251–255.

Loeber, R., & Keenan, K. (1994). Interaction between conduct disorder and its comorbid conditions: Effects of age and gender. *Clinical Psychology Review, 14*, 497–523.

Loeber, R., Keenan, K., Lahey, B. B., Green, S. M., & Thomas, C. (1993). Evidence for developmentally based diagnoses in oppositional defiant disorder and conduct disorder. *Journal of Abnormal Child Psychology, 21*, 377–410.

Lou, H. C., Henriksen, L., & Bruhn, P. (1984). Focal cerebral hypoperfusion in children with dysphasia and/or attention deficit disorder. *Archives of Neurology, 41*, 825–829.

Lovejoy, M. C., Verda, M. R., & Hays, C. E. (1997). Convergent and discriminant validity of measures of parenting efficacy and control. *Journal of Clinical Child Psychology, 26*, 366–376.

Lufi, D., & Parish-Plass, J. (1995). Personality assessment of children with attention-deficit hyperactivity disorder. *Journal of Clinical Psychology, 51*, 94–99.

Luk, S. (1985). Direct observation studies of hyperactive behaviors. *Journal of the American Academy of Child Psychiatry, 24*, 338–344.

Mannuzza, S., Gittelman-Klein, R., Bessler, A., Malloy, P., & LaPadula, M. (1993). Adult outcome of hyperactive boys: Educational achievement, occupational rank, and psychiatric status. *Archives of General Psychiatry, 50*, 565–576.

Mannuzza, S., Klein, R. G., Bessler, A., Malloy, P., & Hynes, M. E. (1997). Educational and occupational outcome of hyperactive boys grown up. *Journal of the American Academy of Child and Adolescent Psychiatry, 36*, 1222–1226.

Mariani, M., & Barkley, R. A. (1997). Neuropsychological and academic functioning in preschool children with attention-deficit hyperactivity disorder. *Developmental Neuropsychology, 13*, 111–129.

Mash, E. J., & Johnston, C. (1982). A comparison of mother–child interactions of younger and older hyperactive and normal children. *Child Development, 53*, 1371–1381.

Mash, E. J., & Johnston, C. (1983). Parental perceptions of child behavior problems, parenting self-esteem, and mothers' reported stress in younger and older hyperactive and normal children. *Journal of Consulting and Clinical Psychology, 51*, 86–99.

Mash, E. J., & Johnston, C. (1990). Determinants of parenting stress: Illustrations from families of hyperactive children and families of physically abused children. *Journal of Clinical Child Psychology, 19*, 313–328.

Matier-Sharma, K., Perachio, N., Newcorn, J. H., Sharma, V., & Halperin, J. M. (1995). Differential diagnosis of ADHD: Are objective measures of attention, impulsivity, and activity level helpful? *Child Neuropsychology, 1*, 118–127.

Matson, J. L., Rotatori, A. F., & Helsel, W. J. (1983). Development of a rating scale to measure social skills in children: The Matson Evaluation of Social Skills with Youngsters (MESSY). *Behavior Research and Therapy, 21*, 335–340.

McBurnett, K., Pfiffner, L. J., Tamm, L., & Capasso, L. (1996). *Clinical correlates of children experimentally classified by DSM-IV Attention-Deficit/Hyperactivity Disorder subtypes: Cross-validation of field trials impairment patterns.* Presented at the 1996 meeting of the Society for Research in Child and Adolescent Psychopathology, Santa Monica, CA.

McCarney, S. B. (1995). *The Attention Deficit Disorders Evaluation Scale* (2nd ed.). Columbia, MO: Hawthorne Educational Services, Inc.

McCarney, S. B., Anderson, P. D., & Jackson, M. T. (1996). *Adult Attention Deficit Disorders Evaluation Scale.* Columbia, MO: Hawthorne Educational Services, Inc.

McConaughy, S. H., & Achenbach, T. M. (1994). *Manual for the Semistructured Clinical Interview for Children and Adolescents.* Burlington, VT: University of Vermont, Department of Psychiatry.

McGee, R., Williams, S., Moffitt, T., & Anderson, J. (1989). A comparison of 13 year-old boys with attention deficit and or reading disorder on neuropsychological measures. *Journal of Abnormal Child Psychology, 17,* 37–53.

McGee, R., Williams, S., & Feehan, M. (1992). Attention deficit disorder and age of onset of problem behaviors. *Journal of Abnormal Child Psychology, 20,* 487–502.

McIntosh, D. E., & Cole-Love, A. S. (1996). Profile comparisons between ADHD and non-ADHD children on the Temperament Assessment Battery for Children. *Journal of Psychoeducational Assessment, 14,* 362–372.

Measelle, J. R., Weinstein, R. S., & Martinez, M. (1998). Parent satisfaction with case-managed systems of care for children and youth with severe emotional disturbance. *Journal of Child and Family Studies, 7,* 451–467.

Meichenbaum, D., & Goodman, J. (1971). Training impulsive children to talk to themselves: A means of developing self-control. *Journal of Abnormal Psychology, 77,* 115-126.

Milberger, S., Beiderman, J., Faraone, S. V., Chen, L., & Jones, J. (1996). Is maternal smoking during pregnancy a risk factor of attention-deficit hyperactivity disorder in children? *American Journal of Psychiatry, 153,* 1138–1142.

Milberger, S., Beiderman, J., Faraone, S. V., Chen, L., & Jones, J. (1997). Further evidence of an association between attention-deficit/hyperactivity disorder and cigarette smoking: Findings from a high-risk sample of siblings. *American Journal on Addictions, 6,* 205–217.

Milich, R., & Kramer, J. (1984). Reflections on impulsivity: An empirical investigation of impulsivity as a construct. In K. D. Gadow & I. Bailer (Eds.), *Advances in learning and behavior disabilities* (Vol. 1, pp. 283–398). Greenwich, CT: JAI Press.

Milich, R., Loney, J., & Landau, S. (1982). The independent dimensions of hyperactivity and aggression: A validation with playroom observation data. *Journal of Abnormal Psychology, 91,* 183–198.

Milich, R., & Okazaki, M. (1991). An examination of learned helplessness among attention-deficit hyperactivity disordered boys. *Journal of Abnormal Child Psychology, 19,* 607–623.

Miller, D. L., & Kelley, M. L. (1992). Treatment acceptability: The effects of parent gender, marital adjustment, and child behavior. *Child and Family Behavior Therapy, 14,* 11–23.

Moos, R. H., & Moos, B. S. (1983). Clinical applications of the Family Environment Scale. In E. E. Filsinger (Ed.), *Marriage and family assessment: A source book for family therapy* (pp. 253–273). Beverly Hills, CA: Sage.

Morrison, J., & Stewart, M. (1973). The psychiatric status of the legal families of adopted hyperactive children. *Archives of General Psychiatry, 28,* 888–891.

Munir, K., Biederman, J., & Knee, D. (1987). Psychiatric comorbidity in patients with attention deficit disorder: A controlled study. *Journal of the American Academy of Child and Adolescent Psychiatry, 26,* 844–848.

Murphy, K., & Barkley, R. A. (1996a). Prevalence of *DSM-IV* symptoms of ADHD in adult licensed drivers: Implication for clinical diagnosis. *Journal of Attention Disorders, 1,* 147–161.

Murphy, K., & Barkley, R. A. (1996b). Attention deficit hyperactivity disorder in adults. *Comprehensive Psychiatry, 37,* 393–401.

Nada-Raja, S., Langley, J. D., McGee, R., Williams, S. M., Begg, D. J., & Reeder, A. I. (1997). Inattentive and hyperactive behaviors and driving offenses in adolescence. *Journal of the American Academy of Child and Adolescent Psychiatry, 36,* 515–522.

Naglieri, J. A., LeBuffe, P. A., & Pfeiffer, S. I. (1994). *The Devereux Scales of Mental Disorders.* San Antonio, TX: The Psychological Corporation.

Nemzer, E. D., Arnold, L. E., Votolato, N. A., & McConnell, H. (1986). Amino acid supplementation as therapy for attention deficit disorder. *Journal of the American Academy of Child Psychiatry, 25*(4), 509–513.

O'Leary, K. D., Vivian, D., & Nisi, A. (1985). Hyperactivity in Italy. *Journal of Abnormal Child Psychology, 13*, 485–500.

Olson, D. H., & Portner, J. (1983). Family Adaptability and Cohesion Evaluation Scales. In E. E. Filsinger (Ed.), *Marriage and family assessment: A source book for family therapy* (pp. 299–315). Beverly Hills, CA: Sage.

Orvaschel, H. (1994). Psychiatric interviews suitable for use in research with children and adolescents. In J. E. Mezzich, J. R. Miguel, & I. M. Salloum (Eds.), *Psychiatric epidemiology: Assessment and concepts and methods* (pp. 509–522). Baltimore, MD: John Hopkins University Press.

Osher, T., deFur, E., Nava, C., Spencer, S., & Toth-Dennis, D. (1999). New roles for families in systems of care. *Systems of Care: Promising Practices in Children's Mental Health, 1998 Series, Volume I.* Washington, DC: Center for Effective Collaboration and Practice, American Institutes for Research.

Ostrander, R., Weinfurt, K. P., Yarnold, P. R., & August, G. J. (1998). Diagnosing Attention Deficit Disorders with the Behavioral Assessment System for Children and the Child Behavior Checklist: Test and construct validity analyses using optimal discriminant classification trees. *Journal of Consulting and Clinical Psychology, 66*, 660–672.

Owens, N., & Owens, B. W. (1993). *Attention Deficit Disorder Behavior Rating Scales.* Garland, TX: Ned Owens, Inc.

Ownby, R. L., & Matthews, C. G. (1985). On the meaning of the WISC-R third factor: Relations to selected neuropsychological measures. *Journal of Consulting and Clinical Psychology, 53*, 531–534.

Paternite, C., Loney, J., & Roberts, M. (1995). External validation of oppositional disorders and attention deficit disorder with hyperactivity. *Journal of Abnormal Child Psychology, 23*, 453–471.

Pekarik E., Prinz, R., Liebert, D., Weintraub, S., & Neil, J. (1976). The Pupil Evaluation Inventory: A sociometric technique for assessing children's social behavior. *Journal of Abnormal Child Psychology, 4*, 83–97.

Pelham, W. E., & Bender, M. E. (1982). Relationships in hyperactive children: Description and treatment. *Advances in Learning and Behavioral Disabilities, 1*, 365–436.

Pelham, W. E., & Lang, A. R. (1993). Parental alcohol consumption and deviant child behavior: Laboratory studies of reciprocal effects. *Clinical Psychology Review, 13*, 763–784.

Pelham, W. E., & Milich, R. (1991). Individual differences in response to Ritalin in classwork and social behavior. In L. L. Greenhill & B. B. Osman (Eds.), *Ritalin: Theory and patient management* (pp. 203–221). New York: Mary Ann Liebert.

Pelham, W. E., Schnedler, R. W., Bender, M. E., Miller J., Nilsson, D., Budrow, M., Ronnei, M., Paluchowski, C., & Marks, D. (1988). The combination of behavior therapy and methylphenidate in the treatment of hyperactivity: A therapy outcome study. In L. Bloomingdale (Ed.), *Attention deficit disorders* (Vol. 3, pp. 29–48). London: Pergamon.

Pelham, W. E., Walker, J. L., Sturges, J., & Hoza, J. (1989). Comparative effects of methylphenidate on ADD girls and ADD boys. *Journal of the American Academy of Child and Adolescent Psychiatry, 28*, 773–776.

Pelham, W. E., McBurnett, K., Harper, G. W., Milich, R., Murphy, D. A., Clinton, J., & Tyiel, C. (1990). Methylphenidate and baseball playing in ADHD children: Who's on first? *Journal of Consulting and Clinical Psychology, 58*, 130–133.

Pelham, W. E., Evans, S. W., Gnagy, E. M., & Greensalde, K. E. (1992). Teacher ratings of *DSM-III-R* symptoms for the disruptive behavior disorders: Prevalence, factor analyses, and conditional probabilities in a special education sample. *School Psychology Review, 21*, 285–299.

Pelham, W. E., Gnagy, E. M., Greenslade, K. E., & Milich, R. (1992). Teacher ratings of *DSM-III-R* symptoms for the disruptive behavior disorders. *Journal of the American Academy of Child and Adolescent Psychiatry, 31*, 210–218.

Pelham, W. E., Wheeler, T., & Chronis, A. (1998). Empirically supported psychosocial treatments for attention-deficit hyperactivity disorder. *Journal of Clinical Child Psychology, 27*, 190–205.

Pfiffner, L. J. (1996). *All about ADHD: The complete practical guide for classroom teachers*. New York: Scholastic.

Pfiffner, L. J., & O'Leary, S. G. (1987). The efficacy of all-positive management as a function of the prior use of negative consequences. *Journal of Applied Behavior Analysis, 20*, 265–271.

Pfiffner, L. J., Rosen, L. A., & O'Leary, S. G. (1985). The efficacy of an all-positive approach to classroom management. *Journal of Applied Behavior Analysis, 18*, 257-261.

Pisterman, S., Firestone, P., McGrath, P., Goodman, J., Webster, I., Mallory, R., & Goffin, B. (1992). The effects of parent training on parenting stress and sense of competence. *Canadian Journal of Behavioural Science, 24*, 41–58.

Pisterman, S., Firestone, P., McGrath, P., Goodman, J., Webster, I., & Mallory, R. (1992). The role of parent training in the treatment of preschoolers with attention deficit disorder with hyperactivity. *American Journal of Orthopsychiatry, 62*, 397–408.

Pisterman, S., McGrath, P., Firestone, P., & Goodman, J.T. (1989). Outcome of parent-mediated treatment of preschoolers with attention deficit disorder with hyperactivity. *Journal of Consulting and Clinical Psychology, 57*, 636–643.

Pliszka, S. R. (1987). Tricyclic antidepressants in the treatment of children with attention deficit disorder. *Journal of the American Academy of Child and Adolescent Psychiatry, 26*, 127-132.

Pliszka, S. R., McCracken, J. T., & Maas, J. W. (1996). Catecholamines in attention-deficit hyperactivity disorder: Current perspectives. *Journal of the American Academy of Child and Adolescent Psychiatry, 35*, 264–272.

Porrino, L. J., Rapoport, J. L., Behar, D., Sceery, W., Ismond, D. R., & Bunney, W. E. (1983). A naturalistic assessment of motor activity of hyperactive boys. *Archives of General Psychiatry, 40*, 681–687.

Porter, J. E., & Rourke, B. P. (1985). Socioemotional functioning of learning-disabled children: A subtypal analysis of personality patterns. In B. P. Rourke (Ed.), *Neuropsychology of learning disabilities: Essentials of subtype analysis* (pp. 257–280). New York: Guilford Press.

Powes, T. J., Hess, L. E., & Bennett, D. S. (1995). The acceptability of interventions for attention-deficit hyperactivity disorder among elementary and middle school teachers. *Journal of Developmental and Behavioral Pediatrics, 16*, 238–243.

Puig-Antich, J., & Chambers, W. (1978). *The Schedule for Affective Disorders and Schizophrenia for School-Age Children*. New York: New York State Psychiatric Institute.

Quay, H. C. (1997). Inhibition and attention-deficit hyperactivity disorder. *Journal of Abnormal Child Psychology, 25*, 7–13.

Quay, H. C., & Peterson, D. R. (1975). *Manual for the Behavior Problem Checklist*. Unpublished manuscript, University of Miami.

Quay, H. C., & Peterson, D. R. (1983). *Interim Manual for the Behavior Problem Checklist*. Unpublished manuscript, University of Miami.

Rapoport, J., & Mikkelsen, E. (1978). Antidepressants. In J. Werry (Ed.), *Pediatric psychopharmacology* (pp. 208–233). New York: Brunner/Mazel.

Rapport, M. D. (1987). Attention-deficit disorder with hyperactivity. In M. Hersen & V. B. Van Hasselt (Eds.), *Behavior therapy with children and adolescents* (pp. 325–361). New York: Wiley.

Rapport, M. D., & Kelly, K. L. (1991). Psychostimulant effects on learning and cognitive function: Findings and implications for children with Attention-Deficit Hyperactivity Disorder. *Clinical Psychology Review, 11*, 61–92.

Rapport, M. D., Tucker, S. B., DuPaul, G. J., Merlo, M., & Stoner, G. (1986). Hyperactivity and frustration: The influence of size and control over rewards in delaying gratification. *Journal of Abnormal Child Psychology, 14*, 191–204.

Rapport, M. D., Jones, J. T., DuPaul, G. J., Kelly, K. L., Gardner, M. J., Tucker, S. B., & Shea, M. S. (1987). Attention Deficit Disorder and methylphenidate: Group and single-subject analyses of dose effects on attention in clinic and classroom settings. *Journal of Clinical Child Psychology, 16*, 329–338.

Rapport, M. D., DuPaul, G. J., & Kelly, K. L. (1989). Attention-Deficit Hyperactivity Disorder and methylphenidate: The relationship between gross body weight and drug response in children. *Psychopharmacology Bulletin, 25*, 285–290.

Rapport, M. D., Denney, C., DuPaul, G. J., & Gardner, M. J. (1994). Attention deficit disorder and methylphenidate: Normalization rates, clinical effectiveness, and response prediction in 76 children. *Journal of the American Academy of Child and Adolescent Psychiatry, 33,* 882–893

Raskin, L. A., Shaywitz, S. E., Shaywitz, B. A., Anderson, G. M., & Cohen, D. J. (1984). Neurochemical correlates of attention deficit disorder. *Pediatric Clinics of North America, 31,* 387–396.

Reich, W., Welner, Z., Herjanic, B., & MHS staff. (1996). *Diagnostic Interview for Children and Adolescents-IV Computer Program (DICA-IV).* New York: MultiHealth Systems.

Reeves, J. C., & Werry, J. S. (1987). Soft signs in hyperactivity. In D. E. Tupper (Ed.), *Soft neurological signs.* New York: Grune & Stratton.

Reich, W., Cottler, L., McCallum, K., Corwin, D., & VanEerdewegh, M. (1995). Computerized interviews as a method of assessing psychopathology in children. *Comprehensive Psychiatry, 36,* 40–45.

Reimers, T. M., Wacker, D. P., Cooper, L. J., & DeRaad, A. O. (1992). Clinical evaluation of the variables associated with treatment acceptability and their relation to compliance. *Behavioral Disorders, 18,* 67–76.

Reinecke, M. A., Beebe, D. W., & Stein, M. A. (1999). The third factor of the WISC-III: It's (probably) not freedom from distractibility. *Journal of the American Academy of Child and Adolescent Psychiatry, 38,* 322–327.

Reynolds, C. R., & Kamphaus, R. W. (1992). *BASC: Behavior Assessment System for Children Manual.* Circle Pines, MN: American Guidance Service.

Riccio, C. A., Hynd, G. W., Cohen, M. J., Hall, J., & Molt, L. (1994). Comorbidity of central auditory processing disorder and attention-deficit hyperactivity disorder. *Journal of the American Academy of Child and Adolescent Psychiatry, 33,* 849–857.

Roberts, M. A. (1990). A behavioral observation method for differentiating hyperactive and aggressive boys. *Journal of Abnormal Psychology, 9,* 183–198.

Roberts, M. A., Ray, R. S., & Roberts, R. J. (1984). A playroom observational procedure for assessing hyperactive boys. *Journal of Pediatric Psychology, 9,* 177–191.

Robin, A. L., & Foster, S. L. (1989). *Negotiating parent–adolescent conflict: A behavioral–family systems approach.* New York: Guilford Press.

Rosenblatt, A. (1996). Bows and ribbons, tape, and twine: Wrapping the wraparound process for children with multi-system needs. *Journal of Child and Family Studies, 5,* 101–116.

Rosvold, H. E., Mirsky, A. F., Sarason, I., Bransome, E. D., Jr., & Beck, L. H. (1956). A continuous performance test of brain damage. *Journal of Consulting Psychology, 20,* 343–350.

Routh, D. K. (1978). Hyperactivity. In P. Magrab (Ed.), *Psychological management of pediatric problems* (pp. 3–48). Baltimore: University Park Press.

Routh, D. K., & Schroeder, C. S. (1976). Standardized playroom measures as indices of hyperactivity. *Journal of Abnormal Child Psychology, 4,* 199–207.

Russo, M. F., & Beidel, D. C. (1994). Comorbidity of childhood anxiety and externalizing disorders: Prevalence, associated characteristics, and validation issues. *Clinical Psychology Review, 14,* 199–221.

Rutter, M. (1983). Introduction: Concepts of brain dysfunction syndromes. In M. Rutter (Ed.), *Developmental neuropsychiatry* (pp. 1–14). New York: Guilford Press.

Sandford, J. A., & Turner, A. (1994). *Intermediate Visual and Auditory Continuous Performance Test.* Richmond, VA: Braintrain.

Satterfield, J. H., Satterfield, B. T., & Cantwell, D. P. (1980). Three-year multimodality treatment study of 100 hyperactive boys. *Journal of Pediatrics, 98,* 650-655.

Satterfield, J. H., & Schell, A. (1997). A prospective study of hyperactive boys with conduct problems and normal boys: Adolescent and adult criminality. *Journal of the American Academy of Child and Adolescent Psychiatry, 36,* 1726–1735.

Schachar, R., & Tannock, R. (1995). Test of four hypotheses for the comorbidity of attention-deficit hyperactivity disorder and conduct disorder. *Journal of the American Academy of Child and Adolescent Psychiatry, 34,* 639–648.

Schachar, R. J., Tannock, R., & Logan, G. (1993). Deficient inhibitory control in attention-deficit hyperactivity disorder. *Journal of Abnormal Child Psychology, 23,* 411–438.

Schwab-Stone, M., Fallon, T., Briggs, M., & Crowther, B. (1994). Reliability of diagnostic reporting for children aged 6–11 years: A test–retest study of the Diagnostic Interview for Children—Revised. *American Journal of Psychiatry, 151,* 1048–1054.

Schwab-Stone, M., Shaffer, D., Dulcan, M., Jensen, P. S., Fisher, P., Bird, H. R., Goodman, S. H., Lahey, B. B., Lichtman, J. H., Canino, G., Rubio-Stipec, M., & Rae, D. S. (1996). Criterion validity of the NIMH Diagnostic Interview Schedule for Children, Version 2.3 (DISC 2.3). *Journal of the American Academy of Child and Adolescent Psychiatry, 35*, 878–888.

Schleifer, M., Weiss, G., Cohen, N. J., Elman, M., Cvejic, H., & Kruger, E. (1975). Hyperactivity in preschoolers and the effect of methylphenidate. *American Journal of Orthopsychiatry, 45*, 38–50.

Sergeant, J. A. (1995). Hyperkinetic disorder revisited. In J. A. Sergeant (Ed.), *Eunnethydis: European approaches to hyperkinetic disorder* (pp. 7–17). Amsterdam: J. A. Sergeant.

Sergeant, J. A., & Scholten, C. A. (1985). On resource strategy limitations in hyperactivity: Cognitive impulsivity reconsidered. *Journal of Abnormal Child Psychology and Psychiatry, 26*, 97–109.

Shaffer, D. (1994). Attention-deficit hyperactivity disorder in adults. *American Journal of Psychiatry, 151*, 633–638.

Shaffer, D., Fisher, P., Dulcan, M. K., Davies, M., Piacentini, J., Schwab-Stone, M. E., Lahey, B. B., Bourdon, K., Jensen, P. S., Bird, H. R., Canino, G., & Regier, D. A. (1996). The NIMH Diagnostic Interview Schedule for Children, Version 2.3 (DISC-2.3): Description, acceptability, prevalence rates, and performance in the MECA study. *Journal of the American Academy of Child and Adolescent Psychiatry, 35*, 865–877.

Shapiro, E. S., & Cole, C. L. (1994). *Behavior change in the classroom: Self-management interventions.* New York: Guilford Press.

Shapiro, E. S., DuPaul, G. J., Bradley, K. L., & Bailey, L. T. (1996). A school-based consultation program for service delivery to middle school students with attention-deficit hyperactivity disorder. *Journal of Emotional and Behavioral Disorders, 4*, 73–81.

Shapiro, J. P., Welker, C. J., & Jacobson, B. J. (1997). The Youth Client Satisfaction Questionnaire: Development, construct validation, and factor structure. *Journal of Clinical Child Psychology, 26*, 87–98.

Shaywitz, B. A., Shaywitz, S. E., Byrne, T., Cohen, D. J., & Rothman, S. (1983). Attention deficit disorder: Quantitative analysis of CT. *Neurology, 33*, 1500–1503.

Shelton, T., Barkley, R., Crosswait, C., Moorehouse, M., Fletcher, K., Barrett, S., Jenkins, L., & Metevia, L. (1998). Psychiatric and psychological morbidity as a function of adaptive disability in preschool children with aggressive and hyperactive-impulsive–inattentive behavior. *Journal of Abnormal Child Psychology, 26*, 475–494.

Shelton, T. L., & Stepanek, J. S. (1994). *Family-centered care for children needing specialized health and developmental services.* Bethesda, MD: Association for the Care of Children's Health.

Sheras, P. L., & Abidin, R. R. (1998). *Stress Index for Parents of Adolescents.* Odessa, FL: Psychological Assessment Resources.

Sherman, D. K., McGue, M. K., & Iacono, W. G. (1997). Twin concordance for attention-deficit hyperactivity disorder: A comparison of teachers' and mothers' reports. *American Journal of Psychiatry, 154*, 532–535.

Shure, M. B., & Spivack, G. (1972). Means–ends thinking, adjustment, and social class among elementary-school-age children. *Journal of Consulting and Clinical Psychology, 38*, 348–350.

Sieg, K. G., Gaffney, G. R., Preston, D. F., & Hellings, J. A. (1995). SPECT brain imaging abnormalities in attention-deficit hyperactivity disorder. *Clinical Nuclear Medicine, 20*, 55–60.

Silberg, J., Rutter, M., Meyer, J., Maes, H., Hewitt, J., Simonoff, E., Pickles, A., Loeber, R., & Eaves, L. (1996). Genetic and environmental influences on the covariation between hyperactivity and conduct disturbance in juvenile twins. *Journal of Child Psychology and Psychiatry, 37*, 803–816.

Simpson, J. S., Koroloff, N., Friesen, B. F., & Gac, J. (1999). Promising practices in family-provider collaboration. *Systems of Care: Promising Practices in Children's Mental Health, 1998 Series, Volume II.* Washington, DC: Center for Effective Collaboration and Practice, American Institutes for Research.

Smith, B., Pelham, W., Evans, S., Gnagy, E., Molina, B., Bukstein, O., Greiner, A., Myak, C., Presness, M., & Willoughby, M. (1998). Dosage effects of methylphenidate on the social behavior of adolescent diagnosed with attention-deficit hyperactivity disorder. *Experimental and Clinical Psychopharmacology, 6*, 187–204.

Smith, B., Pelham, W., Gnagy, E., & Yudell, R. (1998). Equivalent effects of stimulant treatment for attention-deficit hyperactivity disorder during childhood and adolescence. *Journal of the American Academy of Child and Adolescent Psychiatry, 37*, 314–321.

Snyder, D. K. (1981). *Marital Satisfaction Inventory.* Los Angeles, CA: Western Psychological Services.

Solanto, M. V., & Conners, C. K. (1982). A dose–response and time-action analysis of autonomic and behavior effects of methylphenidate in attention deficit disorder with hyperactive children. *Psychophysiology, 19*, 658–667.

Sostek, A. J., Buchsbaum, M. S., & Rapoport, J. L. (1980). Effects of amphetamine on vigilance performance in normal and hyperactive children. *Journal of Abnormal Child Psychology, 8*, 491–500.

Spanier, G. B. (1979). The measure of marital quality. *Journal of Sex and Marital Therapy, 5*, 288–300.

Spanier, G. B. (1989). *Dyadic Adjustment Scale.* Tonawanda, New York: Multi-Health Systems.

Sprafkin, J., Grayson, P., Gadow, K. D., Nolan, E. E., & Paolicelli, L. M. (1986). Code for Observing Social Activity (COSA). Stoney Brook, NY: State University of New York, Department of Psychiatry and Behavioral Science.

Stallard, P. (1996). Validity and reliability of the Parent Satisfaction Questionnaire. *British Journal of Clinical Psychology, 35*, 311–318.

Still, G. F. (1902). Some abnormal physical conditions in children. *Lancet, i*, 1008–1012, 1077–1082, 1163–1168.

Strauss, A. A., & Kephart, N. C. (1955). *Psychopathology and education of the brain-injured child: Vol. 2. Progress in theory and clinic.* New York: Grune & Stratton.

Strauss, A. A., & Lehtinen, L. E. (1947). *Psychopathology and education of the brain-injured child.* New York: Grune & Stratton.

Strayhorn, J. M., & Weidman, C. (1988). A parent-practices scale and its relation to parent and child mental health. *Journal of the American Academy of Child and Adolescent Psychiatry, 27*, 613–618.

Streissguth, A. P., Booksetin, F. L., Sampson, P. D., & Barr, H. M. (1995). Attention: Prenatal alcohol and continuities of vigilance and attentional problems from 4 through 14 years. *Development and Psychopathology, 7*, 419–446.

Sutter, J., & Eyberg, S. M. (1984). *Sutter-Eyberg Student Behavior Inventory.* Unpublished manuscript, University of Florida at Gainesville.

Swanson, J. M. (1992). *School-based assessments and intervention for ADD students.* Irvine, CA: KC Publishing.

Swanson, J., Wigal, S., Greenhill, L., Browne, R., Waslick, B., Lerner, M., Williams, L., Flynn, D., Agler, D., Crowley, K., Fineberg, E., Baren, M., & Cantwell, D. (1998a). Analog classroom assessment of Adderall® in children with ADHD. *Journal of the American Academy of Child and Adolescent Psychiatry, 37*, 519–526.

Swanson, J., Wigal, S., Greenhill, L., Browne, R., Waslick, B., Lerner, M., Williams, L., Flynn, D., Agler, D., Crowley, K., Fineberg, E., Regino, R., Baren, M., & Cantwell, D. (1998b). Objective and subjective measures of the pharmacodynamic effects of Adderall in the treatment of children with ADHD in a controlled laboratory classroom setting. *Psychopharmacology Bulletin, 34*, 55–60.

Szatmari, P. (1992). The epidemiology of attention-deficit hyperactivity disorders. In G. Weiss (Ed.), *Child and adolescent psychiatric clinics of North America: Attention-deficit hyperactivity disorder* (pp. 361–372). Philadelphia: Saunders.

Tannock, R., & Schachar, R. (1996). Executive dysfunction as an underlying mechanism of behavior and language problems in attention-deficit hyperactivity disorder. In J. H. Beitchman, N. J. Cohen, M. M. Konstantareas, & R. Tannock (Eds.), *Language, learning and behavior disorders: Developmental, biological, and clinical perspectives* (pp. 128–155). New York: Cambridge University Press.

Tarnowski, K. J., & Simonian, S. J. (1992). Assessing treatment acceptance: The Abbreviated Acceptability Rating Profile. *Journal of Behavior Therapy and Experimental Psychiatry, 23*, 101–106.

Tarnowski, K. J., Simonian, S. J., Park, A., & Bekeny, P. (1992). Acceptability of treatments for child behavioral disturbance: Race, socioeconomic status, and multicomponent treatment effects. *Child and Family Behavior Therapy, 14*, 25–37.

Taylor, E. A. (1986). Childhood hyperactivity. *British Journal of Psychiatry, 149*, 562–573.

Taylor, E., Chadwick, O., Heptinstall, E., & Danckaerts, M. (1996). Hyperactivity and conduct problems as risk factors for adolescent development. *Journal of the American Academy of Child and Adolescent Psychiatry, 35*, 1213–1226.

Thomasgard, M., & Shonkoff, J. P. (1998). In J. M. Sattler (Ed.), *Clinical and forensic interviewing of children and families.* San Diego: Sattler.

Tyron, W. W. (1984). Measuring activity using actometers: A methodlogical study. *Journal of Behavioral Assessment, 6*(2), 147–153.

Ullmann, R. K. (1985). ACTeRS useful in screening learning disabled from attention-deficit disordered (ADD-H) children. *Psychopharmacology Bulletin, 21*, 339–344.

Ullmann, R. K., & Sleator, E. K. (1985). Attention-deficit disorder children with or without hyperactivity: Which behaviors are helped by stimulants. *Clinical Pediatrics, 24*, 547–551.

Ullmann, R. K., Sleator, E. K., & Sprague, R. L. (1985). Introduction to the use of the ACTeRS. *Psychopharmacology Bulletin, 21*, 915–920.

van den Oord, E. J. C. G., & Rowe, D. C. (1997). Continuity and change in children's social maladjustment: A developmental behavior genetic study. *Developmental Psychology, 33*, 319–332.

Vignoe, D., & Achenbach, T. M. (1999). *Bibliography of published studies using the Child Behavior Checklist and related materials: 1999 edition.* Burlington, VT: University of Vermont Department of Psychiatry.

Voelker, S., Lachar, D., & Gdowski, C. L. (1983). The Personality Inventory for Children and response to methylphenidate: Preliminary evidence for predictive utility. *Journal of Pediatric Psychology, 8*(2), 161–169.

Waldman, I., & Lilienfeld, S. (1991). Diagnostic efficiency of symptoms for oppositional defiant disorder and attention-deficit hyperactivity disorder. *Journal of Consulting and Clinical Psychology, 59*, 732–738.

Waldman, I., Lilienfeld, S., & Lahey, B. (1995). Toward construct validity in the childhood disruptible behavior disorders: Classification and diagnosis in *DSM-IV* and beyond. *Advances in Clinical Child Psychology, 17*, 323–363.

Walker, H. M., & McConnell, S. R. (1988). *Walker–McConnell Scale of Social Competence and School Adjustment.* Austin, TX: Pro-Ed.

Walsh-Allis, G. A., & Orvaschel, H. (1986). Multidimensional assessment of social adaptation children and adolescents. *Advances in Behavioral Assessment of Children and Families, 2*, 207–226.

Wang, Y. C., Chong, M. Y., Chou, W. J., & Yang, J. L. (1993). Prevalence of attention deficit hyperactivity disorder in primary school children in Taiwan. *Journal of Formosa Medical Association, 92*, 133–138.

Waschbusch, D. A., Willoughby, M. T., & Pelham, W. E. (1998). Criterion validity and the utility of reactive and proactive aggression: Comparisons to attention-deficit hyperactivity disorder, oppositional defiant disorder, conduct disorder, and other measures of functioning. *Journal of Clinical Child Psychology, 27*, 396–405.

Webster-Stratton, C. (1984). Randomized trial of two parent training programs for families with conduct-disordered children. *Journal of Consulting and Clinical Psychology, 52*, 666–678.

Webster-Stratton, C. (1998). Preventing conduct problems in Head Start children: Strengthening parenting competencies. *Journal of Consulting and Clinical Psychology, 66*(5), 715–730.

Wechsler, D. (1974). *The Wechsler Intelligence Scale for Children—Revised.* New York: Psychological Corporation.

Wechsler, D. (1991). *Manual for the Wechsler Intelligence Scale for Children—Third Edition.* San Antonio, TX: Psychological Corporation.

Weiss, G., & Hechtman, L. (1986). *Hyperactive children grown up.* New York: Guilford Press.

Weiss, G., & Hechtman, L. (1993). *Hyperactive children grown up* (2nd ed.). New York: Guilford Press.

Welner, Z., Reich, W., Herjanic, B., & Jung, K. G. (1987). Reliability, validity, and parent–child agreement studies of the Diagnostic Interview for Children and Adolescents (DICA). *Journal of the American Academy of Child and Adolescent Psychiatry, 26*(5), 649–653.

Wender, P. H. (1973). Minimal brain dysfunction in children. *Pediatric Clinics of North America, 20*, 187–202.

Wender, P. H. (1983). Some speculations concerning a possible biochemical basis of minimal brain dysfunction. *Annals of the New York Academy of Sciences, 205,* 18–28.

Werry, J. S., & Sprague, R. L. (1970). Hyperactivity. In C. G. Costello (Ed.), *Symptoms of psychopathology* (pp. 397–417). New York: Wiley.

Whalen, C. K., Henker, B., & Dotemoto, S. (1980). Methylphenidate and hyperactivity: Effects of teacher behaviors. *Science, 208,* 1280–1282.

Wielkiewicz, R. M. (1990). Interpreting low scores on the WISC-R third factor: It's more than distractibility. *Psychological Assessment: A Journal of Consulting and Clinical Psychology, 2,* 91–97.

Willis, T. J., & Lovaas, I. (1977). A behavioral approach to treating hyperactive children: The parent's role. In J. B. Millichap (Ed.), *Learning disabilities and related disorders* (pp. 119–140). Chicago: Yearbook Medical Publications.

Wirt, R. D., Lachar, D., Klinedinst, J. K., & Seat, P. D. (1977). *Multidimensional description of child personality: A manual for the Personality Inventory for Children.* Los Angeles: Western Psychological Services.

Witt, J. C., & Elliott, S. N. (1986). Children's Intervention Rating Profile. *Journal of School Psychology, 24,* 23–35.

Wodrich, D. L., & Kush, J. C. (1998). The effect of methylphenidate on teachers' behavioral ratings in specific school situation. *Psychology in the Schools, 35,* 81–88.

Wolf, S. M., & Forsythe, A. (1978). Behavior disturbance, phenobarbital, and febrile seizures. *Pediatrics, 61,* 728–731.

Wolraich, M. L., Hannah, J. N., Pinnock, T. Y., Baumgaertel, A., & Brown, J. (1996). Comparison of diagnostic criteria for attention-deficit hyperactivity disorder in a county-wide sample. *Journal of the American Academy of Child and Adolescent Psychiatry, 35,* 319–324.

Wolraich, M. L., Wilson, D. B., & White, J. W. (1995). The effect of sugar on behavior or cognition in children: A meta-analysis. *Journal of the American Medical Association, 274,* 1617–1621.

Woodcock, R. W., McGrew, K. S., & Mather, N. (2000). *Woodcock Johnson III Complete Battery (WJ III).* Itasca, IL: Riverside Publishing.

Zahn, T. P., Kruesi, M. J. P., & Rapoport, J. L. (1991). Reaction time indices of attention deficits in boys with disruptive behavior disorders. *Journal of Abnormal Child Psychology and Psychiatry, 26,* 233–252.

Zahn-Waxler, C., Schmitz, S., Fulker, D., & Robinson, J. (1996). Behavior problems in 5-year-old monozygotic and dizygotic twins: Genetic and environmental influences, patterns of regulation, and internalization of control. *Development and Psychopathology, 8,* 103–122.

Zametkin, A. J., Liebenauer, L. L., Fitzgerald, G. A., King, A. C., Minkunas, D. V., Herscovitch, P., Yamada, E. M., & Cohen, R. M. (1993). Brain metabolism in teenagers with attention-deficit hyperactivity disorder. *Archives of General Psychiatry, 50,* 333–340.

Zametkin, A. J., Nordahl, T. E., Gross, M., King, A. C., Semple, W. E., Rumsey, J., Hamburger, S., & Cohen, R. M. (1990). Cerebral glucose metabolism in adults with hyperactivity of childhood onset. *New England Journal of Medicine, 323,* 1361–1366.

Zametkin, A. J., & Rapoport, J. L. (1987). Neurobiology of attention deficit disorder with hyperactivity: Where have we come in 50 years? *Journal of the American Academy of Child and Adolescent Psychiatry, 26,* 676–686.

Zeiner, P. (1995). Body growth and cardiovascular function after extended (1.75 years) treatment with methylphenidate in boys with attention-deficit hyperactivity disorder. *Journal of Child and Adolescent Psychopharmacology, 5,* 129–138.

Zentall, S. (1985). A context for hyperactivity. In K. D. Gadox & I. Bialer (Eds.), *Advances in learning and behavioral disabilities* (Vol. 4, pp. 273–343). Greenwich, CT: JAI Press.

Zentall, S. (1993). Research on the educational implications of attention-deficit hyperactivity disorder. *Exceptional Children, 60,* 143–153.

Appendices

A. ADHD Rating Scale—IV (School Version)

B. Academic Performance Rating Scale

C. Parenting Scale

D. Sample Items from the Parenting Stress Index—Short Form

E. Adult AD/HD Rating Scale—Self-Report Version

F. Samples Items from the Symptom Checklist-90—Revised

G. Sample Items from the Dyadic Adjustment Scale—Revised

H. Sample Items from the Parenting Alliance Inventory

I. Sample Items from the Behavior Assessment System for Children (6–11; Teacher Version)

J. Child and Family Information Form

K. Developmental and Health History Information

L. Semi-Structured Background Interview

M. Cover Letter for Parent Rating Scale Packet

N. Instructions for Completing Parent Rating Scale Packet

O. Cover Letter for Teacher Rating Scale Packet

P. Instructions for Completing Teacher Rating Scale Packet

Q. Information Resources

Appendix A

ADHD Rating Scale—IV
(School Version)

ADHD RATING SCALE—IV: SCHOOL VERSION

Child's name ————————————— Sex: M F   Age ————— Grade —————
Completed by: ——————————————————————————————

Circle the number that *best describes* this student's school behavior over the past 6 months (or since the beginning of the school year).

	Never or rarely	Sometimes	Often	Very often
1. Fails to give close attention to details or makes careless mistakes in schoolwork.	0	1	2	3
2. Fidgets with hands or feet or squirms in seat.	0	1	2	3
3. Has difficulty sustaining attention in tasks or play activities.	0	1	2	3
4. Leaves seat in classroom or in other situations in which remaining seated is expected.	0	1	2	3
5. Does not seem to listen when spoken to directly.	0	1	2	3
6. Runs about or climbs excessively in situations in which it is inappropriate.	0	1	2	3
7. Does not follow through on instructions and fails to finish work.	0	1	2	3
8. Has difficulty playing or engaging in leisure activities quietly.	0	1	2	3
9. Has difficulty organizing tasks and activities.	0	1	2	3
10. Is "on the go" or acts as if "driven by a motor."	0	1	2	3
11. Avoids tasks (e.g., schoolwork, homework) that require sustained mental effort.	0	1	2	3
12. Talks excessively.	0	1	2	3
13. Loses things necessary for tasks or activities.	0	1	2	3

14. Blurts out answers before questions have been completed.	0	1	2	3
15. Is easily distracted.	0	1	2	3
16. Has difficulty awaiting turn.	0	1	2	3
17. Is forgetful in daily activities.	0	1	2	3
18. Interrupts or intrudes on others.	0	1	2	3

Appendix B

Academic Performance
Rating Scale

ACADEMIC PERFORMANCE RATING SCALE

Student _____ Date _____

Age _____ Grade _____ Teacher _____

For each of the items below, please estimate the above student's performance over the *past week*. For each item, please circle *one* choice only.

Item	1	2	3	4	5
1. Estimate the percentage of written math work *completed* (regardless of accuracy) relative to classmates.	0–49%	50–69%	70–79%	80–89%	90–100%
2. Estimate the percentage of written language arts work *completed* (regardless of accuracy) relative to classmates.	0–49%	50–69%	70–79%	80–89%	90–100%
3. Estimate the *accuracy* of completed written math work (i.e., percent correct of work done).	0–64%	65–69%	70–79%	80–89%	90–100%
4. Estimate the *accuracy* of completed language arts work (i.e., percent correct of work done).	0–64%	65–69%	70–79%	80–89%	90–100%
5. How consistent has the quality of this child's academic work been over the past week?	Consistently poor	More poor than successful	Variable	More successful than poor	Consistently successful
6. How frequently does the student accurately follow teacher instructions and/or class discussion during *large-group* (i.e., whole class) instruction?	Never	Rarely	Sometimes	Often	Very often

	Never	Rarely	Sometimes	Often	Very often
	1	2	3	4	5
7. How frequently does the student accurately follow teacher instructions and/or class discussion during *small-group* (e.g., reading group) instruction?	Never	Rarely	Sometimes	Often	Very often
	1	2	3	4	5
8. How quickly does this child learn new material (i.e., pick up novel concepts)?	Very slowly	Slowly	Average	Quickly	Very quickly
	1	2	3	4	5
9. What is the quality or neatness of this child's handwriting?	Poor	Fair	Average	Above average	Excellent
	1	2	3	4	5
10. What is the quality of this child's reading skills?	Poor	Fair	Average	Above average	Excellent
	1	2	3	4	5
11. What is the quality of this child's speaking skills?	Poor	Fair	Average	Above average	Excellent
	1	2	3	4	5
12. How often does the child complete written work in a careless, hasty fashion?	Never	Rarely	Sometimes	Often	Very often
	1	2	3	4	5
13. How frequently does the child take more time to complete work than his/her classmates?	Never	Rarely	Sometimes	Often	Very often
	1	2	3	4	5
14. How often is the child able to pay attention without you prompting him/her?	Never	Rarely	Sometimes	Often	Very often
	1	2	3	4	5

	Never	Rarely	Sometimes	Often	Very often
15. How frequently does this child require your assistance to accurately complete his/her academic work?	Never 1	Rarely 2	Sometimes 3	Often 4	Very often 5
16. How often does the child begin written work prior to understanding the directions?	Never 1	Rarely 2	Sometimes 3	Often 4	Very often 5
17. How frequently does this child have difficulty recalling material from a previous day's lessons?	Never 1	Rarely 2	Sometimes 3	Often 4	Very often 5
18. How often does the child appear to be staring excessively or "spaced out"?	Never 1	Rarely 2	Sometimes 3	Often 4	Very often 5
19. How often does the child appear withdrawn or tend to lack an emotional response in a social situation?	Never 1	Rarely 2	Sometimes 3	Often 4	Very often 5

Note. Reprinted with permission of G. J. DuPaul.

Appendix C

Parenting Scale

PARENTING SCALE

Child's Name: _____ Today's Date: _____

Sex: Boy _____ Girl _____ Child's Birthdate: _____

At one time or another, all children misbehave or do things that could be harmful, that are "wrong", or that parents don't like. Examples include:

hitting someone	*whining*	*throwing food*
forgetting homework	*not picking up toys*	*lying*
having a tantrum	*refusing to go to bed*	*wanting a cookie before dinner*
running into the street	*arguing back*	*coming home late*

Parents have many different ways or styles of dealing with these types of problems. Below are items that describe some styles of parenting.

For each item, fill in the circle that best describes your style of parenting during the past two months with the child indicated above.

SAMPLE ITEM

At meal time ...
I let my child decide how much to eat.　　o—o—o—o—o—o—o　　I decide how much my child eats.

1. **When my child misbehaves ...**
I do something right away.　　o—o—o—o—o—o—o　　I do something about it later.

2. **Before I do something about a problem ...**
I give my child several reminders or warnings.　　o—o—o—o—o—o—o　　I use only one reminder or warning.

3. **When I'm upset or under stress ...**
I am picky and on my child's back.　　o—o—o—o—o—o—o　　I am no more picky than usual.

4. **When I tell my child not to do something ...**
I say very little.　　o—o—o—o—o—o—o　　I say alot.

5. **When my child pesters me ...**
I can ignore the pestering.　　o—o—o—o—o—o—o　　I can't ignore the pestering.

6. **When my child misbehaves ...**
I usually get into a long argument with my child.　　o—o—o—o—o—o—o　　I don't get into an argument.

7. **I threaten to do things that ...**
I am sure I can carry out.　　o—o—o—o—o—o—o　　I know I won't actually do.

8. **I am the kind of parent that ...**

sets limits on what my
child is allowed to do.   o—o—o—o—o—o—o   lets my child do whatever
                                                                                        he or she wants.

9. **When my child misbehaves ...**

I give my child a long
lecture.   o—o—o—o—o—o—o   I keep my talks short and
                                                                                        to the point.

10. **When my child misbehaves ...**

I raise my voice or yell.   o—o—o—o—o—o—o   I speak to my child calmly.

11. **If saying no doesn't work right away'...**

I take some other kind of
action.   o—o—o—o—o—o—o   I keep talking and try to
                                                                                        get through to my child.

12. **When I want my child to stop doing something ...**

I firmly tell my child to
stop.   o—o—o—o—o—o—o   I coax or beg my child to
                                                                                        stop.

13. **When my child is out of my sight ...**

I often don't know what
my child is doing.   o—o—o—o—o—o—o   I always have a good idea
                                                                                        of what my child is doing.

14. **After there's been a problem with my child ...**

I often hold a grudge.   o—o—o—o—o—o—o   things get back to normal
                                                                                        quickly.

15. **When we're not at home ...**

I handle my child the way
I do at home.   o—o—o—o—o—o—o   I let my child get away
                                                                                        with alot more.

16. **When my child does something I don't like ...**

I do something about it
every time it happens.   o—o—o—o—o—o—o   I often let it go.

17. **When there's a problem with my child ...**

things build up and I do
things that I don't mean to   o—o—o—o—o—o—o   things don't get out of
do.   hand.

18. **When my child misbehaves, I spank, slap, grab, or hit my child ...**

never or rarely.   o—o—o—o—o—o—o   most of the time.

19. **When my child doesn't do what I ask ...**

I often let it go or end up
doing it myself.   o—o—o—o—o—o—o   I take some other action.

20. **When I give a fair threat or warning ...**

I often don't carry it out.   o—o—o—o—o—o—o   I always do what I said.

21. **If saying no doesn't work ...**

I take some other kind of
action.   o—o—o—o—o—o—o   I offer my child something
                                                                                        nice so he/she will behave.

22. **When my child misbehaves ...**

I handle it without getting
upset.
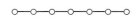
I get so frustrated or angry
that my child can see I'm
upset.

23. **When my child misbehaves ...**

I make my child tell me
why he/she did it.
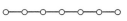
I say "No" or take some
other action.

24. **If my child child misbehaves and then acts sorry ...**

I handle the problem like I
usually would.
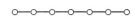
I let it go that time.

25. **When my child misbehaves ...**

I rarely use bad language
or curse.
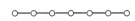
I almost always use bad
language.

26. **When I say my child can't do something ...**

I let my child do it
anyway.
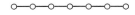
I stick to what I said.

27. **When I have to handle a problem ...**

I tell my child I'm sorry
about it.
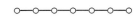
I don't say I'm sorry.

28. **When my child does something I don't like, I insult my child, say mean things, or
call my child names ...**

never or rarely.
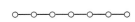
most of the time.

29. **If my child talks back or complains when I handle a problem ...**

I ignore the complaining
and stick to what I said.
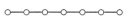
I give my child a talk
about not complaining.

30. **If my child gets upset when I say "No", ...**

I back down and give in to
my child.
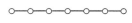
I stick to what I said.

Appendix D

Sample Items from the Parenting Stress Index—Short Form

PARENTING STRESS INDEX
(Short Form)

Richard R. Abidin
University of Virginia

Directions: In answering the following questions, please think about the child you are most concerned about. The questions on the following pages ask you to mark an answer which best describes your feelings. While you may not find an answer which exactly states your feelings, plase mark the answer which comes closest to describing how you feel.

YOUR FIRST REACTION TO EACH QUESTION SHOULD BE YOUR ANSWER

Please mark the degree to which you agree or disagree with the following statements by circling the number which best matches how you feel. If you are not sure, please circle #3.

1	2	3	4	5
Strongly Agree	Agree	Not Sure	Disagree	Strongly Disagree

Sample Items

1. I often have the feeling that I cannot handle things very well.	1	2	3	4	5
2. I find myself giving up more of my life to meet my children's needs than I ever expected.	1	2	3	4	5
3. I feel trapped by my responsibilities as a parent.	1	2	3	4	5
13. My child rarely does things for me that make me feel good.	1	2	3	4	5
14. Most times I feel that my child does not like me and does not want to be close to me.	1	2	3	4	5
27. I feel that my child is very moody and easily upset.	1	2	3	4	5
34. There are some things my child does that really bother me a lot.	1	2	3	4	5
36. My child makes more demands on me than most children.	1	2	3	4	5

Appendix E

Adult AD/HD Rating Scale—
Self-Report Version

ADULT AD/HD RATING SCALE—SELF-REPORT VERSION

<u>Directions</u>: Indicate the number that best describes your behavior during each of the following time periods.

0 = Never or rarely   1 = Sometimes   2 = Often   3 = Very Often

	Before Age 7	8–12 Years	13–18 Years	Past 6 Months
1. Fail to give close attention to details or make careless mistakes in my work.	_____	_____	_____	_____
2. Fidget with hands or feet or squirm in my seat.	_____	_____	_____	_____
3. Difficulty sustaining my attention in tasks or fun activities.	_____	_____	_____	_____
4. Leave my seat in classroom or in other situations in which remaining seated is expected.	_____	_____	_____	_____
5. Don't listen when spoken to directly.	_____	_____	_____	_____
6. Feel restless.	_____	_____	_____	_____
7. Don't follow through on instructions and fail to finish work.	_____	_____	_____	_____
8. Have difficulty engaging in leisure activities or doing fun things quietly.	_____	_____	_____	_____
9. Have difficulty organizing tasks and activities.	_____	_____	_____	_____
10. Feel "on the go" or "driven by a motor."	_____	_____	_____	_____
11. Avoid, dislike, or reluctant to engage in work or schoolwork that requires sustained mental effort.	_____	_____	_____	_____
12. Talk excessively.	_____	_____	_____	_____
13. Lose things necessary for tasks and activities.	_____	_____	_____	_____
14. Blurt out answers before questions have been completed.	_____	_____	_____	_____
15. Easily distracted.	_____	_____	_____	_____
16. Having difficulty awaiting turn.	_____	_____	_____	_____
17. Forgetful in daily activities.	_____	_____	_____	_____
18. Interrupt or intrude on others.	_____	_____	_____	_____

AD/HD criteria are adapted and reprinted with permission from the Diagnostic and Statistical Manual of Mental Disorders, Fourth Edition (pp. 83–85). Copyright 1994 American Psychiatric Association.

Appendix F

Sample Items from the Symptom Checklist-90—Revised

SCL-90-R

Leonard R. Derogatis, Ph.D.

INSTRUCTIONS: Below is a list of problems people sometimes have. Please read each one carefully, and circle the number to the right that best describes HOW MUCH THAT PROBLEM HAS DISTRESSED OR BOTHERED YOU DURING THE PAST 7 DAYS INCLUDING TODAY. Circle only one number for each problem and do not skip any items. If you change your mind, erase your first mark carefully. If you have any questions please ask about them.

Sample Items

HOW MUCH WERE YOU DISTRESSED BY:	Not at all	A Little Bit	Moderately	Quite a Bit	Extremely
30 Feeling blue	0	1	2	3	4
33. Feeling fearful	0	1	2	3	4
44. Trouble falling asleep	0	1	2	3	4

Appendix G

Sample Items from the Dyadic Adjustment Scale—Revised

REVISED DYADIC ADJUSTMENT SCALE

Most persons have disagreements in their relationships. Please indicate below the approximate extent of agreement or disagreement between you and your partner for each item on the following list:

	Always Agree	Almost Always Agree	Occasionally Agree	Frequently Disagree	Almost Always Disagree	Always Disagree
2. Demonstrations of affection	————	————	————	————	————	————
3. Making major decisions	————	————	————	————	————	————
4. Sex relations	————	————	————	————	————	————

	All the time	Most of the time	More often than not	Occasionally	Rarely	Never
8. How often do you and your partner quarrel?	————	————	————	————	————	————
9. Do you ever regret that you married (or live together)?	————	————	————	————	————	————

Appendix H

Sample Items from
the Parenting Alliance Inventory

PARENTING ALLIANCE INVENTORY

Richard R. Abidin
University of Virginia

Directions: The questions listed below concern what happens between you and your child's other parent, or the other adult most involved in the care of your child. While you may not find an answer which exactly describes what you think, please circle the answer that comes closest to what you think. YOUR FIRST REACTION SHOULD BE YOUR ANSWER

Strongly Agree	Agree	Not Sure	Disagree	Strongly Disagree
5	4	3	2	1

Sample Items

	SA	A	NS	D	SD
3. When there is a problem with our child, we work out a good solution together.	5	4	3	2	1
4. My child's other parent and I communicate well about our child.	5	4	3	2	1
8. My child's other parent and I agree on what our child should and should not be permitted to do.	5	4	3	2	1
11. My child's other parent and I are a good team.	5	4	3	2	1
15. My child's other parent sees our child the same way I do.	5	4	3	2	1
17. If our child needs to be punished, my child's other parent and I usually agree on the type of punishment.	5	4	3	2	1
18. I feel good about my child's other parent's judgment about what is right for our child.	5	4	3	2	1
20. My child's other parent and I have the same goals for our child.	5	4	3	2	1

Appendix I

Sample Items from the Behavior Assessment System for Children (6–11; Teacher Version)

BASC
Teacher Rating Scales
TRS-C (6–11)

Instructions
On this form are phrases that describe how children may act. Please read each phrase and mark the response that describes how this child has acted over the last **six months**. If the child's behavior has changed a great deal during this period, describe the child's most recent behavior.

Circle **N** if the behavior **never** occurs.
Circle **S** if the behavior **sometimes** occurs.
Circle **O** if the behavior **often** occurs.
Circle **A** if the behavior **almost always** occurs.

Please mark every item. If you don't know or are unsure, give your best estimate. A "never" response does not mean that a child "never" engages in a behavior, only that you have not observed the child to behave that way.

2.	Argues when denied own way	N	S	O	A
18.	Is easily distracted from classwork	N	S	O	A
37.	Analyzes the nature of a problem before starting to solve it	N	S	O	A
49.	Complains about health	N	S	O	A
59.	Acts without thinking	N	S	O	A
94.	Uses foul language	N	S	O	A
95.	Is easily upset	N	S	O	A
97.	Is good at getting people to work together	N	S	O	A
102.	Has trouble making new friends	N	S	O	A
105.	Has reading problems	N	S	O	A
126.	Has trouble shifting gears from one task to another	N	S	O	A
128.	Says, "I'm not very good at this"	N	S	O	A
130.	Babbles to self	N	S	O	A
136.	Offers help to other children	N	S	O	A

Appendix J

Child and Family
Information Form

CHILD INFORMATION

Child's Name _____ Birthdate _____ Age _____

Address _____
(Street)   (City)   (State)   (Zip)

Home Phone (   ) _____ Work Phone (   ) _____ Mom/Dad
(Circle One)

Child's School _____ Teacher's Name _____

School Address _____
(Street)   (City)   (State)   (Zip)

School Phone (   ) _____ Child's Grade _____

Is child in Special Education?   YES   NO   If so, what type? _____

FAMILY INFORMATION

Mother's Name _____ Age _____ Education _____

Mother's Place of Employment _____

Type of Employment _____ Annual Salary _____

Father's Name _____ Age _____ Education _____

Father's Place of Employment _____

Type of Employment _____ Annual Salary _____

Is the Child Adopted?   YES   NO   If yes, age when adopted _____

Are parents married?   YES   NO   Separated?   YES   NO   Divorced?   YES   NO

Child's Physician _____

Physician's Address _____
(Street)   (City)   (State)   (Zip)

Physician's Telephone Number (   ) _____

Please list all other children in the Family:

Name	Age	School/Grade
_____	_____	_____
_____	_____	_____

Appendix K

Developmental and Health History Information

DEVELOPMENTAL AND HEALTH HISTORY INFORMATION

PREGNANCY AND DELIVERY

A. Length of pregnancy (e.g., full term or 40 weeks, 32 weeks, etc.) _____

B. Length of delivery (number of hours from initial labor pains to birth) _____

C. Mother's age when child was born _____

D. Child's birth weight _____

E. Did any of the following conditions occur during pregnancy/delivery?

	NO	YES
1. Bleeding		
2. Excessive weight gain (more than 30 lbs.)		
3. Toxemia/Preeclampsia		
4. Rh factor incompatibility		
5. Frequent nausea or vomiting		
6. Serious illness or injury		
7. Took prescription medication a.) If yes, name of medication _____		
8. Took illegal drugs		
9. Used alcoholic beverages a.) If yes, approximate # of drinks per week _____		
10. Smoked cigarettes a.) If yes, approximate # of cigarettes/day (e.g., ½ pack) _____		
11. Was given medication to ease labor pains a.) If yes, name of medication _____		
12. Delivery was induced		
13. Forceps were used during delivery		
14. Had a breech delivery		
15. Had a cesarean section delivery		
16. Other problems … please describe _____		

F. Did any of the following affect your child during delivery or within the first few days after birth?

	NO	YES
1. Injured during delivery		
2. Cardiopulmonary distress during delivery		
3. Delivered with cord around neck		
4. Had trouble breathing following delivery		
5. Needed oxygen		
6. Was cyanotic, turned blue		
7. Was jaundiced, turned yellow		
8. Had an infection		
9. Had seizures		
10. Was given medications		
11. Born with a congenital defect		
12. Was in hospital more than 7 days		

INFANT HEALTH AND TEMPERAMENT

A. During the first 12 months, was your child:

	NO	YES
1. Difficult to feed		
2. Difficult to get to sleep		
3. Colicky		
4. Difficult to put on a schedule		
5. Alert		
6. Cheerful		
7. Affectionate		
8. Sociable		
9. Easy to comfort		
10. Difficult to keep busy		
11. Overactive, in constant motion		
12. Very stubborn, challenging		

EARLY DEVELOPMENTAL MILESTONES

A. At what age did your child first accomplish the following:

	Years	Months
1. Sitting without help		
2. Crawling		
3. Walking alone, without assistance		
4. Using single words (e.g., mama, dada, ball, etc.)		
5. Putting two or more words together (e.g., mama up)		
6. Bowel training, day and night		
7. Bladder training, day and night		

HEALTH HISTORY

A. Date of child's last physical exam _____

B. At any time has your child had:

	NEVER	PAST	PRESENT
1. Asthma			
2. Allergies			
3. Diabetes, arthritis, or other chronic illness			
4. Epilepsy or seizure disorder			
5. Febrile seizures			
6. Chicken pox or other common childhood illnesses			
7. Heart or blood pressure problems			
8. High fevers (over 103)			
9. Broken bones			
10. Severe cuts requiring stitches			
11. Head injury with loss of consciousness			
12. Lead poisoning			
13. Surgery			
14. Lengthy hospitalization			
15. Speech or language problems			
16. Chronic ear infections			

	NEVER	PAST	PRESENT
17. Hearing difficulties			
18. Eye or vision problems			
19. Fine motor/handwriting problems			
20. Gross motor difficulties, clumsiness			
21. Appetite problems (overeating or undereating)			
22. Sleep problems (falling asleep, staying asleep)			
23. Soiling problems			
24. Wetting problems			
25. Other health difficulties … please describe			

Appendix L

Semi-Structured
Background Interview

AD/HD CLINIC
SEMI-STRUCTURED BACKGROUND INTERVIEW

I. CLIENT DATA

    Child's Name _____   Informant(s) _____

    Chart Number _____   Interviewer _____

    Date of Birth _____   Date _____

    Age (Months) _____

II. REFERRAL INFORMATION

A. Type of Evaluation

    1. Initial—Psych only   3. Medication Trial   5. Re-evaluation

    2. Initial—Psych/IQ/Ed   4. PT Group Screening   6. Other

B. Reason for Referral

Evaluation being conducted in order to:	NO	YES
1. Address ADHD as primary diagnosis		
2. Address secondary diagnostic concerns		
3. Obtain second opinion		
4. Establish treatment plan		
5. Establish/implement treatment plan		
6. Address need for medication		
7. Other		

C. Referral Source

    1. Parent   3. Family Physician   5. Other

    2. School   4. Mental Health Practitioner

III. SCHOOL HISTORY

A. Preschool Experience

Has child ever attended:	Never	Previously	Presently
1. Early Intervention			
2. Day Care			
3. Head Start Program			
4. Regular Preschool			
5. Developmental Preschool			
6. Special Education Preschool			

B. School Performance & Behavior

Has child ever:	P	K	1	2	3	4	5	6	7	8	9	10	11	12
1. Undergone testing														
2. Had IEP/SPED														
3. Been labeled LD														
4. Worked < potential														
5. Failed a subject														
6. Repeated a grade														
7. Been suspended														
8. Been expelled														

C. Current Educational Program

    1. What is current grade level? _____

    2. Now on an IEP or receiving SPED services   NO   YES

If yes, what type?	NO	YES
a.) Resource room (part-time)		
b.) Self-contained LD room (full time)		
c.) Behavior disorders classroom		
d.) Speech/language therapy		
e.) Occupational therapy		
f.) Physical therapy		
g.) Social skills group therapy		
h.) School counseling		
i.) Other		

    3. Are any other accommodations (e.g., daily report   NO   YES
        system) being used to address your child's classroom
        difficulties?

    4. Is child now enrolled in Advanced Learner   NO   YES
        programming?

IV. FAMILY HISTORY

A. Family Composition

    1. Number of children in immediate family   _____

    2. Ordinal position in immediate family   _____

    3. Nature of relations with siblings?
        a.) Below average   b.) Typical   c.) Above average

B. Composition of Household

Currently living with:	NO	YES
1. Biological mother		
2. Biological father		
3. Step-parent		
4. Adoptive parents		
5. Foster parents		
6. Biological parent's significant other		
7. Full sibling		
8. Half-sibling/step-sibling		
9. Other relatives/friends		

C. Marriage/Caretaker Relationship

1. Stability of parents' current marriage/relationship:
   a.) Generally stable   b.) Sometimes unstable   c.) Often unstable

D. Biological Parents

1. Child's biological parents:
   a.) Never were married, but still together   d.) Once married, now separated
   b.) Never were married, now apart   e.) Once married, now divorced
   c.) Currently married   f.) Once married, now widowed

2. Number of years biological parents married/together   _____

3. Custody of child is held:
   a.) jointly   c.) by father only   e.) other
   b.) by mother only   d.) by DSS

E. Recent Lifestyle Changes/Psychosocial Stressors

1. Over the past year, have there been any major lifestyle changes or stresses affecting immediate family?

   a. Pregnancy   f. Medical problems   k. Job termination/layoff
   b. New sibling   g. Psychiatric problems   l. Serious money strains
   c. Marriage   h. Death of relative/friend   m. Legal problems
   d. Marital tensions   i. Change in residence   n. Other
   e. Separation/   j. Change in work
       divorce   schedule

F. Psychiatric/Medical Characteristics of Biological Relatives

Past/present hx of:	Siblings	Mother	Father	Extended Maternal	Extended Paternal
1. AD/HD symptoms/dx					
2. ODD symptoms/dx					

Past/present hx of:	Siblings	Mother	Father	Extended Maternal	Extended Paternal
3. CD symptoms/dx					
4. Antisocial behavior					
5. LD symptoms/dx					
6. Mental Retardation					
7. Psychosis/Sx					
8. Bipolar Disorder					
9. Depression/suicide					
10. Anxiety disorders					
11. Phobias					
12. Tics/Tourettes					
13. Alcohol abuse					
14. Substance abuse					
15. Physical abuse					
16. Sexual abuse					
17. Seizures/epilepsy					
18. Other medical					
19. Other psychiatric					
20. Outpatient psy. tx					
21. Inpatient psy. tx					

V. MOOD/AFFECT/PSYCHIATRIC STATUS

A. <u>Predominant Mood</u>: What mood is your child in <u>most</u> of the time?
   1. Cheerful/Happy   3. Nervous/Anxious
   2. Sad/Depressed   4. Angry/Irritable
B. <u>Stability of Mood</u>: Do your child's moods change frequently, abruptly, and/or unpredictably?
   1. Yes   2. No
C. <u>Range of Affect</u>: Is your child's range of emotional expression extremely limited? (robot-like?)
   1. Yes   2. No
D. <u>Appropriateness of Affect</u>: Does your child often show inappropriate emotional reactions?
   1. Yes   2. No

E. Other Concerns

Any evidence of:	NEVER	PAST	PRESENT
1. Loose thinking			
2. Disoriented, confused			
3. Delusions			
4. Hallucinations			
5. Diminished interest in peers			
6. Self-injurious behavior			
7. Self-stimulation			
8. Alcohol abuse			
9. Substance abuse			
10. Cigarette smoking			
11. Physical abuse			
12. Sexual abuse			

VI. <u>PEER RELATIONS</u>

A. <u>Making Friends</u>: Does your child have problems making friends?

    1.) Almost never   2.) Some of the time   3.) Most of the time

B. <u>Keeping Friends</u>: Does your child have problems keeping friends?

    1.) Almost never   2.) Some of the time   3.) Most of the time

C. <u>Peer Group Age Range</u>: How old are most of your child's friends?

    1.) Younger   2.) Same age   3.) Older

D. <u>Number of Close Friends</u>: How many close friends does he/she have?

    1.) None   2.) Just a few   3.) Lots

E. <u>Peer Interaction Style</u>: When your child plays with other children, is he/she often ...?

    1.) Inattentive, spacey   4.) Shy, reserved, withdrawn
    2.) Bossy, controlling, aggressive   5.) Appropriate for age
    3.) Combination of 1 & 2

F. <u>Peer Conflict Resolution</u>: When your child has disagreements or conflicts with other children, how well does he/she resolve such situations?

    1.) Not very well   2.) Moderately well   3.) Very well

G. <u>Conflict Resolution Style</u>: What does your child usually do to resolve conflicts?

    1.) Compromises, bargains   4.) Asks an adult for help
    2.) Gives in to others   5.) Avoids conflict
    3.) Threatens, bullies, fights

H. <u>Peer Acceptance:</u> Do most children ...?

    1.) Accept/enjoy being with your child

    2.) Overtly reject/tease your child

    3.) Avoid/ignore your child

I. <u>Child's Self-Perception:</u> How does your child feel about his/her relations with other children?

    1.) Generally happy and satisfied

    2.) Occasionally dissatisfied

    3.) Often upset and distressed

VII. CHILD'S EVALUATION & TREATMENT HISTORY

A. <u>Prior Evaluation/Diagnoses</u>

Has child ever undergone:	NO	YES
1. Psychiatric Evaluation		
2. Pediatric Assessment		
3. Neurologic Work-up		
4. Dietary Analysis		
5. Intelligence Testing		
6. Psychoeducational Testing		
7. Speech/Language/Hearing Evaluation		
8. Neuropsychological Testing		
9. Previously established diagnosis of ADHD?		
10. Other previously established diagnoses?		

B. <u>Psychological/Psychiatric Treatment</u>

Has child ever received:	NEVER	PREVIOUS	PRESENT
1. Individual therapy			
2. Play Therapy			
3. Family Therapy			
4. Group Therapy			
5. Brief Inpatient Treatment			
6. Residential Treatment			
7. Behavioral Parent Training			
8. Social Skills Training			

C. Pharmacotherapy

Has child ever taken:	NEVER	PREVIOUS	PRESENT
1. Ritalin			
2. Dexedrine			
3. Cylert			
4. Adderal			
5. Imipramine			
6. Nortriptyline			
7. Amitriptyline			
8. SSRI			
9. Other Antidepressant			
10. Clonidine			
11. Anticonvulsant			
12. Antihistamine			
13. Major Tranquilizer			
14. Other			

15. If currently taking psychotropic medication ... total daily dosage? _____

16. How often?
    a.) 5 days/week—school year   c.) 7 days/week—year round
    b.) 7 days/week—school year

17. Any improvement?
    a.) None at all   b.) Somewhat   c.) Very much

18. Any side effects?
    1.) None at all   b.) Some   c.) Many

19. Does your child take prescribed medication for any other reason?
    a.) No   b.) Yes   _____
                                 _____
                                 (list name, dosage, reason)

D. Other Forms of Treatment/Support Services

Has child/family ever tried:	NEVER	PREVIOUS	PRESENT
1. Dietary changes			
2. Neurobiofeedback			
3. Parent Support Group			
4. Other			

VIII. HOME MANAGEMENT

A. <u>Compliance</u>:

    1. How often does your child do what you ask on the first request?
        a.) Almost never   b.) Some of the time   c.) Most of the time

    2. How often does your child eventually do what you want them to do?
        a.) Almost never   b.) Some of the time   c.) Most of the time

B. <u>Strategies</u>:

Have you used:	NEVER	PREVIOUS	PRESENT
1. Privilege Removal			
2. Isolation/Time Out			
3. Grounding			
4. Spanking/Physical Punishment			
5. Verbal Reprimands			
6. Allowance System			
7. Special Privileges/Rewards			
8. Star Chart/Token System			
9. Verbal Praise			
10. Other			

C. <u>Parenting Effectivenss/Consistency</u>

    1. Overall, how effectively do you manage your child's behavior?
        a.) Not very well   b.) Moderately well   c.) Very well

    2. Overall, how effectively does your spouse/partner manage your child's behavior?
        a.) Not very well   b.) Moderately well   c.) Very well

    3. Do you & your spouse/partner generally agree on which behaviors to discipline?
        a.) Almost never   b.) Some of the time   c.) Most of the time

    4. Do you & your spouse/partner generally agree on how to discipline?
        a.) Almost never   b.) Some of the time   c.) Most of the time

IX. DIAGNOSTIC CONCLUSIONS & TREATMENT RECOMMENDATIONS

A. <u>Diagnostic Status</u> (enter 999 if no diagnosis)

    1. _____   2. _____   3. _____

B. <u>Treatment Plan</u>

Recommendations for treatment:	NO	YES
1. Intelligence testing		
2. LD screening/psychoeducational testing		

Recommendations for treatment:	NO	YES
3. Neuropsychological evaluation		
4. Other assessment procedures		
5. Classroom modifications		
6. Parent training		
7. Stimulant medication trial		
8. Individual therapy		
9. Family therapy		
10. Social skills training		
11. Other treatment services		

Appendix M

Cover Letter for Parent
Rating Scale Packet

Dear Parent/Legal Guardian:

It is our understanding that you are interested in having your child evaluated through the Attention-Deficit/Hyperactvity Disorder Clinic. Before setting up an appointment for such an evaluation, we would like to have additional information.

Please complete the enclosed questionnaires and return them in the self-addressed envelope that we have provided.

If you have access to previously completed school reports or other types of psychological/medical evaluation reports, please forward copies of these as well.

Once we receive this information, as well as the questionnaires that you gave us permission to send to your child's teacher(s), we will contact you to schedule your evaluation appointment.

In advance, thank you for your cooperation with these procedures.

Sincerely,

_____
Director, AD/HD Clinic

Appendix N

Instructions for Completing Parent Rating Scale Packet

INSTRUCTIONS FOR COMPLETING QUESTIONNAIRES

We very much appreciate your willingness to complete the enclosed questionnaires. Your responses will give us a much better understanding of your child's home behavior. The instructions for filling out these forms are listed below. Please follow these as closely as possible.

Who should complete these forms?

Ideally, this should be the parent who spends the most time with the child. If two or more parents wish to complete these questionnaires, each should do so independently on separate forms, which may be obtained from the AD/HD Clinic upon requeust.

What if my child is already on medication?

If your child is now taking medication (e.g., Ritalin) for behavior management purposes, it is very likely that you observe his/her behavior both on and off medication. Please answer the attached questionnaires based on how you observe your child <u>most</u> of the time. Also, please let us know on what basis you responded, by checking one of the following:

    ____ My child does not take medication for behavior problems.

    ____ My child takes medication, but my ratings reflect how he/she behaves when off medication.

    ____ My child takes medication, and my ratings reflect how he/she behaves when on medication.

Why do I need to answer questions about myself?

When completing the questionnaires pertaining to yourself and to other aspects of your family life, please keep in mind that we are trying to learn as much as we can about the home environment in which your child functions. Having such information allows us to make clinical management recommenations that maximize your child's behavior and performance both at home and at school.

Should you have questions about these instructions, please feel free to call the graduate student clinician assigned to your case for assistance. Once again, thank you for completing these forms.

**PLEASE RETURN THIS FORM
ALONG WITH THE COMPLETED QUESTIONNAIRES**

Appendix O

Cover Letter for Teacher Rating Scale Packet

_____

(Student's Name)

To Whom It May Concern:

The above-named student will soon be scheduled for the evaluation in an Attention-Deficit/Hyperactivity Clinic.

Your observations of this student in school are extremely important to us. Therefore, we very much would like you to complete the enclosed questionnaires and to return them as soon as possible in the self-addressed envelope that we have provided.

We recently received telephone permission from this student's parent(s) to obtain this information from you. If this type of consent is not sufficient, then please let the parent(s) know that you must have additional consent (e.g., written release of information) before returning our materials.

If by chance you are not one of this student's primary academic teachers, we very much would appreciate your forwarding this letter and the enclosed forms to the teacher whom you believe is most familiar with his/her current classroom behavior and performance.

In advance, we thank you for your prompt assistance in this matter.

Sincerely,

_____

Director, AD/HD Clinic

Appendix P

Instructions for Completing Teacher Rating Scale Packet

INSTRUCTIONS FOR COMPLETING QUESTIONNAIRES

We very much appreciate your willingness to complete the enclosed questionnaires. Your responses will provide us with an extremely important source of
information about this student's functioning in school. When completing these
forms, please pay careful attention to the instructions below.

Who should complete these forms?

Ideally, this should be the teacher who spends the most time with the student. If
more than one teacher wishes to respond, each should do so independently on
on separate forms, which may be obtained from the AD/HD Clinic upon requeust.

What if the student is currently taking medication?

If this student now taking medication (e.g., Ritalin) for behavior management
purposes, it is very likely that you have observed his/her behavior both on and
off medication. Please answer the attached questionnaires based on how you
observe this student most of the time. Also, please let us know on what basis you
responded, by checking one of the following:

    ____ This student does not take medication for behavior problems.

    ____ This student takes medication, but my ratings reflect how
          he/she behaves when off medication.

    ____ This student takes medication, and my ratings reflect how
          he/she behaves when on medication.

Why do I need to answer questions about the school setting?

The conditions under which you observe this student can have a significant
impact on our interpretation of your ratings. Having information about the
school setting also allows us to make treatment recommendations that maximize this student's behavior and performance in school. For reasons such as
these, we would appreciate your providing the information requested below:

Name of Teacher Completing Forms: _____

Type of Classroom Setting: Regular _____   Special Education _____

Number of Students in Classroom: _____

Number of Teachers/Aides in Classroom (including yourself): _____

Total Amount of Time (in hours) Spent with Student Each Day: _____

Should you have questions about these instructions, please free to call the AD/
HD Clinic for assistance. Once again, thank you for your time and assistance.

PLEASE RETURN THIS FORM
ALONG WITH THE COMPLETED QUESTIONNAIRES

Appendix Q

Information Resources

RESOURCES

CHADD
8181 Professional Place, Suite 201
Landover, MD 20785
(800) 233-4050
(301) 306-7070
FAX (301) 306-7090
http://www.chadd.org

A.D.D. WareHouse
300 Northwest 70th Avenue, Suite 102
Plantation, FL 33317
(800) 233-9273
(954) 792-8100
FAX (954) 792-8545

Author Index

Subject Index